HANDBOOK OF EVALUATION METHODS
FOR HEALTH INFORMATICS

HANDBOOK OF EVALUATION METHODS FOR HEALTH INFORMATICS

Jytte Brender
University of Aalborg, Denmark

Translated by Lisbeth Carlander

ELSEVIER

AMSTERDAM • BOSTON • HEIDELBERG • LONDON
NEW YORK • OXFORD • PARIS • SAN DIEGO
SAN FRANCISCO • SINGAPORE • SYDNEY • TOKYO

Academic Press is an imprint of Elsevier

Elsevier Academic Press
30 Corporate Drive, Suite 400, Burlington, MA 01803, USA
525 B Street, Suite 1900, San Diego, California 92101-4495, USA
84 Theobald's Road, London WC1X 8RR, UK

The front page illustration has been reprinted from Brender J. Methodology for Assessment of Medical IT-based Systems – in an Organisational Context. Amsterdam: IOS Press, Studies in Health Technology and Informatics 1997; **42**, with permission.

This book is printed on acid-free paper. ∞

Library of Congress Cataloging-in-Publication Data
Brender, Jytte.
 Handbook of evaluation methods in health informatics / Jytte
Brender.
  p. ; cm.
 Includes bibliographical references and index.
 ISBN-13: 978-0-12-370464-1 (pbk. : alk. paper)
 ISBN-10: 0-12-370464-2 (pbk. : alk. paper)
  1. Medical informatics--Methodology. 2. Information storage and
retrieval systems--Medicine--Evaluation. I. Title.
 [DNLM: 1. Information Systems--standards. 2. Medical Informatics
--methods. 3. Decision Support Techniques. W 26.55.I4 B837h
2006]
 R858.B7332 2006
 651.5'04261--dc22
                                     2005025192

British Library Cataloguing in Publication Data
A catalogue record for this book is available from the British Library

ISBN 13: 978-0-12-370464-1
ISBN 10: 0-12-370464-2

For all information on all Elsevier Academic Press publications
visit our Web site at www.books.elsevier.com

Printed in the United States of America
05   06   07   08   09   10   9 8 7 6 5 4 3 2 1

Contents

NOTE TO THE READER

This *Handbook of Evaluation Methods* is a translated and updated version of a combination of the following two publications:

- Brender J. Handbook of Methods in Technology Assessment of IT-based Solutions within Healthcare. Aalborg: EPJ-Observatoriet, ISBN: 87-91424-04-6, June 2004. 238pp (in Danish).
- Brender J. Methodological and methodical perils and pitfalls within assessment studies performed on IT-based solutions in healthcare. Aalborg: Virtual Centre for Health Informatics; 2003 May. Report No.: 03-1 (ISSN 1397-9507). 69pp.

The Aim of the Handbook

"[W]e view evaluation not as the application of a set of tools and techniques, but as a process to be understood. By which we mean an understanding of the functions and nature of evaluation as well as its limitations and problems."

(Symons and Walsham 1988)

The primary aim of this book is to illustrate options for finding appropriate tools within the literature and then to support the user in accomplishing an assessment study without too many disappointments. There are very big differences between what developers and users should assess with regard to an IT-based solution. This book deals solely with assessments as seen from the users' point of view.

Within the literature there are thousands of reports on assessment studies for IT-based systems and solutions specifically for systems within the healthcare sector. However, only a fraction of these are dedicated to a description of assessment activities. Consequently, from an assessment perspective one has to consider them as superficial and rather useless as model examples. Only the best and paradigmatic examples of evaluation methods are included in this book.

The problem in assessment of IT-based solutions lies partly in getting an overview of the very complex domain encompassing topics that range from technical aspects to the soft behavioral and organizational aspects and partly in avoiding pitfalls and perils to obtain valid results, as well as identifying appropriate methods and case studies similar to one's own.

Please note the terminology of the book, which encompasses the notions of evaluation and assessment in Section 2.1. Briefly, *evaluation* means to measure characteristics (in a decision-making context), while *assessment* is used in an overall sense that does not distinguish between retrospective objectives of the study aims and therefore not whether it is evaluation, verification, or validation.

This book deals mainly with current user-oriented assessment methods. It includes methods that give the users a fair chance of accomplishing all or parts of an investigation, which lead to a professionally satisfactory answer to an actual information need.

It is not each and every one of the methods included that were originally developed and presented in the literature as evaluation methods, but nevertheless, they may be applicable either directly – as evaluation methods for specific purposes – or indirectly – as support in an evaluation context. An example is the Delphi method developed for the American military to predict future trends. Another example is diagramming techniques for modelling workflow, which in some instances constitute a practical way of modelling, such as in assessing effect or impact or in field studies, and so forth.

The book is primarily aimed at the health sector, from which the chosen illustrative examples are taken. The contents have been collected from many different specialist areas, and the material has been chosen and put together in order to cover the needs of assessment for IT-based solutions in the health sector. However, this does not preclude its use within other sectors as well.

Target Group

It is important to remember that a handbook of methods is *not* a textbook but a reference book enabling the reader to get inspiration and support when completing a set task and/or as a basis for further self-education. Handbooks, for use in natural sciences for instance, are typically aimed at advanced users and their level of knowledge. The structure of this handbook has similarly been aimed at the level of user with a profile as described below.

The target readers of this book constitute all professionals within the healthcare sector, including IT professionals. However, an evaluation method is not something that one pulls out of a hat, a drawer, or even from books, and then uses without reflection and meticulous care. A list of desirable competences and personal qualifications is therefore listed in the next section.

Skills Required to Evaluate an IT System Appropriately

In the following list, the personal and professional qualifications needed to accomplish assessment studies are briefly discussed. Ultimately, this of course depends on the specific information needs and the complexity of the overall system. In short, it is important to be responsible and independently minded, have a good overview of the subject matter, and be both reflective and self-critical.

- It is critical to be able to disregard the political interests of one's own profession to view the situation in a larger perspective. There is a need to be able to gain an overview and thereby a need to make abstractions and reflections about issues within their larger context before, during, and after an assessment study. Often, activities may be carried out in more than one way, and it is necessary to be able to judge which one is best given the conditions.
- It is necessary to have the skills needed for dealing with methods. One must have the ability and the courage to form one's own opinion and carry it out in terms of variations of known methods and so on. It is also important that one is capable of capturing, handling, and interpreting deviations within the actual investigation and among the factual observations. Such deviations are more or less inevitable in practice.
- There is a need for stringency and persistence, as assessment studies are usually large and involve a great deal of data, the analysis of which must be methodically, cautiously, and exhaustively carried out.
- One must have a degree of understanding of IT-based solutions, enabling one to see through the technology, its conditions and incidents, and so that one dares set limits (without being stubborn) toward professionals with formal credentials. It is necessary to be able to see through the implications of the interaction between the IT systems and their organizational environment, as well as conditions, interactions, and events for the organization and for its individuals.
- There is a need for project management skills and experience. An assessment study is not something that one does single-handedly or as a desk test. Therefore, it is necessary to be able to coordinate and delegate, to perform critical problem solving and decision making, and to have the ability to predict the consequences of one's decisions and initiatives.
- One must have the motivation and desire to acquaint oneself with new material and search for information in the literature, on the Internet, or from professionals in other disciplines.
- It is essential to be able to remain constructively critical, verging on the suspicious, toward verbal or written statements, including one's own approach and results.
- There is a need for thorough insight into the healthcare sector, including the conditions under which such organizations work.

In other words, there is a greater emphasis on functional competences than on academic achievements.

Criteria for Inclusion

Methods that require specific qualifications, such as economic and statistical methods, have been excluded. It requires particular understanding for processing the basis that leads to the methods description in this handbook. Apart from common sense, economic methods fall outside the author's personal area of competence, so they have been consciously omitted from this handbook. Assessing IT-based solutions is a multidisciplinary task, so without the necessary competence in a particular area, the assessor must acknowledge this and ask for advice from experts with that knowledge, specifically in areas such as economics and the law.

Statistical methods are not designed to assess IT-based systems. They are general methods used to support processing results of an assessment activity, for instance. Knowledge of basic statistical methods should be applied conscientiously. When such knowledge is lacking, one should get help from professionals or from the vast number of existing statistical textbooks as early as during the planning stage of the assessment study. Descriptions of these methods are not relevant to this book.

Commercial assessment tools, techniques, and methods based on already implemented software products have been excluded, unless the method or technique has been sufficiently well documented in its own right.

Verification of inference mechanisms, consistency checks of knowledge bases, and so on for knowledge-based systems are subject to the type of verification that specifically falls under development work and is classified as a type of assessment ('debugging'), which normal users are not expected to undertake. Therefore, this aspect has been excluded from this handbook.

There are no distinctions between different types of IT systems, such as EHR, laboratory information systems, hospital information systems, or decision-support systems. The only types of IT systems excluded are embedded IT systems – systems that do not have an independent user interface but that work as integral parts of medico-technical equipment, for example. Some of the methods may be more relevant to one type of IT system than to another type. This would be the case in assessment of the precision of clinical diagnostics, for example. The handbook has been organized in such a way that the choice of methods follows a natural pattern. The keys to the methods are the development stage and an actual need for information rather than for a system type.

Similarly, assessments of knowledge-based IT systems (expert systems and decision-support systems) have not been described separately. In principle these systems are not different from other IT-based systems. The dissimilarity lies in their role within the organization and the consequential variation of the focus (points of measure) in an assessment study. Extraordinary demands are put on the technical correctness (as in diagnostic, prognostic, screening, and monitoring) of (user) assessments of knowledge-based systems, including specificity, sensitivity, and so on. Formally, however, this type of assessment is still classified as *"Technical Verification"* (see below). Other user assessments (i.e., *Usability* and *User Satisfaction*) work in the same way as in other types of IT systems.

Methods specific to embedded systems have also been excluded, such as software components in various monitoring equipment, electronic pumps, and so forth. This does not preclude that some of the methods can be used for ordinary assessment purposes, while other specific information needs are referred to technology assessment approaches within the medico-technical domain.

Acknowledgments

This book is based on the author's knowledge accumulated over a period of thirty years, initially twelve years specializing in Clinical Biochemistry, a medical domain strong in metrology. Subsequently the author gained knowledge from a number of research projects within Health Informatics under various EU Commission Framework Programmers[1], and from a PhD project financed by the Danish Research Council for Technical Science from 1995 to 1996.

All of this has contributed to a process of realization of what evaluation is really all about and what it means in a decision-making context. The author's three most appreciated colleagues during this process – as expert counterparts, collaborators, and coaches – are – in alphabetical order – Marie-Catherine Beuscart-Zéphir, cognitive psychologist from EVALAB, CERIM, Univ. 2, Lille France; Peter McNair, Project Manager at the Copenhagen Hospital Corporation, Denmark; and Jan Talmon, Associate Professor at the Department of Medical Informatics, Maastricht University, Maastricht, Holland.

[1] The projects KAVAS (A1021), KAVAS-2 (A2019), OpenLabs (A2028), ISAR (A2052), and CANTOR (HC 4003), and the concerted actions COMAG-BME and ATIM.

The funding supporting the present synthesis comes from two primary and equal sources: (1) the CANTOR (HC4003) Healthcare Telematics Project under the European Commission's Fourth Framework Programme, leading to an early version of the framework in Part III, and (2) the MUP-IT project under the Danish Institute for Evaluation and Health Technology Assessment (CEMTV) that enabled the finalization of the framework and the analysis of the literature for sample cases. The author owes both of those her sincere gratitude.

The author would also like to thank the panel of reviewers of an early Danish version of this handbook for the effort they have put into reviewing the book. This handbook would not have been nearly as good had it not been for their extremely constructive criticisms and suggestions for improvement. The panel of reviewers consisted of Arne Kverneland, Head of Unit, and Søren Lippert, Consultant, both at the Health Informatics Unit at the National Board of Health; Pia Kopke, IT Project Consultant, the Informatics Department, the Copenhagen Hospital Cooperation; Egil Boisen, Assistant Professor, the Department of Health Science and Technology, Aalborg University; and Hallvard Lærum, PhD Student, Digimed Senter, Trondheim, Norway. The final and formal review was carried out by an anonymous reviewer, whom the author wishes to thank for pointing out the areas where the book may have been unclear.

Furthermore, the author wishes to thank colleagues at the Department of Health Science and Technology and the Department of Social Development and Planning at Aalborg University, who on many occasions listened to expositions of theories, conceptual discussions, metaphors of validation, and the like, and who have all volunteered as professional adversaries. On each occasion they have raised the level and contributed to ensuring the best possible professional foundation. I also thank the Danish Society for Medical Informatics and the EPJ Observatory for giving encouragement and the opportunity to test and discuss some of the ideas of the contents of the *Handbook* with its future users and for financing the printing of the Danish version of the *Handbook*.

Additional Comments

Descriptions of individual methods and techniques are consciously stated with differing levels of detail: The less accessible the original reference, the more detail is given for the method described. This gives the reader a chance to better understand the actual method before deciding whether to disregard it or actively search for it.

Registered trademarks from companies have been used within this document. It is acknowledged here that these trademarks are recognized and this document in no way intends to infringe on any of the rights pertaining to these trademarks, especially copyrights. The document therefore does not contain a registered trademark symbol after any instance of a trademark.

Jytte Brender
University of Aalborg
June 2005

Part I: Introduction

1. Introduction

1.1 What Is Evaluation?

Evaluation can be defined as "acts related to measurement or exploration of a system's properties". In short *system* means "all the components, attributes, and relationships needed to accomplish an objective" (Haimes and Schneiter 1996). Evaluation may be accomplished during planning, development, or operation and maintenance of an IT system. When put to its logical extreme, evaluation simply means to put numbers on some properties of the system, and, consequently, evaluation has little sense as a self-contained and independent activity. The purpose of evaluation is to provide the basis for a decision about the IT system investigated in some decision-making context, and that decision-making context is also the context of the evaluation:

> *"Evaluation can be defined as the act of measuring or exploring properties of a health information system (in planning, development, implementation, or operation), the result of which informs a decision to be made concerning that system in a specific context."*

> (Ammenwerth et al. 2004)

When evaluation is used in the context of controlling whether an IT system – for instance, at delivery – fulfills a previously set agreement, then the activity is called verification. Similarly, the concept of validation is used when the decision-making context is concerned with whether or not the system suffices to fulfill its purpose. The concept of 'assessment' is used as a collective term when it is unnecessary to distinguish between the different types of purpose of an evaluation. For further details on the definitions, see Section 2.1.

It is not yet possible to write a cookbook for the assessment of IT-based systems with step-by-step recipes of "do it this way". The number of aspects to be investigated and types of systems are far too large. Consequently, as Symons and Walsham (1988) express it:

> *"[W]e view evaluation not as the application of a set of tools and techniques, but as a process to be understood. By which we mean an understanding of the functions and nature of evaluation as well as its limitations and problems."*

In short: One has to understand what is going on and what is going to take place.

When addressing the issue of assessing an electronic healthcare record (abbreviated EHR) or another IT system within healthcare, the object of the assessment activity is usually the entire organizational solution and not only the technical construct. The book distinguishes between an 'IT system' and an 'IT-based solution'. The term 'IT system' denotes the technical construct of the whole solution (hardware, software, including basic software, and communication network), while 'IT-based solution' refers to the IT system *plus* its surrounding organization with its mission, conditions, structure, work procedures, and so on. Thus, assessment of an IT-based solution is concerned not only with the IT system, but also its interaction with its organizational environment and its mode of operation within the organization. For instance, it includes actors (physicians, nurses, and other types of healthcare staff, as well as patients), work procedures and structured activities, as well as external stakeholders, and, last but not least, a mandate and a series of internal and external conditions for the organization's operation. Orthogonal to this, evaluation methods need to cope with aspects ranging from the technical ones – via social and behavioral ones – to managerial ones. The assessment activity must act on the basis of this wholeness, but it is of course limited to what is relevant in the specific decision-making context.

The preceding short introduction to the concept of evaluation indicates that to accomplish an evaluation requires more than picking a standard method and using it. The important part is to understand the process within which the future result is going to be used, as well as the premises for obtaining a good result – before one can choose a method at all. Applying a given method in reality is probably the easiest yet most laborious part of an evaluation.

The first thing to make clear, before starting assessment activities at all, is "Why do you want to evaluate?", "What is it going to be used for?", and "What will be the consequence of a given outcome?" The answers to the questions "Why do you want to evaluate?" and "What is it going to be used for?" are significant determinants for which direction and approach one may pursue. Similarly, the intended use of the study results is a significant factor for the commitment and motivation of the involved parties and thereby also for the quality of the data upon which the outcome rests.

There are natural limits to how much actual time one can spend on planning, measuring, documenting, and analyzing, when assessment is an integrated part of an ongoing implementation process (cf. the concept of 'constructive assessment' in Section 2.1.3). Furthermore, if one merely needs the results for internal purposes – for progressing in one decision-making context or another, for example – then the level of ambition required for scientific publications may not necessarily be needed. However, after the event, one has to be very careful in case the option of publication, either as an article in a scientific journal or as a public technical report, is suggested. The results may not be appropriate for publication or may not be generalizable and thereby of no value to others. In this day and age, with strict demands on evidence (cf. 'evidence-based medicine'), one must be aware that the demands on the quality of a study are different when making one's results publicly available.

Answers depend on the questions posed, and if one does not fully realize what is possible and what is not for a given method, there is the risk that the answers will not be very useful. It is rare that one is allowed to evaluate simply to gain more knowledge of something.

A problem often encountered in assessment activities is that they lag behind the overall investment in development or implementation. Some aspects can only be investigated once the system is in use on a day-to-day basis. However, this is when the argument "but it works" normally occurs – at least at a certain level – and "Why invest in an assessment?" when the neighbor will be the one to benefit. There must be an objective or a gain in assessing, or it is meaningless. Choice of method should ensure this objective.

Furthermore, one should refrain from assessing just one part of the system or within narrow premises and then think that the result can be used for an overall political decision-making process. Similarly, it is too late to start measuring the baseline against which a quantitative assessment should be evaluated once the new IT system is installed, or one is totally immersed in the analysis and installation work. By then it will in general be too late, as the organization has already moved on.

It is also necessary to understand just what answers a given method can provide. For instance, a questionnaire study cannot appropriately answer all questions, albeit they are all posed. Questionnaire studies are constrained by a number of psychological factors, which only allow one to scratch the surface, but not to reach valid quantitative results (see Parts II and III). The explanation lies in the difference between (1) what you do, (2) what you think you do, and (3) how you actually do things and how you describe it (see Part III and Brender 1997a and 1999). There is a risk that a questionnaire study will give the first as the outcome, an interview study the second (because you interact with the respondent to increase mutual understanding), while the third outcome can normally only be obtained through thorough observation. This difference does not come out of bad will, but from conditions within the user organization that make it impossible for the users to express themselves precisely and completely. Part III presents several articles where the differences between two of the three aspects are shown by triangulation (Kushniruk et al. 1997; Østbye et al. 1997; Beuscart-Zéphir et al. 1997). However, the phenomenon is known from knowledge engineering (during the development of expert systems) and from many other circumstances (Dreyfus and Dreyfus 1986; Bansler and Havn 1991; Stage 1991; Barry 1995; Dreyfus 1997; and Patel and Kushniruk 1998). For instance, Bansler and Havn (1991) express it quite plainly as follows:

"Approaches for system development implicitly assumes that documents such as a functional specification and a system specification contain all relevant information about the system being developed; developers achieve an operational image (a mental image, a theory) of the solution as a kind of apprenticeship; the programmers' knowledge about the program cannot be expressed and therefore communicated by means of program specifications or other kinds of documentation."

In other words, one has to give the project careful thought before starting. The essence of an assessment is:

There must be accordance between the aim, the premises, the process, and the actual application of the results – otherwise it might go wrong!

1.2   Instructions to the Reader

The *Handbook of Evaluation Methods* is divided into three main parts:
I.   The Introduction is concerned with the terminology and the conceptualization fundamental to this handbook.
II. Part II contains descriptions of methods.
III. Part III comprises an exhaustive review of known perils and pitfalls for experimental investigations with sample cases from the literature on assessment of IT-based solutions in healthcare.

This *Handbook of Evaluation Methods* is not intended to be read like a normal book. It is an encyclopedia, a work of reference to be used when one needs support for accomplishing a specific assessment study or when one needs inspiration for the formulation of candidate themes for investigation. The Handbook exemplifies available options.

It is recommended that one initially reads Chapters 1-3 of the Introduction to ensure an understanding of the terms and concepts. Then, when one has a feeling of what one wants to explore and has recognized the state of the IT system within its life cycle, it may be useful to familiarize oneself with the candidate methods in Part II. Additionally, one should get acquainted with a number of the book references, like (van Gennip and Talmon 1995; Friedman and Wyatt 1996; and Coolican 1999). It is important to be familiar with the terminology, and with the overall meaning of evaluation. The aforementioned references also give instructions on how to get off to a sensible start.

When ready to take the next step, proceed from the beginning of Chapter 4 and onwards, while adjusting the list of candidate methods based on the identified information needs versus details of the specific methods and attributes of the case.

Get hold of the relevant original references from the literature and search for more or newer references on the same methods or problem areas as applicable to you.

When a method (or a combination of several) is selected and planning is going on, look through Part III to verify that everything is up to your needs or even better. Part III is designed for carrying out an overall analysis and judgment of the validity of an assessment study. However, it is primarily written for experienced evaluators, as the information requires prior know-how on the subtlety of experimental work. Nevertheless, in case the description of a given method in Part II mentions a specific pitfall, less experienced evaluators should also get acquainted with these within Part III in order to judge the practical implication and to correct or compensate for weaknesses in the planning.

1.3   Metaphor for the Handbook

As discussed above, the point of departure for this handbook is that one cannot make a cookbook with recipes on how to evaluate. Evaluation is fairly difficult; it depends on one's specific information need (the question to be answered by the evaluation study), on the demands for accuracy and precision, on the project development methods (for constructive assessment), on preexisting material, and so forth.

Descriptions of evaluation methods and their approaches are usually fairly easy to retrieve from the literature, and the target audience is used to make literature searches. This was discussed during meetings with a range of target users at an early stage of the preparation of the handbook. They explicitly stated that they can easily retrieve and read the original literature as long as they have good references.

As a consequence of this and of the huge number of biases in existing reports on assessment studies demonstrated in the review in Part III, it was decided to exclude exhaustive descriptions of the individual methods. Instead the emphasis is on aspects like assumptions for application, tacit built-in perspectives of the methods as well as their perils and pitfalls. Authors of methods rarely describe this kind of information themselves, and it is very difficult for nonexperts to look through methods and cases in the literature to identify potential problems during application.

Consequently, the emphasis of this handbook is on providing the information, which ordinary members of the target group don't have the background and experience to recognize. This includes experimental perils and pitfalls.

The Danish handbook *Politikens Svampeguide* from 1993 by Henning Knudsen served as inspiration for a metaphor for the description of methods. This is a small handbook about mushrooms, designed to be carried in your pocket or basket when you go mushroom picking in the forest. It acts as your guide to distinguish between the poisonous mushrooms and the safe, delicious ones, with the aim of helping you decide what is worth bringing home for dinner.

Corresponding to the metaphor of mushrooms, it is important that users of this handbook learn to distinguish between the values of one method from that of another for different purposes and to be able to judge the dangers in different contexts.

Thus, the *Handbook* is based on a meta-perspective (a bird's eye view) for the representation of the method descriptions. One can easily apply a method incorrectly, and therefore it is important to have an understanding of a method at an abstract level that extends beyond a procedural description. It is the understanding that enables the bird's eye view. It is also the understanding that facilitates juggling with and within the frame of a method's application range while adapting it to local conditions and information needs, and interpreting the results correctly and completely, as compared to the study conditions and acquired data. A method is not something one can just pull out of a drawer or off a shelf and put to use.

Similarly, the art of assessment studies is to know and understand when and how it is possible to make changes or accept that things change, beyond your control, without necessarily ruining your investigation.

Consequently, a profound understanding of a method is more important than a procedural description of when and how to do what. One may acquire the latter through the literature, while quite a lot of experience is needed to advance a profound understanding effortlessly. This is the motivation behind the selected metaphor for this handbook.

2. Conceptual Apparatus

2.1 Evaluation and Related Concepts

There are two basic types of assessment: *summative* and *constructive*. But before we discuss them, we need to define how the concepts of evaluation, verification, validation, and assessment are used in this handbook. This is because they are used in many different ways in the literature, often at random, but also because they are all used in everyday language. Therefore, their current use needs to be outlined.

2.1.1 Definitions

The concepts of *evaluation, validation, verification* and *assessment* are often used somewhat at random in everyday language and in the literature. The term *evaluation* in particular is often used as a collective term for evaluation, validation, and verification. The terminology in this report distinguishes sharply between these concepts; see Table 2.1. The basis for this distinction is the meaning of the words as described in comprehensive English dictionaries and also in (Nykänen 1990 and Hoppe and Meseguer 1993), who review and discuss the use of these concepts with the purpose of synthesizing their definitions. A few details from these discussions and synthesis can be found in the table.

As a note to the definition of evaluation in the table, it is worth mentioning that evaluation as an independent activity does not normally have any meaning, precisely because the concept means just to produce figures regarding some qualities. Nevertheless, it does happen that evaluation is carried out because contractual terms stipulate it, but with no consequence as to the results – for instance, when evaluating a closing task before the project is terminated. Therefore, at the start of the introduction it has been stipulated that "the purpose of evaluation is to provide the basis for a decision about the IT system investigated in some decision-making context, and that decision-making context is also the context of the evaluation".

Constructive evaluation means that an evaluation activity puts figures on some measures, whereupon others (project management, the steering group or the project group for example) pick out the figures and put them into a decision-making context. On the other hand, when the subject is that of validation, the whole process is viewed from when the purpose is defined, through the evaluation of certain qualities in the process to an assessment of whether its objective has been fulfilled.

Table 2.1: Formal definition of some key concepts.

assessment **process** of performing **evaluation, verification** and / or **validation** NOTE - assessment of **quality** of a **system** may e.g. comprise firstly the act of performing measurements (i.e. the **evaluation**) followed by a comparison of these measured qualities with a given frame of reference leading to a conclusion of whether the **system** will suit its purpose (i.e. the **validation**). NOTE - technology assessment is sometimes used when the object for assessment is a physical device or a **system**. The contents of technology assessment in medicine is described as (Perry & Dunlap 1990) as: "Technology assessment in medicine means careful and formal **evaluation** of a technology in terms of safety, efficacy, effectiveness and cost-effectiveness and of its social, economic and ethical implications, both in absolute terms and in comparison with other competing technologies."
evaluation act of measuring quality characteristics NOTE - modified from (Nykänen 1990). (Hoppe & Meseguer 1993) concludes that "Evaluation assesses or measures a KBS's quantitative or qualitative characteristics and compare them with expected or desired values.". As this description overlaps too much with our definition of **validation**, we prefer to adopt the definition above.
validation act of comparing properties of an object with the stated goal as a frame of reference NOTE - modified from a combination of the definitions: 1) (ISO 9000-3) "**validation** for (software): The process of evaluating software to ensure compliance with specified requirements.", 2) (Nykänen 1990) "comparison of quality measures with a frame of reference. Validation means deciding on quality, answering a question "Is it good enough?".."; and 3) (Hoppe & Meseguer 1993) "Validation checks whether a KBS corresponds to the system it is supposed to represent.", i.e. checking whether the right **system** has been built.
verification act of checking well-defined properties of an object against its specification (modified from: Hoppe & Meseguer 1993) NOTE - this definition conforms with the ISO definition (ISO 9000-3): "**verification (for software)**: The process of evaluating the products of a given phase to ensure correctness and consistency with respect to the products and standards provided as input to that phase." EXAMPLE - for instance checking whether an information system (or a KBS) has been built right.

(Reprinted from (Brender 1997a) with permission)[2]

---

[2] Please note that the definition of *evaluation* has been further refined (see the discussion above). Also note that in formal definitions of concepts one should always define the concept in the same syntax as in itself, – that is, a verb should be defined with another verb (plus possibly a specification/description). In day-to-day speech it may sound artificial, but we have chosen to keep it that way.

2.1.2   Summative Assessment

The purpose of summative assessments is to contribute, with a kind of statement of properties of the object in a decision-making context. Typical examples of summative assessments are (1) evaluation of objectives fulfillment or (2) the kind of assessment carried out in a contractual relationship, when an IT system is delivered and one wants to ascertain that the installation functions in accordance with the contract.

In summative assessments of the functional mode of operation it is usually taken for granted that when the users sit down by the IT system in order to evaluate it, it is (reasonably) free of programming bugs. However, this is an unreasonable request in situations when constructive assessment is used precisely to guide the future direction of the development. Instead one has to handle errors as a necessary evil.

In its philosophy the Health Technology Assessment (HTA) is summative by nature: An analysis is carried out of a number of qualities in a device, a technology, or a service with the aim of providing a basis for a political or administrative decision. Once the results of an HTA are ready, these can form part of a negotiation process with a vendor, thereby giving it a constructive (sub) role.

2.1.3   Constructive Assessment

Constructive assessment or formative assessment is the kind of assessment activity that aims at giving direction for decision making with regard to subsequent development or implementation tasks – that is, to control a dynamically changeable development process. Most IT projects constitute a compromise between an ideal solution and something realizable, controlled by local concerns, considerations, and limiting factors. Furthermore, irrespective of whether it is an off-the-shelf system or not, most IT projects are both large and unpredictable, one of the reasons being organizational conditions and changes. Such dynamically changing conditions for assessments imply huge demands on the handling of evaluation methods to establish an ongoing decision-making basis

When looking at an 'ideal' IT development project, the philosophy should be that whenever one encounters a significant problem that cannot be rectified, patched, or compensated for immediately one must take one step back in the plan and go ahead with what is called 'interim corrective activities' – that is, a 'feed-back loop'. Analyzing and making the causality explicit will strengthen the possibilities of an optimal correction in the plans instead of just providing a temporary remedy. Most development projects are compromises between the ideal and something practicable, steered by local conditions, regardless of whether the limits are put down for budgetary reasons, technological limitations, the users' imagination, or traditions, and so forth.

One drawback of these interim corrections is that the development object may become a moving target. The moving target phenomenon portrays the situation in which the final and overall solution for the complete system changes as a factor of time. This could unintentionally be caused by the fact that you learn as you go or that conditions change and one chooses to accept the consequences. It has consequences for the basis of the assessment – for instance, if one, prior to the development project, starts measuring base values of the qualities to which one wants to compare the end product. This phenomenon is inevitable in actual development projects of IT-based solutions, as opposed to just getting an off-the-shelf product. It is of course possible to disregard the problems encountered, but then the outcome may not be an optimized solution.

Such dynamically changing circumstances of assessments imply big demands on the ability to handle and adapt assessment methods to the continuous information needs. The assessment activities provide the input for the system development process regardless of what they are called. This type is called *constructive assessment* or *formative assessment*.

Constructive assessment activities adapt to the value norms of the organization. For instance, if the conditions of responsibility and competence have to be left unchanged, then the assessment must take these conditions into account in order to direct the development in accordance with this value norm. When rationalizing, focus naturally has to be on efficiency as well as effectiveness. If it is the quality of the operation or service of the department that needs improvement through a development project, one has to make it clear how to observe or assess precisely these aspects while keeping them in focus during the assessment activities. It is worth mentioning here that there will always be a number of aspects that have to be looked at in parallel, making it necessary to weigh them jointly against each other for each decision instance.

2.2 Methodology, Method, Technique, and Framework

The strategy of developing a methodology for assessment activities during an IT development or implementation project is based on a framework called "The Metrology Framework". *Metrology* means "the science of measurement" (BIPM et al. 1993). This section examines the related concepts as they are used in this book.

2.2.1 Method

A method is a formal description of the procedure involved in how to carry out an actual task. A method is based on a well-defined theory and includes a consistent set of techniques, tools, and principles to organize it. A method is also characterized by its application area and perspectives (see the latter concept in Section 2.4). Methods are realized with the aid of a chain of goal-oriented actions (subtasks), each with its underlying philosophy or theory and strategy, and they are carried out by means of appertaining techniques, tools, and principles. It is important to remember that a method can be misunderstood (misconstrued) or misused, should it be outside its normal context and assumptions.

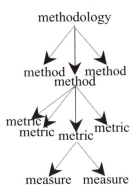

Another important point is that methods are normally abstract (i.e., described in an anonymous way) and must be instantiated and probably also adapted to the concrete conditions. An instantiated method is a method where all tools, techniques, and descriptions of procedures are operationalized to suit the actual task.

2.2.2 Technique

The author has been asked why she does not distinguish between techniques and methods in the descriptions in this book. The author had to go through several Danish and English dictionaries without finding good definitions of the two concepts that would once and for all clarify the difference. Here is an example.

> *Technique: "a practical **method**, skill or art applied to a particular task".*
>
> *Method: "1. a way of proceeding or doing something, especially a systematic or regular one. 2. orderliness of thought, action, etc. 3. (often pl.) the **techniques** or arrangement of work for a particular field or subject."*

(Collins English Dictionary 1995).

In other words, the two concepts are mutually defined by the opposite party. Neither does it help that the literature does not agree on the difference between the two concepts (see, for instance, Arbnor and Bjerke 1997, page 8). The author's own understanding of the two concepts is that a method in connection with an assessment procedure is the formal and abstract description of what to do together with the underlying description of theory, assumptions, and suppositions, among others, while a technique is the practical and concrete instruction or implementation of how to carry out an assessment. A technique can in itself have underlying theories, assumptions, and suppositions, and be worked out in an abstract form, whereby it works as a method. Or a technique could represent the practical implementation of a concrete method, such as in the shape of a tool, a formula, a procedure, and so on. A method can, in the same way, be so simple – for instance, how to open a carton of juice– to render it more appropriate to call it a technique. In other words, there is a very large gray area between the understandings of the two concepts. Hence the understanding of a method as a context and a safeguard for the (correct) use of techniques. Nevertheless, it has been decided to use the authors' original terms (method, technique) in descriptions of methods from the literature.

2.2.3   *Measures and Metrics*

The concept of *metric* in assessment methods is used as a concrete measurement technique or tool, usually just a formula to calculate, or a device for measuring something. In other words, metrics are those concepts that allow measures to be given a concrete value. The equation for a straight line is one example of a metric, and in the equation $y = ax + b$, y is the concrete measure. Another example of this 'concrete' could be a measurable characteristic of an IT system, such as response time.

Sometimes, a measure will have an implicit metric. This is, for instance, the case in assessing the esthetics of an object, while a subject such as user satisfaction can be measured both qualitatively and subjectively (here without equation) or quantitatively and objectively with the aid of a questionnaire study. In a questionnaire study, for example, the metric is equal to the equations used to calculate averages and dispersion of responses.

2.2.4   *Methodology*

The term *methodology* signifies "the science of methods" (BIPM et al. 1993) from the Greek *logos*, which means "the science of". In functional terms it relates to the knowledge of how to prepare and use methods. Expressed in structural terms a methodology consists of "a coherent set of methods covering all the subtasks necessary for a given undertaking". In other words, a methodology is supposed to (1) provide the answer to what to do next, when to do what, and how to do it, and (2) to describe the ideas behind such choices and the suppositions (for instance, the philosophical background) behind them.

An essential point concerning the structural understanding of methodology is that the set of methods used include all necessary tools to fulfill a task. Hence (in practical terms) a methodology also encompasses the strategy of how to split up a task into smaller subtasks, and how to choose and construct a combination of methods in such a way that they make a coherent entirety that can lead to the fulfillment of the objective – taking the underlying philosophy of the kind of problem areas and their context and qualities into consideration. Therefore, the list of prescribed tasks of a methodology includes at minimum of the three following tasks: (1) analysis and delimitation of the problem and the task, (2) definition of the overall strategy and procedure, and (3) selection and combination of a set of methods to achieve the objective.

Apart from the above, a methodology must (in order to be complete and coherent) comprise:

- The basic philosophies and theories, so that a user of the methodology can judge the validity of its use
- Perspective (see below)
- Assumptions
- Areas of use
- Applicable methods, tools, and techniques

A methodology can refer to (or include) several methods and a method can have several metrics, which separately can deliver different measures of success or characteristics of the problem areas. In order that a method can be called useable in connection with a given methodology, its philosophy, theories, and perspectives need to comply with the aspects of the methodology; the assumptions and suppositions for its use and its application areas all have to be fulfilled.

2.2.5 Framework

A framework is best expressed by the functional definition provided by Hornby et al. 1963: "*that part of a structure that gives shape and support*". In other words, a framework corresponds to a rack on which one can hang concepts in a structural way, giving significance in a previously defined context. A framework can be very abstract or quite concrete, simple or very elaborate, but all frameworks that are based on a philosophy, a theory, and assumptions have limited areas of application. Thus, frameworks look quite a lot like methodologies. The difference is that a framework is a passive, descriptive, or structuring tool, while a methodology is a prescriptive tool to carry out a given task.

A (very concrete) framework can include a lot of details and guidelines and, depending on how it is being used, thereby increase the analogy to a methodology. A couple of examples are the references (*Handbook of Objectives-Oriented Planning* 1992; Preece and Rombach 1994), which with slight modification or expansion can be used as methodologies. The first reference describes a process of project planning in developing countries, much used for aid projects; the reference calls it a framework, but it does contain a number of examples and recommendations on how to carry out the planning and thus resembles a methodology quite a lot. In a similar way the latter reference consists of a taxonomy combined with a recommendation of how to use it. This continuum between the two terms is the reason why these two concepts are often confounded.

2.3   Quality Management

Commentary: The description of the theoretical background for this subsection is aimed at bringing a better understanding of the principles behind how to develop and use methods, and thereby enabling the readers to use the results of the report in more detail in other connections. However, understanding this section is not a necessity for the use of the methods and metrics described.

The aim of *Quality Management* (QM) is to ensure the best possible process and outcome of a given activity or of the overall functionality and service level of an organization.

The three component concepts – Quality Assurance (QA), Quality Control (QC), and Quality Inspection (QI) – are used here in the context that forms the basis for the ISO900x standards (ISO-8402). The latest version of ISO-900x, ISO-9000: 2000, defines the concepts less sharply (see ISO-9000:2000), but in essence there is no marked difference in their interpretation. The idea is the same. In the context of planning, this can be explained in an abstract and brief way as follows:

QA: The QA activity comprises an analysis of the actual objective, its circumstances or conditions, and establishment of principles, plan of action and strategy for a solution including the overall choice of method. This corresponds to analysis and selection at a strategic level to ensure that the conditions and the objective are turned into guidelines for the process in such a way that an optimal outcome is achieved.

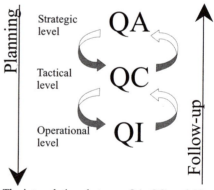

The interrelations between QA, QC, and QI
(from Brender 1997a)

QC: The QC activity transforms the result of QA into use for the actual case – that is, guidelines for the actual process of organizing and adapting the chosen methods, corresponding to a tactical level.

QI: The QI activity implements the results of QA and QC in terms of preparation and installation of pragmatic instructions, tools, and work procedures. For instance, the tools could be tables to complete, checklists, or operationalized methods such as concrete instructions corresponding to an operational level.

As seen in the illustration, these three levels naturally reflect a traditional distribution of responsibility and competence from a 'Steering Group' (the strategic level) through a 'Project Group' (the tactical level) to the practical working group (the operational level). The functions of QA, QC, and QI, as described above, correspond to the planning function alone. The follow-up of the QM activities is supposed to analyze whether the decisions made during planning have resulted in the desired level of quality for the ongoing or completed task.

Metrology means "the science of measurement", as shown above. There is an important interaction between the QM dimension and the metrology dimension, although they are independent: QM defines the way in which one can prepare and achieve quality, while metrology concretizes how to integrate the process of measure into the entirety. QA corresponds to the concretization that takes place at the methodology level, QC corresponds to concretization at a method level, and QI corresponds to implementation and carrying out of measures and metrics.

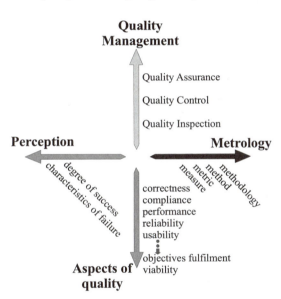

Overview of the elements in the framework for quality management

Quality Aspects contain a list of the characteristics defined as relevant for the object studied – here an EHR, for instance. From a legal perspective the quality is defined in terms of the requirements specification's individual requirements, while for a user in everyday work there can be a number of other aspects that are relevant, such as how user friendly is the dialogue between the system and the user. A typical example of a quality aspect in a requirements specification is the performance of the system with the response time as a concrete example of how the performance can be measured. The synthesis of information from quality aspects that have been measured and analyzed forms the decision-making basis.

The last dimension of the conceptual apparatus in this respect is the 'Perception' of quality. It deals with the implicit understanding of the concept of quality. Quality is usually measured as the compliance with the requirements specified (i.e., the degree of success as, for example, the medical term PV_{pos}). A number of assessment methods use balanced weightings based on prioritization of the individual requirements to summarize the level of compliance. The author's interpretation is that the 'degree of success' is not the only thing of importance when assessing IT-based solutions, but that it can be at least as important to obtain characteristics of the 'consequences of deviance' – that is, failure points. An important example of this is how patients categorized under 'misclassification' for a given diagnostic method are distributed over the different subcategories and what will be the consequence for the patient of such a misclassification with respect to prognosis and further examinations.

Another example of a failure characteristic better known from IT systems is an aspect of a tender that, if not fulfilled, will stop the client from choosing that particular solution or that particular supplier (a showstopper).

2.4 Perspective

The concept of 'perspective' stands for hidden aspects and assumptions deeply buried in the design and application of methods (see, for instance, Mathiassen and Munk-Madsen 1986; Arbnor and Bjerke 1997; Brender 1997a). In a generalized version, the perspective is the implicit assumptions of (cause-effect relations within) the object of study. So, the perspective is synonymous with "that aggregation of (conscious or unconscious, epistemological) assumptions of how things relate in combination with imprinted attitudes guiding our decision making – for example in a problem-solving situation".

The concept of perspective is defined within the systems development domain as "assumptions on the nature of the working processes and how people interact in an organizational setting" (Mathiassen and Munk-Madsen 1986) – that is, assumptions on the nature of work procedures and how people interact in an organizational context, implicit or nonconscious models of understanding behind the principles forming the basis for our development methods and management principles, and thus for how we deal with elements in a project.

In a generalized version perspective can be interpreted as "(implicit) assumptions of a given object, for instance, cause-effect relationships ". In other words, the perspective is a collection of (conscious, subconscious epistemological and ontological[3]) assumptions of how a given point functions. This must also be seen in the light of the (unconscious) cultural influences on how we perceive things, which again forms the background for how we make decisions.

Some people will probably ask what this concept has to do with assessment. This is mainly because the term perspective is not used in the same sense as we know it from daily use. The concept of *perspective* in its present use comes from system development and is something hidden in most methods, and not often noticed – not even by their originators. Through their implicit nature (i.e., completely unknown to first time users) some perspectives can contain pitfalls, where the perspective of the method conflicts with the actual purpose the method is intended to be used for. This is why this concept is so prominent in this handbook.

This should be seen in the context of our – often subconscious – culturally conditioned way of perceiving a situation, which in turn forms the basis for how we make decisions. Few method designers are aware that our cultural background (professional, religious, and national) alone maintains a series of tacit assumptions affecting our way of doing things (see, for instance, Hampden-Turner and Trompenaars 1993, 1997; Trompenaars and Hampden-Turner 1997; Schneider and Barsoux 2003; and Arbnor and Bjerke 1997, page 6ff; as well as a brief overview in Cabrera et al. 2001). Thus, in a similar way, one can, simply through greater attentiveness when picking from the literature, capture some of these conditions of the methods, thereby avoiding certain pitfalls in the assessment project. This is why it is worth discussing the concept in this book. But the understanding of this section is not strictly necessary for using the methods described here, because the perspectives of the methods are outlined and discussed individually for each method.

Now we will look more closely at some examples of actual perspectives in system development and assessment.

2.4.1   *Example: Cultural Dependence on Management Principles*

A concrete example of a perspective is management principles, which will form the basis for how we construct a project organization and who is selected to take

---

[3] Epistemology = theory of knowledge; ontology = theory of the true nature of things. In other words, in epistemology it is knowledge as a concept that is the object of the study (i.e., its validity and area of application), while ontology deals with the actual correlation between parts (e.g., understanding the causality) of an object.

part in a development project. In Denmark it is the **right** of the work force to be consulted in matters of technological project development, and it is becoming quite natural for staff to get deeply involved in development projects. But you don't have to go very far south in Europe before you find a different balance between management and staff that is just as natural (Fröhlich et al. 1993). And in Asian countries, such as Thailand, you cannot make the work force get involved at all – they simply do not want to (Malling 1992). Thus, methods in the 'participatory design' category cannot be used in Asia. This also means that we cannot just use any method designed by others. Nevertheless, one should not just discard everything not invented in one's own country or in the health sector but should think carefully and consciously of possible hidden assumptions when choosing a method.

2.4.2   Example: Diagramming Techniques

Another example is that many diagramming techniques assume that the work procedures that the diagram depicts are carried out sequentially or, if this is not the case, that such an omission does not have any consequences when the technique is being used (for instance, in terms of incorrectly organized functions in an IT-based system) (Brender 1999).

2.4.3   Example: Value Norms in Quality Development

A third example is the description of the model for the controlling indicators in 'Quality of Care' in (Chilingerian 2000):

1. Patient satisfaction (% very satisfied and why, pain management, % willing to recommend the place)
2. Information and emotional support (the amount and the clarity of the information, time spent listening, time spent encouraging)
3. Amenities (cleanliness, punctuality, respect for the patient, service on demand)
4. Efficiency in decision making (sufficient clinical resources to obtain a constant level of service, quick diagnosis, and treatment)
5. Outcome (mortality and morbidity, changes to the functional status, health status, and degree of illness)

Where is the staff in this quality model? Clearly staff is there indirectly as they provide the service. But, for example, the job satisfaction of staff is not an explicit parameter in this quality model. Staff satisfaction and well-being in the organization is an indicator of the long-term quality level of the organization, as it expresses something about the stability of the organization and its value norms and also its ability to enter into and contribute to development processes in order to achieve lasting solutions. Again, this is a European (Scandinavian) perspective, while the book referred to above is American. Quite another model for quality development would probably be found in the Asian and African cultures because their value norms are different.

2.4.4   Example: Assumptions of People's Abilities

The traditional way of carrying out systems development or purchase (i.e., preparation of a detailed requirements specification and completion of a tender as stipulated by EU regulations for public institutions when a project is over a certain size), includes some of the following assumptions:

1. That the users are able to express their demands correctly and completely and in accordance with the technological possibilities. In the literature it is quite well documented that the users find it difficult to describe or express their demands (see, for example, Cunningham et al. 1985; Beuschel 1991; Brender 1997a; and Beuscart-Zéphir et al. 1997).

2. That the introduction of nontrivial IT solutions often requires important restructuring of work procedures and the structure of the organization and that the users are the real experts when it comes to knowledge of how the organization functions. The literature, however, shows (1) that things do not always happen in the way the users specify them, (2) that all work procedures vary greatly in the way they are carried out, and (3) that rules are generally broken and procedures not followed; cf. "work-to-rule" (see the discussions in (Beuscart-Zéphir et al. 1997; and Brender 1997a).

2.4.5   Example: The User Concept

The concept of 'user' is rather complex. The author's definition is:

> *"[A] user is any or all persons, organisations or establishments who's work processes are part of the activities connected with the operation of the computer-based (or computer-supported) system"*.

(Brender 1997a)

In this definition, apart from the end user (who has the actual interaction with the IT system), the concept comprises all stakeholders, including decision makers and management in the organization where the IT system is to be implemented. For example, the general manager of a hospital is responsible for services and budgets for his/her hospital; therefore, anything that might influence these is also his/her area of responsibility, and it is something that he/she has to account for to his/her superiors and in the end to the politicians. In that way he/she is an essential piece of the puzzle that as an overall concept is called *users* in the organization implementing the system. Of course, this does not mean that the person concerned has to be part of all the working groups, but it shows that the concept of user is a very complex concept that changes from one project decision to the next.

Please note also that this interpretation is derived from a Danish perspective – that is, an interpretation that has evolved against a background of Danish culture and the legislation and trade union agreements, and so on, derived from it. This is precisely where user involvement works differently in Thailand, as discussed in Section 2.4.1.

2.4.6   Example: The Administrative Perspective

The author's experience is that users in the healthcare sector have an inflated confidence, verging on the naive, in the provision of IT systems. Many user organizations in healthcare are relatively inexperienced with regard to IT-based systems and seem to expect that this type of system is just as thoroughly tested as IT hardware and medico-technical equipment, for instance. This is not always the case, and there are great differences between IT off-the-shelf products and IT systems custom made to the actual purpose, as is currently the case with a number of EHR projects. It is reasonable to expect off-the-shelf products (like Microsoft's Word) to be virtually free of errors, but this is not automatically the case for IT systems or those parts of the system functionalities that are either new developments or adaptations.

With regard to the development and introduction of IT systems (whole systems and/or single new modules) it is important that the management responsible in the user organization can and will undertake responsibility for running the system – that is, that management can trust that the system works correctly, completely, and coherently. They must also be confident that it functions efficiently and according to its purpose in such a way that the system does not have any medical side effects in patient treatment. In the case of development projects, where one does not know the product beforehand and therefore cannot make a choice, it is by no means a foregone conclusion that the final solution will work satisfactorily in day-to-day clinical practice. It is of no use that the IT people say that it works, because they do not have the administrative competence and responsibility to judge this. The introduction of an IT system is a very responsible task, especially when or if something goes wrong – regardless of whether it is a pilot run or it is fully operational.

This is, therefore, an important perspective when planning and organizing assessment activities, both prior to its introduction and in connection with all subsequent changes and adjustments. The traditional HTA falls a little short with regard to the four traditional aspects of economy, technology, patient, and organization: The administrative aspect must be explicitly included in the analysis of all four aspects.

The administrative perspective is further complicated in healthcare by the present division of competence between different administrative, clinical, and para-clinical functions. The conditions of competence and responsibility become very complex when one deals with integrated IT solutions, such as the implementation of EHR, and this still has to find its practical solution in an administrative context. For example, the para-clinics have been responsible for the contents and presentation of information in their result reports to the clinics, whereas should an element in the report be taken out of its original context and used in another context (such as in a scientific article), the performer of this act undertakes the responsibility for the use of the new, composite information and its correctness in the use context. Who will then have the responsibility for the presentation of the para-clinical data in an EHR and thereby the decision-making competence of such conditions in the development and implementation project?

2.4.7 Example: Interaction between Development and Assessment Activities

Truex and Klein (1991) also show, for instance, that *"human systems are not deterministic"* and *"human systems are always in the process of change"*. In other words, and as Rector (1996) states, when a development or implementation project spans over a period of time, even though the requirements are set out in the requirements specification, technical changes will often make it impossible to avoid implementing changes to an IT-based solution.

This illustrates that there is not much point in fixing the requirements specification too stringently. There must be room for evolution. The final consequence is that a development or implementation project is indeterministic (unpredictable in all details) and undergoes dynamic change. Although there will normally be a continuum of variations between the poles indeterministic and deterministic, or dynamic and static, respectively, only some aspects change, while others remain quite stable.

The consequence of indeterminism and dynamism in IT development projects is the need for supporting activities during the development process:

1. Proactive opportunities in terms of *feed-forward loops*[4] so that conditions that entail changes are immediately incorporated into the plans, taking into account and making room for changes in subsequent activities. An example could be a risk factor that shows up at some point and that would need subsequent monitoring. Or it could be completely new initiatives and

---

[4] The term is borrowed from biology and biochemistry inasmuch as nature contains a lot of regulating mechanisms, some of which hinder or promote subsequent steps in a process (feed-forward loops), while others influence earlier steps in the process, in such a way that the process itself is inhibited (*feed-back loops*).

functions that need to be incorporated into the development project and therefore need to be taken into account in the assessment activities (e.g., in the baseline studies that serve as the frame of reference of the assessment).

2. Adaptation to changes in terms and conditions. Apart from budget changes, with which we are all familiar, technological changes in the domain will also take place during large projects, making it necessary to make some revisions to the assessment plan. It could, for instance, be changing one analytical instrument in the laboratory or one clinical examination method for another.

3. Flexibility: Assessment activities have to follow suit when things in the project change or assessment methods have to be modified or new ones invented, giving way to ad hoc assessments and context related assessments. This can be quite a challenge.

The evaluation methods are the tools that will help the project management to maximize or optimize the features of success and to minimize errors and shortcomings.

2.4.8 Example: Interaction between Human and Technical Aspects

Human and organizational factors are very important in the development and introduction of IT-based solutions. According to a large international study of 500 cases carried out by Price-Waterhouse and Mori (*Without change . . .* 1997) and indications from a recent Delphi study (Brender et al. 2006), these aspects are commonly the cause of things going wrong. These include psychological and social aspects (including political and trade union) and are therefore very dependent on the local culture. Demarcation lines, for example: If a physician or a nurse is employed in a new place, it is taken for granted that this person will quickly adapt to local conditions and the ways in which things are done, including who does what, when, and how. But if an IT-based system introduced in an organization forces through changes of local trade union demarcations, everyone will be against it.

A metaphor can serve as an abstract illustration of the interaction between the human and the technical aspects of an IT-based solution. The metaphor is a pyramid, and each of the two aspects can be illustrated as a pyramid, but in different colors. If just one of the pyramids is solid and an arrow is shot at it, then both the arrow and the pyramid will get damaged, depending on which is harder. This is the same for both pyramids. To introduce a technical pyramid, an IT system, into an organization is a drastic step for the organization and means that the users' situation is turned upside-down, figuratively speaking. Try to turn the human pyramid on its head. How does that feel? Out of control! Vulnerable! You get the feeling that you would fall over at the slightest nudge. You react emotionally to it and you will do anything to defend yourself. Figuratively, this corresponds to shooting an arrow at the other pyramid. What are the characteristics of an IT system that make it seem solid? It could, for instance, be that the IT system is introduced and functions on its own premises or those of a third party. Both parties will get hurt when they clash in this situation.

However, if the pyramids are open (transparent) in every way – meaning that you only experience the edges (the demarcation) – then most attacks will go straight through and exit on the other side of the structure. This corresponds to openness and willingness to accept – well worth it for both parties! Should you now introduce a transparent pyramide into an organization (i.e., an IT system adapted to and respecting the user situation), then you have a totally different situation. Should the organization or the users also be transparent (i.e., open and willing to stand on their heads to accommodate the system and willing to make an effort in spite of being vulnerable due to the new, unknown situation), then only one thing is needed for them to cooperate: that one of the two parties opens up for a while, and instantly you have two superimposed pyramids. When they are viewed together from the side, they are no longer two separate pyramids but a hexagonal star structure with each part supporting the other (try it yourself: when you turn one 90 degrees in relation to the other, they literally support each other). Both are unchanged – but together they amount to more than the sum of their parts.

It is in the interaction and the cooperation that technology and human beings are made to give their utmost in respect of each others' tasks and purposes.

2.5 Evaluation Viewed in the Light of the IT System's Life Cycle

The life cycle of an IT-based solution is the time span from conceiving the idea of a solution to meeting a given objective until that solution is finally abandoned. The solution may be a complete IT system, but it may also just relate to a specific change in an existing IT system.

An IT system's, as well as an IT-based solution's, life cycle consists of a series of phases, where, according to the international standardization organization (ISO), the concept of *phase* means "a defined segment of work" (ISO 9000-3). This definition suggests that the distribution in time for activities in a given phase may well be accomplished in parallel with activities of other phases. At the same time the definition signifies that there may be other equally useful ways of dividing the time axis into phases of the IT system's life. The argument is that it depends on the global approach and the methods chosen to accomplish the major tasks, such as the method of analysis that leads to a requirements specification: A spiral approach has a different set of phases than a waterfall model for systems development, or the same concepts are interpreted differently.

However, this is just one way of graduating time from the very first idea of a (new) IT system until the system (solution) or the idea of it no longer exists. Other models can be equally good. In other words, the life cycle model described below should be seen as just one way of structuring time for a project. Please note that regardless of whether the life cycle model described below, other life cycle models, or development methods are used, the same assessment methods and techniques can be used, but under all circumstances it is necessary to select them with care and adapt them to the purpose or situation at hand.

The present life cycle model merely has the purpose of providing a framework for this handbook to link evaluation methods to typical tasks and activities in a system development or implementation project. For this purpose and irrespective of the system development methodology, we will use four main phases for the life cycle of an IT-based solution, as outlined in the following.

Please note that the assessment activities of the first two phases are only carried out under experimental conditions, while the activities in the following phases are carried out under real routine operations.

The *Explorative Phase* is concerned with the strategic aspects related to the global task, addressing issues like objective, intentions for the solution, basic principles for the solution model, as well as feasibility of realization (technically and organizationally). Typically, this phase ends with a requirements specification and a contract or another kind of specification of what the users want to achieve. The matching material also contains the necessary background information and relevant frames of reference for later assessments.

The *Technical Development Phase* comprises the development and/or adaptation of the IT system, followed by its installation in the organization, also in terms of changed work procedures. User assessment in this phase typically constitutes constructive assessment activities, concluding with a summative verification addressing whether the IT system/IT-based solution is good enough to be put into daily operation and whether the contractual agreement has been fulfilled. The assessment activities during this phase are carried out under experimental conditions – that is, not under real operations. Thus, assessment activities in the pilot phase belong to the next phase.

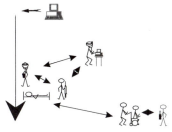

The *Adaptation Phase* (called the Maintenance Phase in Brender 1997a) includes the period immediately after the IT system has been put into daily operation, partially or in full. It is a phase during which extensive adaptations in the IT system, its setup and/or the work procedures take place, until a stable situation is achieved. It is assumed that all significant errors (bugs) and omissions found in the previous phase have been corrected prior to daily operations. This phase is, therefore, concerned with corrections, adaptations, and refinements of all the types of errors, omissions, and shortcomings identified after the system was put into operation and that are necessary for the organization to become effective (again).

This phase ought to be fairly short if the solution implemented functions relatively well and work procedures have been adapted prior to introduction. The transition to the next phase will usually be gradual.

The *Evolution Phase* begins when the worst problem areas in the IT systems and its surrounding work procedures have been overcome, and the operation has entered a state of (reasonable) stability. During the Evolution Phase a number of new developments or changes in activities will usually be initiated, each of which will have a life cycle corresponding to the present life cycle model. Also, measures of the effect or impact of the IT system or solution may take place during this phase. It ends when the IT system/solution is replaced with another system or solution.

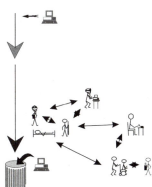

3. Types of User Assessments of IT-based Solutions

What is it that makes the difference between different assessment investigations? And why is it difficult to identify articles within the literature that one can benefit from? Could it be the degree of complexity of the domain of assessment? This complexity will be briefly illustrated in this chapter

There are many different, more or less independent, ways to categorize evaluation, which are called dimensions. For instance, there are two main focuses on the object of study:

- The technical construct (i.e., whether the construction of the IT system is satisfactory)
- The functional mode of operation (i.e., whether the IT system has the right functions and executes these in an appropriate way)

There are two main assessment approaches orthogonal to this dimension:

- Explorative – that is, for clarification purposes (within the social sector this is called 'goal-free evaluation'). The aim of this type of assessment is to obtain a rich picture of what takes place in an organization, how, and why. Typically there is no frame of reference in this situation. This type of investigation is often psychological or sociological in nature.
- Verifying – that is, of a confirmatory nature. This includes validation of objectives fulfillment or attainment. For this type of assessment investigation one always uses a frame of reference (such as a contract or a specification) as a point of comparison. Natural science investigations are often of this type; that is, an investigation is founded on a specific understanding (a model and/or a hypothesis), which the researcher attempts to reject.

The spectrum of assessments further adds to this complexity and ranges from:

- Quantitative to qualitative. This is concerned with whether there is a measuring scale available for putting the results into a metric context or, at the other extreme, whether the result is purely descriptive. A far more thorough account of the distinction between the two is provided in (Silverman 2001), also describing the features of the 'positivism', 'constructionism', and 'emotionalism' perspectives, and many other of the concepts of qualitative research methods.
- Objective and subjective: Objectivity is concerned with rational measurement of physical properties (like response time in a dialogue between a user and the

IT system), while subjectivity is concerned with aspects that are emotionally based (like user satisfaction and job quality). It is not always feasible to separate these aspects from those within the next point (see, for instance, Moehr 2002), but the author prefers this distinction.

- Reductionism and holism: Reductionism is an expression of the perspective that everything consists of parts, which may be taken out of their context and measured or otherwise investigated individually, and that afterwards one may draw conclusions about the wholeness on the basis of the outcome of these individualized measurements of its component parts. The holistic perspective is based on the understanding that the wholeness comprises not only its component elements, but also other aspects that in a mutual interaction con-tribute to the creation of the wholeness. Synergy among members of a team is an example of this add-on element. The holistic perspective implies that, as an investigator, one cannot separate the human factors from the understanding of an organization and its IT-based solution; see, for instance, myth number one in (Berg 2001).

Yet another dimension in the understanding of ways to assess IT-based solutions is the distinction between constructive and summative assessments. See Sections 2.1.2 and 2.1.3.

Furthermore, assessments may support and thereby adhere to a prognostic, a diagnostic (including screening), or a monitoring purpose. While assessment activities cannot be of a treating nature in itself, each one of the others will for that purpose support treatment by providing a decision-making basis for the ongoing process.

It would be inaccurate to say that one of the aspects described in the list above is better than another, as they answer different questions when applied. Furthermore, if it is not feasible to accomplish a quantitative and objective investigation, one could just as well get valuable information from a subjective and qualitative investigation. Still, one should not answer a quantitative question by applying a qualitative method. Similarly, one should not unconditionally reject the reductionistic approach that has been dominant within natural science research for centuries because this may sometimes be the only way forward in an investigation. What is important is that one realizes the guiding perspective behind one's statements and choices, as well as the pitfalls and perils inherent in each method.

It is the many choices of evaluation methods and the multiple dimensions adding to the complexity that make it difficult to get a quick overview identifying relevant articles in the literature.

3.1 Types of User Assessment during the Phases of a System's Life Cycle

In principle, all aspects will be assessed during all phases of system development, but the assessment activities can be either prognostic (during the planning), or screening and diagnostic (prior to introduction) for curative or preventive purposes.

3.1.1 The Explorative Phase

During the analysis and planning phase (called the Explorative Phase in the life cycle model above) the assessment activities will, for example, address the aspects mentioned below, both as an ongoing activity during planning and as a final activity before concluding the task:

- *Relevance*: An assessment of whether the solution in question or a combination of solutions is at all able to solve the current problems and meet the demands and requirements of the organization.

- *Problem Areas*: Where are the weaknesses and the elements of risk in the model solution? For instance, an off-the-shelf product may have to be chosen because the old IT system is so unreliable that it is not possible to wait for a development project to be carried out. Or the plans may be based on a given operational situation even though a knowledge gap would occur should certain employees leave the company and so forth.

- *Feasibility*: Does the organization have the resources needed to implement the chosen solution (structurally in the organization, in terms of competence and financially, for example), as well as the support of management, staff, and politicians?

- *Completeness and consistency*: Is the solution a coherent entity that is neither over- nor undersized?

- *Verifiability*: One must consider whether and how to verify that every small requirement and function in the model solution has been fulfilled once the complete system is implemented and ready to be put to use.

- *Elements of Risk*: Are there any external conditions outside organizational control that will involve a substantial risk to the project should it/they occur? This could, for instance, be dependence on a technology that is not yet fully developed, or dependence on (establishment or functional level of) the parent organization's technical or organizational infrastructure that has to fall into place first, or dependence on coordination and integration with other projects.

3.1.2   *The Technical Development Phase*

During this phase, assessment activities are typically carried out under experimental conditions (i.e., not under real operations). In this phase, the user assessment can be either a constructive one and/or a summative one, depending on the type of development project. It is not just the technical and common* functional aspects that are relevant to assess during this phase, but also the ergonomic and cognitive aspects ending with a complete technical verification. Technical verification means checking whether all the functions of the IT-based system are present and function correctly and in accordance with the agreement (usually a contract).

Constructive assessments are useful in actual development projects as tools to secure desirable development choices, while the acquisition of an off-the-shelf IT system has far smaller, if any, need for the constructive element. One of the focal points in current systems development approaches is the ergonomic and cognitive aspects, and these will typically be of a constructive nature during a development project. The ergonomic aspects address the user dialog with the IT-based system and focuses on the practical and mental strains on the users during the dialog. The cognitive aspects are concerned with the degree of accordance between the users' mental processes while carrying out an activity (work procedure) and the way in which the IT system works. One example of a typical ergonomic aspect is how many actions a user has to perform to carry out an activity – for instance, how many screens one has to go through to move a patient from one ward to another, or how many mouse clicks. An example of a function where the cognitive aspects are important is a physician's diagnostic work when seeing a new patient and having to question the patient at the same time as taking notes of all relevant information in an electronic healthcare record.

Finally, in this phase, a technical verification has to be carried out to provide a basis for making the decision of whether or not to take the IT system into operations. Technical verifications are very work intensive indeed, and they include the aspects of integration and performance and capacity requirements, all in all corresponding to verification of whether the contractual basis has been fulfilled (if the development work is based on a contract) and whether the system as it works is suited for that operation. The former purpose is usually a contractual decision point, while the latter is concerned with the management's responsibility for the department's quality of service. In other words, are all the functions present, are they complete, and do they function correctly and appropriately? Probably the most difficult to assess in this respect is the interoperability aspects – that is, how several integrated IT systems (such as an EHR and a laboratory information system (LIS)) work together, particularly with regard to the time aspects. For example, what happens in the LIS at different points during the analytical and administrative procedures when a ward modifies or cancels an order or moves a patient to another ward?

Normally ordinary technical verification will only be carried out in a summative way. However, when developing decision-support systems or expert systems (knowledge-based systems) the concept of correctness (the technical verification) has a further dimension, which also is relevant to assess constructively: assessment of precision and accuracy in diagnostics, therapies, or screenings (corresponding to all the traditional metrics from medical clinical and pharmaceutical studies).

3.1.3   The Adaptation Phase

The purpose of this phase is to adjust any remaining problems in work procedures as well as in the IT system itself to ensure that the two work together to an optimal level in everyday operations. Each technical change will involve the same assessment activities as during the previous phase, but only to the extent necessary.

Contrary to the Technical Development Phase, which took place under experimental conditions, potential problems of the ergonomic or cognitive aspects will now show up as operational problems when many people and possibly changing staff, temps, and so on are using the system. For instance, ergonomic problems could show up as an operational error or when staff resort to jotting down data on scraps of paper to enter into the system later when there is more peace and quiet. Cognitive problems will show up as operational errors in a similar way, but also as what is known as human errors in the old paper-based system. Cognitive problems will occur when the relevant information is not available at the time the user needs it or when he or she spends much more time to get the information and thus may believe there is no more relevant information.

Problems in the interaction between the functions of the IT system and the work procedures in the surrounding organization will show as operational errors, unfinished activities, delayed tasks, and so on. Typically when this type of problem occurs, the surrounding organization will start to establish new, extra activities in the work processes and procedures in order to compensate for the problems – that is, sprouting activities where the real problem could be the functionality of the IT system.

As this phase is fairly unstable by nature, its purpose being precisely that of adjusting the IT system and/or the organization to each other, there is a limit to the types of assessments that are relevant, other than the three types already mentioned (ergonomic, cognitive, and functional assessment).

3.1.4 *The Evolution Phase*

This phase normally starts when the complete IT solution has achieved reasonable stability (with regard to faults and adaptation) of operations and when actual new developments or major revisions are being started.

Only when the system has reached a certain stability should assessment activities concerning effect and efficiency of the system be started. They could, for instance, address whether the desired effect or purpose has been achieved, the unintentional side effects the system may have, or its impact on operations and services (e.g., mortality and morbidity), training, or the organizational structure (distribution of responsibility and competence). Dedicated methods have to be used for each of these assessment activities.

3.2 Assessment Activities in a Holistic Perspective

Figure 3.1 shows the dynamic aspects of assessment, related to the present life cycle model. The impact of constructive assessment is illustrated by arrows pointing forward and backward to other phases, while the summative assessment is not visible in terms of arrows, as it is totally contained within a given phase. In the case of constructive assessment, the figure therefore shows the entire complexity and illustrates why assessment may be a task for dedicated, experienced professionals. The arrows comprising feed-back loops (pointing upward in the downward directionality of overall progress) illustrate that some decisions implied by the outcome of an assessment may be radical and may even imply changes in previous decisions. Thus, the figure shows the whole complexity of constructive assessment. This is dealt with in more detail in Chapter 4.

Even if the summative assessment, seen from an external point of view, seems rather simple and static, the constantly changing situations also complicate such assessment tasks. For instance, if one has carried out a baseline investigation to be used as the frame of reference for a planned future assessment study, there is still the risk that the foundation for the study may change, implying that the frame of reference becomes more or less invalid or inaccurate. Normally the implementation of an IT-based solution takes years, from defining one's requirements, getting the budget allocated, finding the right vendor, until the chosen system is taken into daily operation - even if it is an off-the-shelf system that is to be implemented. During this period a number of aspects may change drastically: Departments may fuse or restructure; new technology may appear for one or more of the department's normal activities; the department may get more, new, or altered tasks or may be the victim of general budget cuts. All of this could change the conditions for an assessment investigation. The frame of reference is particularly vulnerable under certain summative assessment investigations.

The many arrows in Figure 3.1 illustrate all of the above. The figure also illustrates that it may be risky to stick too stringently to a plan just because it was once decided upon. The reason is – again – that the conditions for the assessment may have changed considerably: The resources allocated may have partially or completely dried up – for instance, if things turn out to be more expensive than anticipated at the planning stage. Further, it may be that one is able to catch up with parts of the delays or that the residual study may be rationalized to achieve a higher effectiveness. However, bear in mind that it might be more beneficial to move a deadline rather than to stick to it. Another option is to be a little less ambitious in general should the project turn out to be more wide-ranging or costly than anticipated.

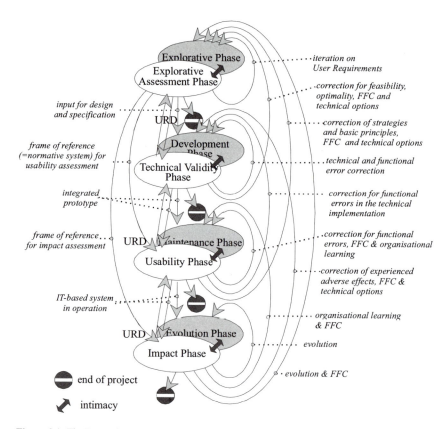

Figure 3.1: The Dynamic Assessment Methodology, complete with descriptions of feed-forward loops (providing frames of reference and preventive measures) and feed-back loops (initiating corrective activities) and indicating the contents of this information flow. The shaded ellipses illustrate the technical activities, whereas the white ellipses illustrate the corresponding constructive assessment activities in a four-phased structure. The thick arrows between the technical development and assessment activities indicate unspecified interaction (coordination and collaboration). (URD = User Requirements Document; FFC = Four Founding Capacities – that is, characteristics regarding the capability and capacity of accommodating changes).

NB: Please note that the shaded ellipses show the development phases and the white ellipses show the corresponding parallel evaluation phases. Also note the slight change in the names of the phases.

(The figure is reprinted from (Brender 1997a) with permission)

4. Choosing or Constructing Methods

To start with:

1. There is no one way to do evaluation.
2. There is no generic logical structure that will ensure a unique right method of choice.
3. Evaluation ultimately becomes judgment and will remain so, as long as there is no ultimate criterion for monotonic ordering of priorities.

The author is unconditionally convinced of these points (see the discussions in Brender 1997a and 1999). Consequently, it is not yet feasible to make a cookbook for assessment, and hence, the following statement is still valid:

> *"[W]e view evaluation not as the application of a set of tools and techniques, but as a process to be understood. By which we mean an understanding of the functions and nature of evaluation as well as its limitations and problems."*
>
> (Symons and Walsham 1988)

4.1 How Do You Do It?

This chapter outlines a series of factors that determine the success of an assessment project.

4.1.1 *Where in Its Life Cycle Is the IT Project?*

The very first issue one has to consider is where the assessment study is positioned in terms of the life cycle of the IT system – in other words, its development or implementation stage. Based on this information, one can identify some candidate methods using the tables listing the methods (see Part II), or one can get inspiration for one's own further progress.

4.1.2   What Is the Information Need?

"[T]he question being asked determines the appropriate research architecture, strategy, and tactics to be used – not tradition, authority, experts, paradigms, or schools of thought."

(Sackett and Wennberg 1997)

There is a clear correlation between the actual information need and the method applicable. Examples of this relationship are described by Anderson and Aydin (1997) and Fernandez et al. (1997). They may be incomplete, but they are perfect to bring an understanding, as well as inspiration, for the further progress of planning. Therefore, the next step is to identify and delimit the strategic objective of the investigation, discussing what it is you really want to know. It is essential to get a complete match between the purpose, the approach, and the actual use of the result.

If you don't know the purpose of evaluating, don't evaluate!

The next question is whether the outcome of the investigation is intended to:
- Establish the foundation for:
    - Ongoing work on the development project?
    - Administrative or political decision making?
    - Healthcare professional or IT professional decision making?
- Establish arguments for a sales promotion of the IT system? A good assessment study can always be used in a marketing context, provided that the system is good (enough) and one dares to be objective
- Establish the basis for a scientific publication? Those who have got as far as considering this do not need to read the rest of this Introduction part, apart from familiarizing themselves with the terminology used and then reading Part III carefully
- To find out about something? That is, exploration of the IT-based solution with the aim of investigating what changes are taking place, have taken place, or are likely to take place within the organization. Very often this scope has a research purpose
- Is the purpose of the study to make a prognosis for the future or to measure reality?

The first two scopes listed do not normally require the same accuracy and stringency as required for scientific research. Be careful when starting with one of the other scopes and subsequently trying to write a scientific article based on the outcome of the investigation. The risk of aiming in parallel at more than one of the above scopes is either that one falls between two stools or that one cracks a nut with a sledgehammer. However, with caution, it may be feasible.

Write down what the information need is and the purpose of the assessment as the starting point of the subsequent planning. It should be published in a way that allows everyone access and makes it possible to refer to the information. An assessment study often requires extra effort from staff, and it is important, therefore, that they understand the task and are committed to it. One gets the best results if there is transparency, and everyone is motivated to work toward the same goal as the one delegating and authorizing the task. Vigorous discussions may arise in connection with such clarification, as the issue is about the reasoning behind carrying out the investigation and hence for taking on the extra burden – that is, the motivation.

It is also important that one realizes whether one's object of study is the IT-based wholeness within the organization or any part thereof, such as the IT-based solution (the organization and the work procedures around the IT system, including the IT system) or the IT-based system itself (the technical construction). In this case, it is often important to reduce the objective to something realistic (financially, in terms of resources, time, and practicality) while being clear about what is cut.

While discussing the purpose, it is also important to realize who the stakeholders are and, thus, who will subsequently be involved in the project from the time of planning. In this connection it is important to analyze the administrative aspects of the project. (See, for instance, how it can go terribly wrong in Part III.)

4.1.3   *Establishing a Methodology*

While methods constitute specific instructions on how to accomplish a certain task, a methodology is the superior wholeness bringing different methods to work together, also enabling a method distributed over several phases to function in a practical wholeness. In the light of major IT projects, selecting a methodology will lead to the global plan for division of the project into phases as well as the overall approach for each of the subtasks, the plan for user participation, for method selection, and so forth or the overall approach for a before-and-after investigation of the system's effect on specific parameters of the organization.

The selection of a methodology is usually implicitly described within the original description of a method. Establishment of a methodology comprises taking a well-organized step from knowing what the information need is, through the conditions for carrying out the study (including policy for the accomplishment and the solution), to value norms, via consequences and assumptions that one must contemplate, to an action plan. The methodology then defines certain limits in the choice of methods. If you have a simple, small, and very specific information need, for which you may apply a specific, well-documented method having detailed instructions, the methodology may not need to be explicit. Otherwise, it may be wise to think in terms of the wholeness.

The point of time within the life cycle is a significant factor for the selection of a methodology: If one has entered the Adaptation Phase before even considering measuring something, then forget making a before-and-after investigation for identifying the effects of the IT system on the organization and its service level, unless a baseline investigation of some sort already exists, which may serve as the frame of reference for interpretation. In the same way, questionnaires can also be used for many things, but questionnaire studies require expertise to formulate the questions, and even with expertise or experience one must be aware of the fact that it is a subjective investigation method with built-in problems of precision and accuracy (see Part III). But the discussion of whether to choose a subjective or an objective method depends on the question that needs answering.

The nature of an assessment study – that is, the distinction between constructive and summative assessments – is the first and crucial issue when establishing a methodology. These are usually larger, but also easier, because there will be enough time for careful planning. In constructive assessment, one constantly has to be at the leading edge and be prepared to adapt to specific needs, while obeying the timeliness and budget constraints, as well as the terms of responsibility and authority within the project.

Anticipated areas of effect influence the choice of methodology and methods in combination with whether it is a constructive or a summative assessment. There may be many issues in this respect. Where the technology introduced inevitably and significantly affects the aspects of responsibility and authority in an organization (changes the structure, the relationships, the coordination or collaboration transversely within the organization), management issues should obviously be addressed. On the other hand, if a purely 'mechanical' effect for the work procedures is anticipated, methods dealing with these would normally be in focus. If one aims at drawing a lesson from the investigation, a third type of methods would be relevant.

4.1.4   Choosing a Method

Be critical about the selection of method(s).

1. Pick methods that comply with the objectives of the project (purpose of the assessment, including the need for accuracy and precision). Make a distinction

between a practical and down-to-earth, internal purpose and a more formal, external-oriented purpose, including those initiated as scientific investigations.

2. Be aware that one should not choose to carry out a qualitative investigation only because there is not enough energy or budget to carry out the quantitative investigation that the information need points at.

3. Choose methods that meet the terms of those using them. It makes little sense to pick a method that technically or professionally is too difficult to handle for those who are supposed to carry out the investigation.

4. Choose methods for which the perspectives are in harmony with your own perspectives; otherwise it may be difficult to interpret the results (see the term perspective in a previous section). We all have a series of assumptions with which we are indoctrinated during our education and in our professional environment and that, unfortunately, is tacit (see Section 2.4 and Arbnor and Bjerke 1997, page 6ff). Therefore, the best thing you can do, is to carefully get acquainted with the methods before making the final choice.

5. Preferably choose methods that are validated and whose advantages and disadvantages are documented within the literature. However, note that "being validated" does not necessarily mean the same as being valid for your purpose. One has to subject the original literature to detailed inspection and reflection, as only the best articles adequately analyze and criticize their method.

6. Carefully check the list of perils and pitfalls in Part III so that no bias is overlooked should a high level of accuracy and precision be needed.

Then note that methods usually applied to analysis and design work in connection with system development can sometimes be valuable for assessment tasks as well, especially for qualitative and explorative investigations. This is the case, for instance, where there is a need to ascertain how things actually work as opposed to the anticipated mode of operation in terms of an investigation of effect or objectives realization.

One can easily apply a method the wrong way. It is therefore important that prior to its use one has insight into the method – that is, understands it at an abstract level. Don't rush at using a method from its instructions. It is the understanding that facilitates a meta-level (bird's eye view), enabling one to juggle with and within the frame of a method as well as to interpret the results correctly and completely, compared to the conditions of the study and the data gathered. A method is not something that one picks out of a drawer. It can be looked at in the same way a chef knows how to get a better and quicker result from a given recipe: The chef knows it is the qualities of the raw materials and their preparation that make the difference, and may use shortcuts where nonprofessionals would fail.

4.1.5 Choosing Metrics and Measures

There is a close connection between metrics, measures (see the explanation of these concepts in Section 2.2), and choice of method, and this must be respected. Every method has its focus area, and typically it leads to certain types of information, requiring special expertise to change.

Select measures carefully.

1. Focusing on visible measures bears a risk of implying a changed behavior or performance by the employees. It is a well-known phenomenon already from the early era of assembly lines and mass production that people change when they know that they are being observed: the Hawthorne effect.

2. Fixation on specific measures may imply that these get special attention by the staff, precipitating a focus on them during daily practice at the expense of the wholeness. This is particularly relevant in the case of constructive assessment where the focus is on something specific during a prolonged process (such as avoiding organizational changes or changes in the interaction between various groups of staff) rather than having a superior objective represented by many varied measures that describe the different characteristics of a solution.

3. One may find invisible measures. For instance, a measure of the effectiveness of an IT system may be as simple as, retrospectively, monitoring the consumption of coffee or the length of the coffee breaks before and after its introduction. Or if one wants to look at the effectiveness of communication, one may register the number of phone calls between specific numbers. This kind of information may be elicited without the users noticing.

4.1.6 Execution of the Method

Keep an eye on what happens within the organization while you are assessing. That way you will know whether something (unforeseen) has to be taken into account during the analysis and interpretation of the results.

1. An organization changes: As soon as its staff gets access to different or new tools and is confident with them, they will invent shortcuts. However, not all of these shortcuts will be compliant with the prescribed procedures, and some may even be contrary to the interests of the organization.

2. The indicators change: What one believed to know about certain variables used during the investigation may suddenly turn out to have unknown limitations. This may be caused by users dynamically changing their way of

> using the system or by previously unknown aspects of the IT system. Or the work procedures may cause the indicators to change: 'Working to rules' is not the norm, but the introduction of an IT system may temporarily make it necessary.
>
> 3. One's scope may change while accomplishing the assessment: An answer to one question may lead to ten new questions. Digging into a topic makes one wiser, and that alone may change one's information need.
>
> 4. It is quite certain that the IT system will change while being assessed – at least newly developed IT systems, because of the correction of bugs and organizational adaptations, or if the assessment lasts for a period of several months.

To some extent the method can/should keep pace with the above-mentioned changes. Occasionally, it is necessary to introduce modifications. The art of assessment means having sufficient overview to be able to know and understand when and how it is feasible to change or accept that things change by themselves, without ruining the outcome of one's investigation. The art is also to observe, note, and deal appropriately with such changes. Be honest about them in a publication context, as some of them may affect the interpretation of one's results and conclusions and thereby also influence the benefit others may gain from using the same method.

4.1.7 *Interpreting Results*

Be critical about what your name is associated with.

> 1. Be fair and objective; be open about unwanted and unexpected results; and, when relevant, accept their implied consequences. It may sometimes be hard to face unwanted or unexpected results, but for constructive assessment, this is essential.
>
> 2. Be self-critical and show that you are aware of the weaknesses of both the method and the interpretation. This is invaluable to others who consider applying the same method or IT solution because it shows that you are sufficiently in control of the investigation that the outcome can be trusted.
>
> 3. Be objective while presenting the results; show both the good and the bad news at a relevant level of detail and in a balanced way. Excluding significant information in the synthesis of a conclusion may strain belief or even be akin to fraud. Normally it is difficult to get negative results published in journals. But to focus on the parts of the results that suit one's own business is untrustworthy.

4.2 From Strategy to Tactics: An Example

The most important thing to note in the example below is the illustration of how value norms can become a conscious part of a process and thereby an integrated element in preparing an assessment method.

The example is from Brender et al. (2002a; 2002b) and deals with a constructive assessment in connection with tendering and selection of a bid. The case is concerned with one common laboratory information system for six independent, clinical biochemistry laboratories. When preparing the requirements specification, the basis for choosing a selection methodology and method was already partly determined, and thereby parts of the strategy, inasmuch as the requirements specification included a Traceability Matrix that the bidders had to complete with the objectives fulfillment.

The strategy was finally determined by a conscious choice based on the value norms and perspectives of the process (the quality management model in Section 2.3), such as:

- To support user responsibility and to interfere as little as possible in the decision-making process. It is not the external consultant but the user organization, with its own structure and culture, which has to make the decision. The consultant only has to facilitate the process.

- To preempt subjective manipulation and hidden agendas; this is a very conscious element of the strategy because hidden agendas can be virtually ruinous for the future cooperation around the system. However, had there just been one laboratory involved, then the criteria behind the selection of vendor and solution would not nearly have had the same significance because it would be a concrete choice reliant on the local organizational culture.

- Gradual elimination of bids combined with a risk analysis and assessment of consequences of elements within the bids. The step-by-step approach is a practical choice, while the last two are important when assessing objectives fulfillment.

The tactical implementation of this strategy consisted of:

- To design a decision-making process with extensive user involvement at all levels. A characteristic of technology developments in Denmark is extensive user involvement at all levels, not just management, although they have the ultimate responsibility and competence. Therefore, the structure was implemented as a network organization with a bottom-up synthesis of information.

- To challenge the decision-making process of the users at all relevant decision-making points.
- By continuous improvement of the information material as a decision-making base – that is, the material was produced in such a way that a decision at a given level was not unequivocally made just to be confirmed, but it introduced choices and/or options to verify the information and the observations.

There were no prefabricated methods and metrics (other than summations and calculation of average values), and, therefore, these methods and metrics had to continuously adapt to the actual need and to the situation in which the information need existed – that is, that the operational level was totally dependent on the context and could not finally be determined beforehand. The Traceability Matrix was used to make a number of tabulator metrics to illustrate the level of objectives fulfillment, but the method foundation developed as a function of time.

The primary principle behind the design of the assessment techniques and tools was built upon the strategic value norms and perspectives and resulted in a hierarchical design of the decision material: The decision basis was created in a synthesis process by the staff, giving them a sense of ownership of the result while the (always busy) management representatives could choose to rely on the judgment of their staff or gradually work their way down the level of detail from overview to information to data.

4.3   Another (Abstract) Example

If the result of an assessment is to be used as a decision-making basis in a political or administrative context, as, for instance, choice of an EHR to be implemented in all departments of a hospital or a region, it is important that there are no awkward surprises after the decision has been made and the contract with the vendor has been signed. Therefore, it is important in this situation to make a stakeholder analysis before starting to plan the assessment in order to include all vital aspects of the system under investigation. On the other hand, whether all observations are accurate to the tenth degree is not at all as important. The chosen method, with its metrics (quantitative or qualitative) and measures, must encompass all relevant aspects for all stakeholders. If just one important point is left out, it could, for instance, be a para-clinical aspect of the EHR, the extreme consequence could then be that the whole solution has to be abandoned or that it could cost a small fortune to rectify the EHR solution.

4.4 A Practical Example of a Procedure

4.4.1 Planning at the Strategic Level

1. Ascertain the real purpose of the task. What is the actual question that needs answering? Limit the task. Determine the organizational and project-related working conditions and value norms, and make sure that they are the same conditions and norms that cover the solution of the assessment task. What are the limits of the procedure and the solution model of the assessment task? What policy covers problem solving in the organization and/or covers this actual task? What is the real object to be investigated?

2. Choose an overall strategy and procedure, and thereby the methodology, depending on the overall purpose of the result. Is a stakeholder analysis necessary prior to choice of methods? Divide the actual information needs into smaller and plainer elements.

3. Choose a set of methods that are suitable, together and separately, to the conditions and assumptions that obviously cover the project and that are in accordance with the philosophy, perspectives, and assumptions, and so on of the methodology. Learn to understand the assumptions of the methods and techniques.

4. Establish an overall implementation plan for the assessment project.

4.4.2 Planning at the Tactical Level

1. Adjust the methods to the actual task, including choice of concrete metrics and measures. Analyze whether the assumptions of the method are applicable to the actual case and, if not, whether they (method and/or metrics) can be adapted to fulfill the assumptions or that the consequences will be without significance for the conclusion and its use.

2. Verify what perils and pitfalls there might be (see Part III), and estimate their consequences on the future result. Analyze whether existing perils and pitfalls – given the premises for carrying out and using the result – constitute a risk (your own or that of others) for using the result according to the objective. If necessary, the choice of method, metrics, measures, and/or the overall choice that lead to the assessment plan will have to be revised, or parts of the process will have to be started all over again.

3. Establish all resources and agreements needed to carry out the assessment project.

4. What are the binding elements with regard to establishing a frame of reference for judging the result of the evaluation activities? If necessary, the frame of reference has to be established already at this point.

4.4.3 Planning at the Operational Level

1. Metrics and measures are prepared and incorporated into the organizational work procedures, instruction material and documentation, and/or in the functions of the IT system.
2. Logistics are prepared, and all necessary agreements are made (i.e., who does what and when).
3. All relevant staff are instructed so that everybody knows exactly what to do.

4.5 Frame of Reference for Assessment

The difference between evaluation and verification or validation (see the definitions in Section 2.1) is that evaluation simply means measuring certain characteristics or properties of the IT-based solution, while the other two types of assessment put the properties measured into some sort of perspective – for example, compare what has been measured with a specification in verification and with a purpose in validation. This 'something' to which the item measured is compared is called the frame of reference.

If during verification or validation activities proper consideration of the establishment of a valid frame of reference is not made, there is a risk of a serious bias in the conclusion. The frame of reference is therefore closely connected to the question, which the whole assessment activity strives to answer. If the benefits of an IT system are to be measured, it is essential that the frame of reference is in order or fully considered before the properties of the new system are measured. Otherwise there is a risk that something quite different is being measured, such as the placebo effect (the effect of just doing something or other) or the Hawthorne effect (the effect of observing people while they perform a task) (Wyatt and Spiegelhalter 1991).

The frame of reference for assessment is totally dependent on what is being assessed. In constructive assessment the frame of reference can, for example, be the actual project objective and value norms or possibly an earlier measurement of the same property. During the first phase of the development or implementation project (the Explorative Phase) the frame of reference will often be the organization's vision, aims, and objectives with the project overall, but as soon as the requirements specification has become the project basis, it will also form an important part of the frame of reference for assessment (see Technical Verification in Part II for references), and possibly so will the resulting material during subsequent phases. Either the documentation needs or the need of an effective operation will often be the driving force, and the frame of reference will depend completely on the information need set out.

When choosing a frame of reference there are several questions that need to be taken into account: Are the users comparable? Are the situations comparable (the control group and the intervention group have to be exposed to the same set of circumstances, which is not easy in a system development project)? Are the organizations comparable? Does the plan secure sufficient data as a basis to make an assessment of a possible effect? Is the time span of such a length that the organization, the users, or the IT system itself will change considerably during the process? They are all matters that one has to consider before, during, and after an assessment study, with the objective of analyzing the consequences on the result and the interpretation of possible unexpected deviations. In other words, the premises upon which the project has been built and carried out need, if at all possible, to be reassessed.

The frame of reference for ergonomic and cognitive assessments of an IT-based system is another matter, because how do you set criteria for what is good and what is bad, and where is the dividing point? Some models will be outlined in Part II.

4.6   Perils and Pitfalls

An investigation into known perils and pitfalls in medical and humanistic research documented that there are analogues for assessments of IT-based solutions and that they certainly are relevant (see Part III). The practical impact of these perils and pitfalls can be enormous or insignificant, depending on the objective of the investigation and the purpose of the result. And please note that they are not all relevant for all assessment studies.

First, it has been convincingly documented in the literature that "users do not do as they say they do, and do what they say they do not do . . ." (see the discussion in Brender 1997a and 1999). In other words, the analysis of work procedures carried out as a basis for the assessment activities is not necessarily absolutely correct. However, depending on what one wants to learn from the assessment, it will probably be precisely everyday work, as it really functions, against which one would want to assess the IT-based solution.

Second, depending on the actual study and what the result will finally be used for, some of the perils and pitfalls will only have marginal impact. If the study is to be used for a scientific publication, the presence of perils and pitfalls will drastically reduce the trustworthiness of the publication, but if it is impossible to avoid the problem, this might be overcome if the error, as well as its size and its consequences, is properly acknowledged and discussed. But if it concerns successive measures with a concrete method for optimizing the development (i.e., constructive assessment), then it is exactly the relative gain of each step that is significant and not the true value of a measure.

Last, but not least, if the users of an IT-based solution are happy with the system, why should you bother to show that the system has problems (ergonomic ones, for instance)?

Part III investigates the perils and pitfalls one at the time. It is therefore possible during planning and interpretation of an assessment study to use the review as a checklist to avoid or possibly compensate for the worst errors encountered.

PART II: Methods and Techniques

5. Introduction

This part presents descriptions of a number of methods that should be feasible for a user organization to perform by itself, although some of them with support from experienced assessors. The descriptions are organized in a way that leads the reader from a given method's relevant application areas through its conditions for a successful application to a list of references to the international literature that contains further information and the complete instructions for application.

It has been decided to use the actual names of references used by the original authors (method and technique, respectively). Similarly, there is no distinction of whether what is described is a method or a methodology: A methodology can be described with such a degree of detail that it will in practice work as both, although the authors have not kept method-related aspects separate. The principal aspect in an evaluation and assessment context is the practical relevance of what is described versus the users' needs.

Also note: The *Handbook* does not distinguish methods according to 'subjectivist' and 'objectivist' approaches. Instead, the focus is on the area of application of the method, relating to the purpose of the assessment.

Furthermore, for various reasons, some of the method descriptions in this handbook provide an overview rather than giving pure method descriptions. Examples of method overviews are *Work Procedures Analysis*, *Impact Assessment*, and *Assessment of Bids*, while examples of method descriptions are *Delphi* and *Balanced Scorecard*. The former are of a problem-oriented nature, while the latter are of a technology-oriented nature. There are many reasons for this variation, and the intention in all of these cases has been to provide inspiration for the reader to identify his or her best approach. The methods mentioned under *Work Procedure Analysis* are not dedicated to, nor specifically designed for, evaluation studies but could clearly have a role as part of an evaluation study. In *Assessment of Bids* a variety of approaches are outlined because no one good method that covers the variety of bid procedures exists. As the solution space in *Impact Assessment* is huge, it may require one method or another or a combination of several, and hence it is more valuable for the reader to get a view of the options, which, by the way, could be a combination of methods described elsewhere in the handbook, and so on.

5.1 Signature Explanations

Please see the conceptual apparatus in the Introduction.

5.1.1 Application Range within the IT System's Life Cycle

Depending on what information a given method is supposed to provide, it could be used in one or more life cycles of a system. Graphic icons are used to illustrate which phase(s) is/are primarily of relevance to the method.

Phase icon　　**Phase outline**

The Explorative Phase: This phase begins with the conception of an idea for a solution and addresses the strategic issues related to its future development, such as objectives, intentions, basic principles, relevance, and feasibility (both technically and within the organization). This phase usually concludes with a User Requirements Specification and a contractual arrangement.

The methods included in this phase are particularly relevant in the assessment of the issues raised during the establishment of a User Requirements Specification – for example, objectives, requirements, and expectations. The evaluation addresses issues such as feasibility, coverage, and compliance of the system with the organization, as well as viability of the solution anticipated in terms of the requirements specification and its ability to serve as an operational frame of reference for later evaluations.

The Technical Development Phase: The Technical Development Phase is concerned with the technical implementation – from systems analysis to technical installation and setting up of daily practices within the context of the new IT system.

The methods included for this phase are particularly suited for user activities during the development and installation of an IT-based solution and may be used to provide feed-back for the technical development or implementation.

Assessment in this phase is typically carried out under experimental conditions and not during real operation. This phase is usually completed with technical verification (verification of the IT construct against a technical specification or the contract) and early ergonomic and cognitive assessments prior to the application of the system into real practice in order to make certain that all necessary functions and features are present and work properly in compliance with the established agreement or contract.

The Adaptation Phase: The Adaptation Phase covers the early stages of real practice of the IT system in daily operation and is concerned with adapting work procedures and system functions to one another.

User assessment in this phase turns much more tangible and substantial in terms of ergonomic assessment, cognitive assessment, and validation of the functionality. Ergonomic assessment is concerned with users' practical and mental workload when physically operating the IT system. Cognitive assessment is concerned with the compatibility of an IT system with the real cognitive processes involved in the user's accomplishment of an activity, such as a physician's mental processing when diagnosing a patient. Functionality assessment addresses the compliance of an IT system to the work processes of the organization in which it is operating (see Brender 1997a and 1999).

Evaluation in this phase has the purpose of providing support for the modification or refinement of the IT-based solution to make the work procedures and the functions implemented within the IT system work optimally as an entirety during daily operation. This phase should be fairly short, provided that the implemented solution functions well from the beginning.

The Evolution Phase: The Evolution Phase includes long-term maintenance and further development of the system, both in technical and organizational terms. The assessment activities in this phase are concerned with assessment of unforeseen or adverse effects and long-term effects in a broad organizational perspective, including fulfillment of objectives and impact assessment.

The starting point of this phase usually coincides with the point in time when the entire IT-based solution has reached a stage of sufficient stability with respect to bugs and corrections and when evolutionary activities have started. Consequently, the shift between this and the previous phase may be fluid.

5.1.2 *Applicability in Different Contexts*

A method's usefulness (i.e., applicability within a given context) is usually a function of its reliability (addressing strengths and weaknesses of the method), its degree of difficulty, as well as its resource requirements. Applicability in this respect shall be interpreted in a practical perspective rather than for research purposes and is illustrated by means of a number of icons. Each icon may comprise one, two, or three symbols of the same kind as seen below. The rating of quality in terms of number of symbols expresses an overall judgment, and consequently, the number may vary for specific investigation purposes. For instance, the efforts put into a questionnaire depend on the number of questions needed to fulfill your specific study purpose or on whether you can find a ready-made questionnaire in the literature.

Note that a sign in brackets indicates that the given method – depending on how accurate and precise the conclusion needs to be – may be accomplished either very simply or more or less stringently, while other methods require the same level of stringency irrespective of the precision needed.

Reliability of the method and its results

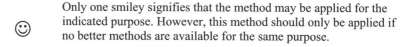 Only one smiley signifies that the method may be applied for the indicated purpose. However, this method should only be applied if no better methods are available for the same purpose.

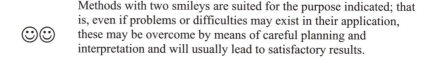 Methods with two smileys are suited for the purpose indicated; that is, even if problems or difficulties may exist in their application, these may be overcome by means of careful planning and interpretation and will usually lead to satisfactory results.

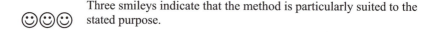 Three smileys indicate that the method is particularly suited to the stated purpose.

Degree of difficulty

§ *Simple* – that is, people with only little prior knowledge of or experience with the given method may apply it. It is, however, assumed that the user of the method has a general insight into and experience of planning experimental investigations, needing only to get acquainted with the principles and approach as well as potential pitfalls and perils of that particular method.

§§ *Medium difficulty* – methods with this level of difficulty presuppose a fairly deep understanding of the method's theory, principles, approaches, pitfalls, and perils, as well as assumptions regarding its application based on prior experience with the method. Alternatively, one may call for assistance from professionals or by active and intensive self-tuition. The latter may sometimes be risky, depending on the level of accuracy and precision needed.

§§§ *Difficult* – valid application of a method with three article symbols assumes fulfillment of special prerequisites with respect to professional background in order to be able to accomplish a satisfactory outcome from such an evaluation study.

Resource requirements

€ The symbol of the Euro currency illustrates the relative magnitude of economic resources needed for carrying out an assessment by means of this method. It is not feasible to put a more specific rating on this aspect of a method, since it depends heavily on the type of system, the specific need for accuracy and precision, and other local conditions.

€€

€€€ The more Euros, the more expensive. Included are all types of resources, which in the end involve one kind of expenditure or another, such as direct and indirect labor resources, external consultants, and other expenses related to the carrying out of the study.

5.1.3   *Type of Assessment*

Constructive assessment. Constructive assessment addresses the so-called 'wh' questions, like when, where, what, why, and which, plus, of course, how. For instance, "In what way does the system behave in this respect?" and "How will it work in (simulated) real practice?" Questions like "Will it fulfill given requirements?" and similar questions are also relevant.

⟷

The double arrow illustrates the interactivity between assessment and technical development activities implied by the role of constructive assessment as a provider of a decision-making basis within a given context.

☑ *Summative Assessment.* This type of assessment corresponds to evaluation or exploration of state-of-affairs (illustrated by the symbol of a tick box). That is, this kind of assessment compares to an information need formulated as "verify that . . .", "explore the qualities in this respect . . .", or "judge whether . . .".

5.1.4 Use of Italics in the Method Descriptions

Italics applied for a name or noun within the textual description of a method signifies that a method of that name is described elsewhere in Part II of this handbook.

5.2 Structure of Methods' Descriptions

A number of icons are shown that together and overall characterize the assessment method's applicability within the IT system's life cycle, as well as its suitability for the purpose described and the types of assessment.

METHOD NAME   <icons>

Areas of application
*A short verbal description of the method's areas of application – for
example, the kind of information that the method will provide*   <icons>

Description
A summary of the method's principles and approaches   <icons>

Assumptions for application
*A description of necessary (nontrivial) conditions for application of the
method in order to obtain a useful result. This includes the necessary skills
or background experiences*

Perspectives
*A description of aspects of importance for attaining or interpreting results,
including the philosophy behind the method and its hidden assumptions*

Frame of reference for interpretation
*Outline of what might serve as the frame of reference and how this will be
applied*

Perils and pitfalls

An outline of where, how, and why one may risk specific pitfalls or perils

Advice and comments

Small tricks/advice that may help to carry out the investigation or how to modify the method

References

A complete list of references used from the literature, plus, for instance, valuable supplementary references on case studies

6. Overview of Assessment Methods

In principle all aspects of a system are candidates for assessment in all phases of the system's development. In practice, some aspects are more prominent in some of the phases than in others. During its life cycle, the assessment may change in nature from being prognostic (during planning), to screening and diagnosing (prior to switching over to daily operation), to treating (in the handling of known error situations or shortcomings). Be aware, therefore, that even if a method is not listed under a specific phase, an information need may arise that requires inspiration from the methods listed under other phases.

Note that few of the references given include a discussion of the weaknesses, perils, and pitfalls of the method described.

6.1 Overview of Assessment Methods: Explorative Phase

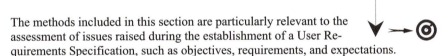

The methods included in this section are particularly relevant to the assessment of issues raised during the establishment of a User Requirements Specification, such as objectives, requirements, and expectations.

Method	Areas of application	Page no
Analysis of Work Procedures	Elucidation of how things are actually carried out within an organization.	73
Assessment of Bids	Comparative assessment of a number of offers from one or more bidders/vendors.	78
Balanced Scorecard	Ongoing optimization of the outcome of a development project by balancing focus areas by means of a set of indicators for a set of strategic objectives.	85
BIKVA	Critical, subjective assessment of an existing practice.	88

Delphi	• (Qualitative) assessment of an effect – for instance, where the solution space is otherwise too big to handle • Exploration of development trends • Elucidation of a problem area – for instance, prior to strategic planning.	106
Field Study	Observation of an organization to identify its practice and to clarify mechanisms controlling change.	111
Focus Group Interview	This is in principle used for the same purposes as other interview methods. In practice, the method is most relevant during the early Explorative Phase – for instance, where attitudes or problems of social groups need elucidation or when a model solution is being established.	116
Future Workshop	Evaluation and analysis of an (existing) situation in order to identify and focus on areas for change – that is, aiming at designing future practices.	125
Grounded Theory	Supportive analytical method for data acquisition methods that generate textual data, such as some open questionnaire methods and interviews (individual and group interviews).	128
Heuristic Evaluation	This is used when no other realizable possibilities exist – for instance, when: • The organization does not have the necessary time or expertise • There are no formalized methods • There is nothing tangible to assess yet.	132
Interview (nonstandardized)	This is particularly suited for elucidation of individuals' opinions, attitudes, and perceptions regarding phenomena and observations.	142
KUBI	Optimization of the outcome of a long-term development project, based on a set of user or customer/client-defined value norms and objectives.	147
Logical Framework Approach	Situation analysis to support the choice of focus for a development but at the same time a simple technique for incorporation of risk handling within project planning.	149
Organizational Readiness	Assessment of the readiness of a healthcare organization for a clinical information system.	154

Pardlzlpp	Preparation of future scenarios.	156
Questionnaire (nonstandardized)	Questionnaires are used to answer a wide range of questions, but its main area of application is (qualitative) investigations of subjective aspects requiring a high level of accuracy.	163
Requirements Assessment	Within the European culture the User Requirements Specification is the basis for purchasing an IT-based solution or engaging in a development project. Consequently, the User Requirements Specification is a highly significant legal document that needs thorough assessment.	180
Risk Assessment	Identification and subsequent monitoring of risk factors, making it possible to take preemptive action.	185
Social Network Analysis	Assessment of relations between elements within an organization (such as individuals, professions, departments or other organizations), which influence the acceptance and use of an IT-based solution.	190
Stakeholder Analysis	Assessment of stakeholder features and their inner dynamics, aiming to identify participants for the completion of a given task, problem-solving activity, or project.	192
SWOT	Situation analysis: establishment of a holistic view of a situation or a model solution.	196
Usability	Assessment of user friendliness in terms of ergonomic and cognitive aspects of the interaction (dialogue) between an IT system and its users. In this phase the concern is a planning or purchasing situation.	207
Videorecording	Monitoring and documenting as a means of analysis of what/how the work procedures or the users' activities are actually carried out or for investigation of complex patterns of interaction.	219
WHO: Framework for Assessment of Strategies	Assessment of different (development) strategies either individually or as a comparative analysis.	222

6.2 Overview of Assessment Methods: Technical Development Phase

The methods listed in this section are particularly suited to user activities during the development and installation of an IT-based solution and may be used to provide feed-back for the technical development.

Assessment in this phase is typically carried out under experimental conditions and not during real operation. The phase is usually completed with a technical verification to make certain that all necessary functions and features are present and work properly in compliance with the established agreement.

Method	Areas of application	Page no
Balanced Scorecard	Ongoing optimization of the outcome of a development project by balancing focus areas by means of a set of indicators for a set of strategic objectives.	85
Clinical/Diagnostic Performance	Measurement of diagnostic 'correctness' (for instance, measures of accuracy and precision) of IT-based expert systems and decision-support systems.	91
Cognitive Assessment	Assessment of cognitive aspects of the interaction between an IT system and its users – for instance: • Identification of where and why operational errors occur • Identification of areas to be focused on for improvement in user friendliness.	96
Cognitive Walkthrough	Assessment of user 'friendliness' on the basis of system design, from specifications, muck-ups, or prototypes, aimed at judging how well the system complies with the users' way of thinking – for instance: • Identification of where and why operational errors occur • Identification of causes behind problems with respect to user friendliness and consequently identification of areas for improvement.	102

Heuristic Evaluation	This is used when no other realizable possibilities exist – for instance, when: • The organization does not have the necessary time or expertise • There are no formalized methods • There is not something tangible to assess yet.	132
Risk Assessment	Identification and subsequent monitoring of risk factors, making it possible to take preemptive action.	185
SWOT	Situation analysis: establishment of a holistic view of a situation or a model solution.	196
Technical Verification	Verification that the agreed functions are present, and work correctly and in compliance with the agreement. This may take place, for instance, in connection with delivery of an IT system or prior to daily operations and at any subsequent change of the IT system (releases, versions, and patches).	199
Think Aloud	An instrument for gaining insight into the cognitive processes as feed-back to the implementation and adaptation of IT-based systems.	204
Usability	Assessment of user friendliness in terms of ergonomic and cognitive aspects of the interaction (dialogue) between an IT system and its users.	207

6.3 Overview of Assessment Methods: Adaptation Phase

In this phase, evaluation has the purpose of providing support for the modification or refinement of the IT-based solution, work procedures, and functions implemented within the IT system to make them work optimally as a whole during daily operations. This phase should be fairly short, provided that the implemented solution is functioning well from the beginning.

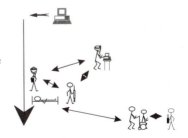

Now that real operational assessment can take place, ergonomic, cognitive, and functionality assessment will gain much more focus, as potential inadequacies or shortcomings will show themselves as operational errors, misuse, or the like.

Method	Areas of application	Page no
Analysis of Work Procedures	Elucidation of how things are actually carried out, in comparison with the expected. This includes the actual use of the IT system in relation to its anticipated use.	73
BIKVA	Critical, subjective assessment of an existing practice.	88
Clinical/Diagnostic Performance	Measurement of diagnostic 'correctness' (for instance, measures of accuracy and precision) in IT-based expert systems and decision-support systems.	91
Cognitive Assessment	Assessment of cognitive aspects of the interaction between an IT system and its users – for instance: • Identification of where and why operational errors occur • Identification of areas to be focused on for improvement in user friendliness.	96
Cognitive Walkthrough	Assessment of user 'friendliness' on the basis of system design, from specifications, muck-ups, or prototypes, aimed at judging how well the system complies with the users' way of thinking – for instance: • Identification of where and why operational errors occur • Identification of causes behind problems with respect to user friendliness and consequently identification of areas for improvement.	102
Equity Implementation Model	Examine users' reaction to the implementation of a new system, focusing on the impact of the changes such a system brings about for the users.	109
Field Study	Observation of an organization to identify its practices and to expose mechanisms that control change.	111
Focus Group Interview	This is in principle used for the same purposes as other interview methods. In practice, the method is most relevant during the early Explorative Phase – for instance, where the attitudes or problems of social groups need elucidation or when a model solution is being established.	116

Functionality Assessment	1. Validation of fulfillment of objectives (realization of objectives) – that is, the degree of compliance between the desired effect and the actual solution 2. Impact Assessment (also called effect assessment) 3. Identification of problems in the relationship between work procedures and the IT system's functional solution The method will expose severe ergonomic and cognitive problems, but it is not dedicated to capture details of this type.	120
Grounded Theory	Supportive analytical method for data acquisition methods that generate textual data, such as some open questionnaire methods and interviews (individual and group interviews).	128
Heuristic Evaluation	This is used when no other realizable possibilities exist – for instance, when: • The organization does not have the necessary time or expertise • There are no formalized methods • There is not something tangible to assess yet.	132
Interview (nonstandardized)	Is in particular suited for the elucidation of individual opinions, attitudes, and perceptions regarding phenomena and observations.	142
Prospective Time Series	Measurement of development trends, including the effect of an intervention.	159
Questionnaire (nonstandardized)	Questionnaires are used to answer a wide range of questions, but its main area of application is (qualitative) investigations of subjective aspects requiring a high level of accuracy.	163
RCT, Randomized Controlled Trial	Verification of efficacy – that is, that the IT system – under ideal conditions – makes a difference to patient care. Particularly used in studies of decision-support systems and expert systems.	172
Risk Assessment	Identification and subsequent monitoring of risk factors, making it possible to take preemptive action.	185
Root Causes Analysis	Exploration of what, how, and why a given incident occurred to identify the root cause of undesirable events.	188

Social Network Analysis	Assessment of relations between elements within an organization (such as individuals, professions, departments, or other organizations), which influence the acceptance and use of an IT-based solution.	190
SWOT	Situation analysis: establishing a holistic view of a situation or a model solution.	196
Technical Verification	Verification that the agreed functions are present, and work correctly and in compliance with the agreement. This may take place, for instance, in connection with delivery of an IT system or prior to daily operations and at any subsequent change of the IT system (releases, versions, and patches).	199
Think Aloud	An instrument for gaining insight into the cognitive processes as feed-back to the implementation and adaptation of IT-based systems.	204
Usability	Assessment of user friendliness in terms of ergonomic and cognitive aspects of the interaction (dialogue) between an IT system and its users.	207
User Acceptance and Satisfaction	Assessment of user opinion, attitudes, and perception of an IT system during daily operation.	215
Videorecording	Monitoring and documenting as a means of analyzing how work procedures and user activities, respectively, are actually carried out or for investigation of complex patterns of interaction.	219

6.4 Overview of Assessment Methods: Evolution Phase

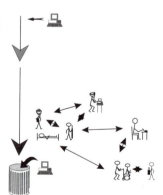

The starting point in time of this phase is usually considered to be when the entire IT-based solution has reached a state of sufficient stability with respect to bugs and corrections and when evolutionary activities are started. Consequently, the shift between this and the previous phase may be fluid.

Method	Areas of application	Page no
Analysis of Work Procedures	Elucidation of how things are actually carried out, in comparison with the expected. This includes its use in relation to measures of effect.	73
Balanced Scorecard	Ongoing optimization of the outcome of a development project by balancing focus areas by means of a set of indicators for a set of strategic objectives.	85
BIKVA	Critical, subjective assessment of an existing practice.	88
Clinical/Diagnostic Performance	Measurement of diagnostic 'correctness' (for instance, measures of accuracy and precision) of IT-based expert systems and decision-support systems.	91
Cognitive Assessment	Assessment of the cognitive aspects of the interaction between an IT system and its users – for instance: • Identification of where and why operational errors occur • Identification of areas to be focused on for improvement in user friendliness.	96
Cognitive Walkthrough	Assessment of the user 'friendliness' on the basis of system design, from specifications, muck-ups, or prototypes of the system, aimed at judging how well the system complies with the users' way of thinking – for instance: • Identification of where and why operational errors occur • Identification of causes behind problems with respect to user friendliness and consequently identification of areas for improvement.	102
Delphi	1. (Qualitative) assessment of an effect – for instance, where the solution space is otherwise too big to handle 2. Exploration of development trends 3. Elucidation of a problem area – for instance, prior to strategic planning.	106
Equity Implementation Model	Examine users' reaction to the implementation of a new system, focusing on the impact of the changes such a system brings about for the users.	109
Field Study	Observation of an organization to identify its practices and to expose mechanisms that control change.	111

Focus Group Interview	It is in principle used for the same purposes as other interview methods. In practice, the method is most relevant during the early analysis stage – for instance, where attitudes or problems of social groups need clarification or elucidation or when a model solution is being established.	116
Functionality Assessment	1. Validation of fulfillment of objectives (realization of objectives) – that is, the degree of compliance between the desired effect and the actual solution 2. Impact Assessment (also called effect assessment) 3. Identification of problems in the relationship between work procedures and the IT system's functional solution The method will expose severe ergonomic and cognitive problems, but it is not dedicated to capture details of this type.	120
Grounded Theory	Supportive analytical method for data acquisition methods that generate textual data, such as some open questionnaire methods and interviews (individual and group interviews).	128
Heuristic Evaluation	This is used when no other realizable possibilities exist – for instance, when: • The organization does not have the necessary time or expertise • There are no formalized methods • There is not something tangible to assess yet.	132
Impact Assessment	Measurement of the effect – that is, the consequence or impact in its broadest sense – of an IT-based solution, with or without the original objective as a frame of reference.	135
Interview (nonstandardized)	This is in particular suited for elucidation of individual opinions, attitudes, and perceptions regarding phenomena and observations.	142
KUBI	Optimization of the outcome of a long-term development project, based on a set of user or customer/client defined value norms and objectives.	147
Prospective Time Series	Measurement of development trends, including the effect of an intervention.	159

Questionnaire (nonstandardized)	Questionnaires are used to answer a wide range of questions, but its main area of application is (qualitative) investigations of subjective aspects requiring a high level of accuracy.	163
RCT, Randomized Controlled Trial	Verification of efficacy – that is, that the IT system – under ideal conditions – makes a difference to patient care. In particular used for studies of decision-support systems and expert systems.	172
Risk Assessment	Identification and subsequent monitoring of risk factors, making it possible to take preemptive action.	185
Root Causes Analysis	Exploration of what, how, and why a given incident occurred to identify the root cause of undesirable events.	188
Social Network Analysis	Assessment of relations between elements within an organization (such as individuals, professions, departments, or other organizations), which influence the acceptance and use of an IT-based solution.	190
Stakeholder Analysis	Assessment of stakeholder features and their inner dynamics, aiming to identify participants for the completion of a given task, problem-solving activity, or project.	192
SWOT	Situation analysis: establishment of a holistic view of a situation or a model solution.	196
Technical Verification	Verification that the agreed functions are present, work correctly, and are in compliance with the agreement. This may take place, for instance, in connection with delivery of an IT system or prior to daily operations, and at any subsequent change of the IT system (releases, versions, and patches).	199
Think Aloud	An instrument for gaining insight into the cognitive processes as feed-back to the implementation and adaptation of IT-based systems.	204
Usability	Assessment of user friendliness in terms of ergonomic and cognitive aspects of the interaction (dialogue) between an IT system and its users.	207
User Acceptance and Satisfaction	Assessment of users' opinion, attitudes, and perception of an IT system at daily operation.	215

Videorecording	Monitoring and documenting as a means of analyzing how work procedures and user activities, respectively, are actually carried out or for investigation of complex patterns of interaction.	219
WHO: Framework for Assessment of Strategies	Assessment of different (development) strategies either individually or as a comparative analysis.	222

6.5   Other Useful Information

There is certain information that cannot be categorized under 'methods' but that should be included nevertheless because an understanding of these issues is valuable. In general, the areas of application outlined in the table below are valid for all phases within the life cycle.

Information	Areas of application	Page no
Documentation in an Accreditation Situation	Planning of assessment activities in connection with the purchase of a 'standard' IT system when the user organization is or considers becoming certified or accredited.	227
Measures and Metrics	Measures and metrics are used throughout evaluation, irrespective of whether it is constructive or summative. Planning of an assessment/evaluation study includes the conversion of an evaluation purpose to specific measures and subsequent establishing metrics for their measurement.	232
Standards	A number of de facto and de jure standards exists, which each defines a series of issues such as the contents of a User Requirements Specification, verification of an IT system, quality aspects of an IT system, as well as roles and relations between a user organization and a vendor in connection with assessment.	238

7. Descriptions of Methods and Techniques

(Shown in alphabetical order by name of method or technique)

Analysis of Work Procedures

☺☺☺
§§
€€€

Areas of Application

When assessing what actually happens compared to the expectations of what should happen, for instance, with respect to:

- Analysis of the extent to which an IT system is being used as expected (during the implementation phase)
- Impact assessment (during the Evolution Phase)

Description

The methods listed here are not dedicated or designed specifically for evaluation studies, but they may clearly have a role as part of an evaluation study. The intention thus is to provide an overview of some well-known options:

- The Learning Organization: This paradigm theory and its strategies focus on analysis of work procedures to ascertain whether the organization has the ability consciously to incorporate experiences, whereby new or changed structures and work process are continuously established (see Argyris and Schön 1996).
- Enterprise modeling: A number of diagramming techniques are used for enterprise modeling. A recent overview of some of these is provided by Shen et al. (2004).
- Business Process Reengineering: Here the focus of the work process analysis is aimed at radical innovation and changes in work processes within the organization (see, for instance, the review in Willcocks 1996).
- Use Cases and scenarios: Use Cases describe the expectations of

what the IT system should accomplish in a given situation but not *how* – that is, the method aims at capturing the essence of the activities in a purpose-oriented way. Some variations of Use Cases use a combination of present and future cases. For further details, see, for instance, (Alexander and Maiden 2004). A scenario is another way of capturing the essence of activities. See, for instance, (Carroll 1995; and Alexander and Maiden 2004).

- Total Quality Management: This focuses on flaws and shortcomings in an organization with the specific aim of redressing them.
- Health Technology Assessment (HTA): Here it is the framework for assessment rather than the actual methods and techniques that are used. Goodman and Ahn (1999) provide a basic overview of HTA principles and methods.
- Computer-Supported Cooperative Work (CSCW): The focus on the work process analysis here is on the interaction between co-operating partners. As Monk et al. (1996) state, *"[A]ll work is cooperative, and so any work supported is computer-supported cooperative work (CSCW)"*. These can be either person-to-person or person-to-machine relationships. An important aspect of this form of analysis is to define tasks and delegate responsibility according to competencies. See, for instance, (Andriessen 1996) and other chapters in the same book.
- Cognitive Task Analysis: This approach, which is addressing the cognitive aspects of work procedures, is an emerging approach to the evaluation of health informatics applications. Kushniruk and Patel (2004) review this field.

Assumptions for Application

The use of diagramming techniques and other forms of graphical modeling requires experience, including that of understanding the principles and procedures involved, their pitfalls, perils, and assumptions. Often it also requires the ability to conceptualize, as it is impossible to include all the details and variations of the organizational work processes. On the other hand, users have special means of interpretation and conception – thereby capturing what goes on and what is and is not important.

Perspectives

Virtually all traditional diagramming techniques or scenarios for the descriptions of work processes are based on the assumption that work processes are either accomplished sequentially with little variation or that all relevant aspects can, nevertheless, be safely represented by means of the diagramming technique in question. Variations of work processes are exactly the aspects that are often not shown in diagram techniques and scenarios:

> "[W]ork processes can usually be described in two ways: the way things are supposed to work and the way they do work . . . People know when the 'spirit of the law' takes precedence over the 'letter of the law'".

(Gruding 1991)

It is still outside the capability of diagramming techniques to distinguish and incorporate ergonomic and cognitive aspects of the work processes, including the difference between how beginners and experts work and think. See, for instance, the discussion in (Dreyfus 1997) or the résumé in (Brender 1999).

Frame of Reference for Interpretation

If one wishes to measure the effect of an IT system from a work process point of view, it is a prerequisite that there be an explicit and unambiguous frame of reference, also called baseline values. Depending on the questions of the study, the frame of reference could, for instance, be the description of the work process for the 'old' system or for the intended new system (from a preliminary analysis or from the User Requirements Specification). The frame of reference could also be what was prescribed for the new or changed work processes prepared before the 'new' system was put into operation.

A frame of reference is normally not used during the Explorative Phase of an investigative study of work processes.

Perils and Pitfalls

Pitfalls in connection with descriptions of work procedures are indirectly evident from the aspects mentioned under Perspectives above. In other words, the most important thing is to find the method that will best describe exactly the information needs you have in connection with the context given.

As the methods described are so different, careful attention should focus on the objective of the study before choosing a method, while searching for descriptions of advantages and disadvantages.

Advice and Comments

Methods normally used for analysis and design work during systems development could potentially be used for assessment studies in cases of qualitative and explorative assessments. However, it often requires some lateral thinking, and maybe the process needs to be adjusted to the project in hand.

In principle many of the systems analysis methods can be used for this purpose. It could certainly be an advantage to employ a technique that has already been used in the organization. This way you will draw on existing experiences of the method while getting the opportunity to apply useful existing material as a frame of reference for evaluating the effect. See also under *Functionality Assessment*, for example.

References

Alexander IF, Maiden N. Scenarios, stories, use cases, through the systems development life-cycle. Chichester: John Wiley & Sons Ltd.; 2004.

Andriessen JHE. The why, how and what to evaluate of interaction technology: a review and proposed integration. In: Thomas P, editor. CSCW requirements and evaluation. London: Springer; 1996. p. 107-24.

Argyris C, Schön DA. Organisational learning II, theory, method, and practice. Reading: Addison-Wesley Publishing Company; 1996.

Brender J. Methodology for constructive assessment of IT-based systems in an organisational context. Int J Med Informatics 1999;56:67-86.

Carroll JM, editor. Scenario-based design, envisioning work and technology in system development. New York: John Wiley & Sons, Inc.; 1995.

Dreyfus HL. Intuitive, deliberative and calculative models of expert performance. In: Zsambok CE, Klein G, editors. Naturalistic decision making. Mahwah: Lawrence Erlbaum Associates, Publishers; 1997. p. 17-28.

Goodman CS, Ahn R. Methodological approaches of health technology assessment. Int J Med Inform 1999;56(1-3):97-105.

Gruding J. Groupware and social dynamics: eight challenges for developers. Scientific American 1991;Sept:762-74.

Kushniruk AW, Patel VL. Cognitive and usability engineering methods for the evaluation of clinical information systems. J Biomed Inform 2004;37:56-76.

Monk A, McCarthy J, Watts L, Daly-Jones O. Measures of process. In: Thomas P, editor. CSCW requirements and evaluation. London: Springer; 1996. p. 125-39.

The publication deals with features of conversation and is thereby a valuable contribution for all assessments that address conversations.

Shen H, Wall B, Zaremba M, Chen Y, Browne J. Integration of business modeling methods for enterprise information system gathering and user requirements gathering. Comput Industry 2004;54(3):307-23.

Willcocks L. Does IT-enabled business process re-engineering pay off? Recent findings on economics and impacts. In: Willcock L, editor. Investing in information systems, evaluation and management. London: Chapman & Hall; 1996. p. 171-92.

Supplementary Reading

Eason K, Olphert W. Early evaluation of the organisational implications of CSCW systems. In: Thomas P, editor. CSCW requirements and evaluation. London: Springer; 1996. p. 75-89.

Provides an arbitrary rating approach to assess cost and benefit for the different user groups and stakeholders.

Assessment of Bids

Areas of Application

Comparative assessment of a number of offers from one or more bidders/vendors

Description

There is not yet a really good method for the assessment of bids from one of more vendors that covers the variety of bid procedures. Thus, the existing approaches need to be adapted to the requirements specification upon which the bids have been made. The consequences are that all the procedures described use a multimethod approach. Therefore, the following points are meant only to be inspirational examples and food for thought.

A. (Brender and McNair 2002; Brender et al. 2002): The method described uses a spreadsheet-based bid table, where each single requirement is numbered and given a value in accordance with the level of need (compulsory, desirable) and with the bidders indication of fulfillment in their offer (0, 1, ..., 3). Initially an analysis will be made of whether the offers overall indicate that there could be problems with one or more of the requirements. Then, each bid is evaluated overall against the client's interpretation of the same contingency table, based on a demo and a hands-on test, and so forth. Finally, an assessment of all deviations is made, specifically with regard to an evaluation of the overall potential to meet the objectives and the consequences of any shortfalls.

B. (Beuscart-Zéphir et al. 2002, 2003, and 2005): The usability aspects (see description in separate section) are used as a point of focus for a practical assessment of the offer, combined with a heuristic evaluation or a multimethod approach to assess other aspects, both emanating from a week-long, on-site, hands-on demo test.

C. Rating & Weighting Techniques: The procedure of techniques for rating & weighting is to give each requirement a priority, then to multiply its degree of fulfillment in the bid solution with the priority. Finally, all numbers are summed into a single figure for all requirements – the objectives fulfillment. See, for instance, (Jeanrenaud and Romanazzi 1994; and Celli et al. 1998).

D. *Balanced Scorecard:* See separate description of this method.

E. Structured product demonstrations (Stausberg 1999): This methodology entails a gradual selection based on a strategic objective and technical functionality requirements, followed by a combination of three activities: (1) demos with quantitative assessments, (2) benefit analysis, and (3) test installation.

Assumptions for Application

Before the preparation of a requirements specification, it is important to be clear on which assessment method will be used. This is because the chosen method has to comply with the type of the requirements specification and with the principles used to prepare it.

Several of the methods need full or part installation of the systems and products that are to be assessed. This necessitates that the supplier is willing to install the product and also that it is possible to do so in the organization, as well as within its technical infrastructure. In itself, this may require a substantial demand on resources.

Method A assumes a stringent and formalized bid, which either is or can be converted to distinct response categories, as in '0' for "not included and not possible", . . . to '3' for "fully achieved by the offer". It needs to be possible for the categories to be converted into objects for either mathematical or logical operations in a spreadsheet.

Method B assumes (1) that the bids are based on ready-made products; (2) that the aspects of usability in the requirements specification are either operational or that professional assessors can assist with the rating; and (3) that the task and activity descriptions of the organization are included as part of the domain description in a requirements specification and therefore can be part of the frame of reference for the assessment.

Method C above assumes (1) that the requirements are mutually independent; (2) that different, equal, and equally desired solutions for a (partial) function will obtain the same outcome; and (3) that the assessment of the degree to which each requirement fulfills the evaluation criteria can be converted into mathematical calculations.

From the methods mentioned above, it is only method B that requires special experience of methods.

Perspectives

Cultural factors are significant not only for the choice of the actual IT solution and how users at different levels within the organization get involved, but also for organizing the procedure and thereby the methods applied for the acquisition of IT systems. As a matter of fact, within the EU tenders are required for the procurement of purchases in excess of a certain financial limit, and there are regulations for instance in Denmark for the involvement of personnel with regard to technological developments. This is markedly different in other parts of the world, as, for instance, in the United States and Asia. These differences have a decisive influence on the choice of method for the preparation of a requirements specification and for a bid assessment. The methods described are all useful within the Western culture.

It is rare that an offer from a vendor meets all the demands from the start and at a reasonable price. In other words, making a choice will need to be some 'give and take'.

All the methods are based on the notion that one cannot rely completely on vendors' statements, so one has to check the suitability for its actual use to make sure that the bidder cannot get around any problems (Rind 1997). This is not necessarily lack of honesty but could be due to too little understanding of the actual use – hence ignorance.

In the same way there may be hidden agendas in the user organization, or individuals among the stakeholders involved may have formed certain preconceptions. The choice of method should help to ensure objectivity.

Frame of Reference for Interpretation

The formal frame of reference for the assessment is the basis of the offer that is, a requirements specification or similar, in which – according to European regulations (in case of tendering) – the assessment model and its criteria have to be specified.

Perils and Pitfalls

It is important not just to select the bid with the highest score and 'jump to it', but to optimize the objectives fulfillment (at strategic and tactical levels) and to minimize potential problems and risks in the deviation between the requirements and in the future model solution. Beuscart-Zéphir et al. (2002) document how easily one can be duped by first impressions.

One pitfall that all the outlined methods have in common is that there can be decisive cultural differences – for example, in how users can or cannot be involved (at various levels within the organization) when selecting the future solution.

Advice and Comments

There is not much literature about methods for choosing bids, probably because (1) it is very difficult to validate the suitability, so they are rarely published and because (2) it is inherently difficult to judge whether one has actually chosen the right solution. To further complicate matters, the fact is that the method publications found about the subject in the literature do not follow up with a causal analysis of unexpected and unintentional occurrences in the future system against the method of choice. For example, the Rating & Weighting method is mentioned several times in the literature, but the consequence of the demand for mutual independence of the requirement items is not sufficiently discussed. And common to the three methods A, B, and E is the fact that the conclusions and thereby their suitability have not been verified by a third party.

In order to optimize the objectives fulfillment it is important to acquire a thorough understanding of the solution by means of demos, hands-on, conversations with the vendor and reference clients, as well as site visits, and so forth. The reason being that the vendor's sales and marketing people are trained to camouflage or avoid possible shortcomings in the solution offered (Rind 1997).

Regarding method B, the week-long hands-on test of the system turned out to be decisive for the final choice of bid because it was not until then that the nitty-gritty details were discussed.

Bevan (2000) deals with human error in the use of IT systems. It is a valuable source of inspiration – for instance, as a checklist when assessing system design, and thus also when assessing a vendor's bid.

See also under the description of *Standards*.

References

Beuscart-Zéphir M-C, Menu H, Evrard F, Guerlinger S, Watbled L, Anceaux F. Multidimensional evaluation of a clinical information system for anaesthesiology: quality management, usability, and performances. In: Baud R, Fieschi M, Le Beux P, Ruch P, editors. The new navigators: from professionals to patients. Proceedings of the MIE2003; 2003 May; St. Malo, France. Amsterdam: IOS Press. Stud Health Technol Inform 2003;95:649-54.

Beuscart-Zéphir MC, Watbled L, Carpentier AM, Degroisse M, Alao O. A rapid usability assessment methodology to support the choice of clinical information systems: a case study. In: Kohane I, editor. Proc AMIA 2002 Symp on Bio*medical Informatics: One Discipline; 2002 Nov; San Antonio, Texas; 2002. p. 46-50.

Beuscart-Zéphir M-C, Anceaux F, Menu H, Guerlinger S, Watbled L, Evrard F. User-centred, multidimensional assessment method of clinical information systems: a case study in anaesthesiology. Int J Med Inform 2005;74(2-4):179-89.

Bevan N. Cost effective user centred design. London: Serco Ltd. 2000. *(Available from http://www.usability.serco.com/trump/. The website was last visited 15.6.2005.)*

Brender J, Schou-Christensen J, McNair P. A case study on constructive assessment of bids to a call for tender. In: Surján G, Engelbrecht R, McNair P, editors. Health data in the information society. Proceedings of the MIE2002 Congress; 2002; Budapest, Hungary. Amsterdam: IOS Press. Stud Health Technol Inform 2002;90:533-38.

Brender J, McNair P. Tools for constructive assessment of bids to a call for tender – some experiences. In: Surján G, Engelbrecht R, McNair P, editors. Health data in the information society. Proceedings of the MIE2002 Congress; 2002; Budapest, Hungary. Amsterdam: IOS Press. Stud Health Technol Inform 2002;90:527-32.

Celli M, Ryberg DE, Leaderman AV. Supporting CPR development with the commercial off-the-shelf systems evaluation technique: defining requirements, setting priorities, and evaluating choices. J Healthc Inf Manag 1998;12(4):11-9.
A fairly thorough case study using the rating & weighting method.

Jeanrenaud A, Romanazzi P. Software product evaluation metrics: a methodological approach. In: Ross M, Brebbia CA, Staples G, Stapleton J, editors. Proceedings of the Software Quality Management II

Conference "Building Quality into Software". Southampton: Comp. Mech. Publications; 1994. p. 59-69.

Rind DM. Evaluating commercial computing systems. [Editorial]. M.D. Computing 1997;14(1):6-7.
Editorial comment pointing out the bias in vendors' sales talk.

Stausberg J. Selection of hospital information systems: user participation. In: Kokol P, Zupan B, Stare J, Premik M, Engelbrecht R, editors. Medical Informatics Europe '99. Amsterdam: IOS Press. Stud Health Technol Inform 1999;68:106-9.

Supplementary Reading
Please note the legislative difference between the United States and the European Union. In the EU all purchases over a certain value have to be submitted to tender. Nevertheless, the references all contain inspiration and good advice for one's own evaluation.

Beebe J. The request for proposal and vendor selection process. Top Health Inform Manag 1992;13(1):11-9.
A case study using a simple rating & weighting technique to preselect vendors and products.

Einbinder LH, Remz JB, Cochran D. Mapping clinical scenarios to functional requirements: a tool for evaluating clinical information systems. Proc AMIA Annu Fall Symp 1996;747-51.
A case study using a simple rating technique, but instead of a weighted summation it simply uses a summary principle.

Feltham RKA. Procurement of information systems effectively (POISE): using the new UK guidelines to purchase an integrated clinical laboratory system. In: Greenes RA, Peterson HE, Protti DJ, editors. Medinfo'95. Proceedings of the Eighth World Congress on Medical Informatics; 1995 July 23-27; Vancouver, Canada. Edmonton: Healthcare Computing & Communications Canada Inc; 1995. p. 549-53.
Brief description of a standardized procedure regarding IT acquisition based on a weighting score mechanism.

Friedman BA, Mitchell W. An analysis of the relationship between a pathology department and its laboratory information system vendor. Am J Clin Path 1992;97(3):363-68.
Discusses perils in the different types of relationships between a vendor of an IT system and the client.

Gell G, Madjaric M, Leodolter W, Köle W, Leitner H. HIS purchase projects in public hospitals of Styria, Austria. Int J Med Inform 2000;58-9:147-55.

> *Outlines an approach to select one from a group of bids by means of a combination of established criteria, functional requirements, and on-site trials.*

Madjaric M, Leodolter W, Leitner H, Gell G. HIS purchase project: preliminary report. In: Kokol P, Zupan B, Stare J, Premik M, Engelbrecht R, editors. Medical Informatics Europe '99. Amsterdam: IOS Press. Stud Health Technol Inform 1999;68:115-20.

> *A case study and some of their experiences.*

Balanced Scorecard

Areas of Application

Ongoing optimization of the outcome of a development project by balancing focus areas by means of a set of indicators for a set of strategic objectives.

Description

Balanced Scorecard (BSC) is based on a principle of critical success factors in terms of a limited set of performance indices. These are continuously monitored and are balanced against each other in an attempt to create an appropriate relation between their results (Shulkin and Joshi 2000; Protti 2002). Normally the success factor relates to the strategic objective at management level, hence the method is classified as being a strategic management tool. There is, however, nothing wrong in having the performance-related index focusing on other areas (Shulkin and Joshi 2000) – for instance, to obtain a better service profile toward service users or even taking it down to a personal level to assess performance.

The philosophy behind BSC is that of a constructive assessment, as the method can be used through group dynamics to create understanding and awareness of how certain aspects of the organization works externally and internally (Protti 1999 and 2002).

Assumptions for Application

The method requires some experience before it can be used in a larger context because, for instance:

1. Good results from this method depend on a good and detailed understanding of the causal relationship relating to the success factors in the model, and thereby also to the practical insight into the organization.

2. It requires the ability to handle the method in a dynamic project situation and in an organization undergoing change. This is because development projects involve constant changes in the object being monitored. In other words, it means that the object under investigation is a moving target or, as expressed by Gordon and Geiger (1999), the organization is in a double-loop learning.

Perspectives

The value norms of the project will inevitably become apparent from the discussion of how to prioritize the strategic success factors. The Scandinavian culture is particularly able to harmonize this with the intentions behind a broad user involvement, because of their national regulations, and can consequently be used to create openness, commitment and motivation through a mutual understanding. For the same reason this method is less valid in some other cultures.

Frame of Reference for Interpretation

(Not applicable)

Perils and Pitfalls

Within cultures and organizations where there is a tradition of top-heavy management, a schism may occur between the management style and the need to get a detailed understanding of work processes and motivation from staff. Hence, it may in certain situations be difficult to get the necessary support and understanding from staff to carry the method through without it hampering the outcome from a management perspective.

Advice and Comments

It is important to be aware that this is a project management tool to obtain a basis for decision making in a constructive development process, rather than a method that can stand completely on its own as an assessment tool.

References

Gordon D, Geiger G. Strategic management of an electronic patient record project using the balanced scorecard. J Healthc Inf Manag 1999;13:113-23.

Quite a good article to learn from should you wish to use this method.

Protti D. An assessment of the state of readiness and a suggested approach to evaluating 'information for health': an information strategy for the modern NHS (1998-2005). University of Victoria; 1999.

Protti D. A proposal to use a balanced scorecard to evaluate *Information for Health*: an information strategy for the modern NHS (1998-2005). Comput Biol Med 2002;32:221-36.
> *Protti argues in favor of the use of BSC and shows how to do it – in both short and long versions.*

Shulkin D, Joshi M. Quality management at the University of Pennsylvania health system. In: Kimberly JR, Minvielle E, editors. The quality imperative, measurement and management of quality in healthcare. London: Imperial College Press; 2000. p. 113-38.
> *The book is an anthology in quality management, and the chapter referenced gives a good description of BSC (Scorecard Measurement and Improvement System) as a method.*

Supplementary Reading

Kaplan R, Norton D. The balanced scorecard – measures that drive performance. Harvard Business Review 1992;70(1):71-9.

Kaplan R, Norton D. Strategic learning & the balanced scorecard. Strategy Leadership 1996;24(5):18.
> *These authors are the originators of the method.*

Niss K. The use of the Balanced ScoreCard (BSC) in the model for investment and evaluation of medical information systems. In: Kokol P, Zupan B, Stare J, Premik M, Engelbrecht R, editors. Medical Informatics Europe '99. Amsterdam: IOS Press. Stud Health Technol Inform 1999;68:110-14.

BIKVA

(from Danish: "**Bruger**Inddragelse i **KVA**litetsudvikling"; translated: User Involvement in Quality Development)

Areas of Application

The method is used as a tool for making critical, subjective decisions about an existing practice.

Description

Like *KUBI*, this method originates from the social sector, where it has been developed as a constructive tool to improve conditions within the socio-medical sector with regard to specific action or problem areas (Krogstrup 2003; Dahler-Larsen and Krogstrup 2003).

The method is based on a reflective process in the sense of getting food for thought. Users of an initiative, which can, for instance, be service functions or an IT-based solution, are the source of information. Its procedure consists of the following steps:

1. During group interviews, users are asked to indicate and justify "why they are either satisfied or not satisfied" with a given service function or an IT function. The users, who are the primary stakeholders in connection with the service function or the IT function, will typically describe incidents and interactions.

2. Summarizing the information obtained during the group interview.

3. Field workers (in IT projects probably the project management or vendor of the service or IT function) are confronted with the users' statements and are encouraged to identify the reasons behind the incidents and interactions referred to. This is

incorporated into the observations previously summarized.

4. In a second group interview management goes through the connections between the observations and the explanations in order to get the points of view of the user group.

. . . and possibly lead to an iterative process with the objective of clarifying all the disparities that relate to the issues of quality identified by the users.

5. The overall conclusion will then be presented to the decision makers in preparation for an assessment of the conclusion and possible initiatives.

Assumptions for Application

It can be a particularly unpleasant experience for an individual or an organization to uncover all its skeletons. It requires a psychologically and socially skilled moderator to facilitate the various processes to avoid being unnecessarily hard on anybody.

Perspectives

The built-in value norm of the BIKVA method is the user attitudes and perceptions. However, this should not be seen as though user attitudes alone determine the criteria. The philosophy behind it is to force the parties concerned to speak to one another in a formalized way to gather material as input for a process of change and learning.

Quite clearly, this method is primarily of use in cultures with a strong tradition of user participation and openness, as is the case in the Scandinavian countries. The principle of user participation would not work in, say, Asian cultures. However, you don't have to go far south in Europe before user participation is far less common than in Scandinavia (Fröhlich et al. 1993) and before openness stops at managements' (or others') desire for a good image and self-respect, 'la belle figure'. In other words, cultural circumstances can make it impossible to apply this method, even in Denmark.

The undisputed advantage of this method is that it gives the user on the ground a formal voice to express that something does not work without this being understood as negativism or lack of constructive cooperation.

Frame of Reference for Interpretation

The frame of reference is the users' view of where the problems lie. Having said that, it is of course also those who wear the shoes who can best feel if the shoes pinch.

Perils and Pitfalls

The pitfall is the representativeness of those involved, technically and functionally, as it is not guaranteed that *everybody* can participate. However, the most pressing problems in an organization will, under all circumstances, become evident from the start. Therefore, a minor bias in the representativeness does not necessarily have consequences in the long term. Consideration should, however, also be given to psychological factors in the representation of an organization with a broad user participation. Should the organization be large and complex, a *Stakeholder Analysis* method could be used to assess the issues regarding participation.

Advice and Comments

The amount of data resulting from this method can turn out to be overwhelming.

References

Dahler-Larsen P, Krogstrup HK. Nye veje i evaluering. Århus: Systime. 2003 (in Danish)

Fröhlich D, Gill C, Krieger H. Workplace involvement in technological innovation in the European Community, vol I: roads to participation. Dublin: European Foundation for the Improvement of Living and Working Conditions; 1993.

Krogstrup HK. Evalueringsmodeller. Århus: Systime; 2003. (in Danish)
   Even if this reference and (Dahler-Larsen and Krogstrup 2003) are both in Danish, the description above should enable experienced evaluators to apply the method or apply it in their own version, with benefit.

Clinical/Diagnostic Performance

§§
€€[5]

Areas of Application

- Measurement of the diagnostic performance (as in measures of accuracy and precision, etc.) of IT-based expert systems and decision-support systems.

This type of assessment falls under the Technical Development Phase – before an expert system or decision-support system is implemented, but it can continue during the operational phase (the Adaptation Phase and eventually also the Evolution Phase).

Description

The clinical performance of the systems (for diagnostic, prognostic, screening tasks, etc.) is typically measured with the help of a number of traditional measures from medicine, such as accuracy, precision, sensitivity, specificity, and predictive values. Also see *Measures and Metrics* for some specific concepts and measures.

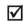

There are thousands of references to clinical performance of an IT-based decision-support system, including case studies. Smith et al. (2003) provide a valuable overview of the literature, although it is limited to neural networks and to the use of purely statistical tools. The advantage of this reference is the authors' summary of metrics and measures for binary as well as multiple categorical and continuous decision problems – that is, when the diagnostic problem consists of two or more diagnoses or diagnoses on a continuous scale.

Assumptions for Application

This depends on the actual measures and (statistical) tools applied. Refer, therefore, to their original literature.

Perspectives

One of the perspectives of decision-support systems and specialist systems is that of being able to measure the diagnostic performance

---

[5] If looked upon as an independent activity, expenditure can be quite large, but if the elements of the study can be included in the usual clinical work, one can equally have the chance of it becoming close to cost-free, apart from the planning stage and data analysis.

of an IT system just as if the IT system were a human being expressing the same.

The measures can without doubt give a significant statement of the value of an expert system's assertions (such as conclusion, recommendations, or similar). But the IT systems are characterized by not knowing their own limitations in such a way that they can adjust their assertions in accordance with the actual situation. Similarly, these systems are unable to take on a holistic view to the clinical object (the patient) in a way that a human being can. In other words, such systems may possibly be able to function with very high clinical, diagnostic performances within a narrow range of cases, but they cannot sensibly know when to abstain from all other cases.

Frame of Reference for Interpretation

The frame of reference is typically either a (predefined) 'golden standard' or a consensus reached by a panel of experts.

Perils and Pitfalls

The sources of error and pitfalls include partly general errors related to the use of concrete methods or metrics and partly problems related to the technology used for the development of clinical decision aids.

The first type of problems in assessing diagnostic performance is closely related to problems of getting a study design, which precludes a number of the pitfalls mentioned in Part III, such as the carryover effect (contamination), co-intervention, the Hawthorne effect, and so on. Friedman and Wyatt (1996) give a number of useful, overriding instructions for the organization of a clinical diagnostic performance study in order to avoid a number of the perils and pitfalls mentioned in Part III.

The other type of error is related to the technology used for the development of the decision-support system. All technology has its assumptions and limitations. When we deal with decision-support systems, there may be a requirement for mutual independence of the variables included or that there must be an adequate number of learning cases to avoid overfitting. Schwartzer et al. (2002) explore a number of these problems by using neural networks, some of which are general and also are valid for other types of decision-support systems.

Advice and Comments

The fact that an article like that of Kaplan (2001) only finds one single publication on decision-support systems and system performance illustrates how difficult it is to capture all relevant articles through a literature search and how difficult it is to go beyond one's own professional background (in this case the healthcare sector). The article together with other references is recommended as an introduction to the literature on clinical diagnostic performance.

References

Friedman CP, Wyatt JC. Evaluation methods in medical informatics. New York: Springer-Verlag; 1996.
> *Contains a really good introduction to assessments.*

Kaplan B. Evaluating informatics applications – clinical decision support systems literature review. Int J Med Inform 2001;64:15-37.
> *Kaplan reviews the literature (although only for the years 1997-1998) on clinical performance of decision-support systems for the period and includes other review articles on the subject.*

Schwartzer G, Vach W, Schumacher M. On the misuses of artificial neural networks for prognostic and diagnostic classifications in oncology. In: Haux R, Kulikowski C, editors. Yearbook of Medical Informatics 2002:501-21.

Smith AE, Nugent CD, McClean SI. Evaluation of inherent performance of intelligent medical decision support systems: utilizing neural networks as an example. Int J Med Inform 2003;27:1-27.

Supplementary Reading

Brender J. Methodology for assessment of medical IT-based systems – in an organisational context. Amsterdam: IOS Press, Stud Health Technol Inform 1997;42.
> *Includes a review of literature relating to assessment of medical knowledge-based decision-support systems and expert systems.*

Brender J, Talmon J, Egmont-Petersen M, McNair P. Measuring quality of medical knowledge. In: Barahona P, Veloso M, Bryant J, editors. MIE 94 Proceedings of the Twelfth International Congress of the European Federation for Medical Informatics; 1994 May; Lisbon, Portugal. 1994. p. 69-74.

Discusses concepts of correctness from traditional medicine, when used for an n * n + 1 contingency table. The authors suggest generalized metrics for, among others, dispersion (random distribution) and bias (systematic variance) together with kappa values.

Egmont-Petersen M, Talmon J, Brender J, McNair P. On the quality of neural net classifiers. AIM 1994;6 (5):359-81.

Uses similar metrics as in (Brender et al. 1994), but specifically designed for neural networks.

Egmont-Petersen M, Talmon JL, Hasman A. Robustness metrics for measuring the influence of additive noise on the performance of statistical classifiers. Int J Med Inform 1997;46(2):103-12.

It is important to keep in mind that (changes in) variations of one's data source influence the results of one's own studies. That is the topic of this article.

Ellenius J, Groth T. Transferability of neural network-based decision support algorithms for early assessment of chest-pain patients. Int J Med Inform 2000;60:1-20.

A thorough paper providing measures and corrective functions to obtain transferability of decision-support systems.

Elstein AS, Friedman CP, Wolf FM, Murphy G, Miller J, Fine P, Heckerling P, Maisiak RS, Berner ES. Comparison of measures to assess change in diagnostic performance due to a decision support system. Proc Annu Symp Comput Appl Med Care 2000:532-36.

The authors make an empirical comparative investigation of ten different measures for diagnostic performance.

Jaeschke R, Sackett DL. Research methods for obtaining primary evidence. Int J Technology Assessment 1989;5:503-19.

Some of the methods (and the rationale for their use) for evaluation studies of therapeutic and diagnostic technologies are discussed with regard to the handling of the placebo effect, confounders, and biases. Advantages and risk in using RCT, case control, and cohort studies are discussed.

Kors JA, Sittig AC, van Bemmel JH. The Delphi Method to validate diagnostic knowledge in computerized ECG interpretation. Methods Inf Med 1990;29: 44-50.

A case study using the Delphi method to validate diagnostic performance.

Malchow-Møller A. An evaluation of computer-aided differential diagnostic models in jaundice [Doctoral dissertation]. Copenhagen: Lægeforeningens Forlag; 1994.

Describes the development and gives a comparative evaluation of diagnostic performances with three different types of decision-support systems.

Miller T, Sisson J, Barlas S, Biolsi K, Ng M, Mei X, Franz T, Capitano A. Effects of a decision support system on diagnostic accuracy of users: a preliminary report. JAMIA 1996;6(3):422-28.

A pilot case study.

Nolan J, McNair P, Brender J. Factors influencing transferability of knowledge-based systems. Int J Biomed Comput 1991;27:7-26.

A study of factors that influence the clinical diagnostic performance of decision-support systems and expert systems.

O'Moore R, Clarke K, Smeets R, Brender J, Nykänen P, McNair P, Grimson J, Barber B. Items of relevance for evaluation of knowledge-based systems and influence from domain characteristics. Public report. Dublin: KAVAS (A1021) AIM Project; 1990. Report No.: EM-1.1.

The report, which is a freely available public technical report, contains a detailed description of which aspects of knowledge-based systems have been assessed in the literature.

O'Moore R, Clarke K, Brender J, McNair P, Nykänen P, Smeets R, Talmon J, Grimson J, Barber B. Methodology for evaluation of knowledge-based systems. Public report. Dublin: KAVAS (A1021) AIM Project; 1990. Report No.: EM-1.2.

The report, which is a publicly available technical report, contains an in-depth description of how to assess knowledge-based systems.

Tusch G. Evaluation of partial classification algorithms using ROC curves. In: Greenes RA, Peterson HE, Protti DJ, editors. Medinfo'95. Proceedings of the Eighth World Congress on Medical Informatics; 1995 Jul; Vancouver, Canada. Edmonton: Healthcare Computing & Communications Canada Inc; 1995. p. 904-8.

A methodological study of the use of ROC for decision-support systems.

Wyatt J, Spiegelhalter D. Field trials of medical decision-aids: potential problems and solutions. In: Clayton P, editor. Proc Annu Symp Comput Appl Med Care 1991:3-7.

Based on the literature, the authors describe a number of biases related to the assessment of medical decision-support systems.

Cognitive Assessment

Areas of Application

Assessment of the cognitive aspects of the interaction between an IT system and its users, such as:

- Identification of where and why operational errors occur
- Identification of focus areas requiring improvement in user friendliness

(See also under *Cognitive Walkthrough* and *Usability.*)

Description

Cognitive aspects deal with the extent to which the system functions in accordance with the way the users think and work in respect of user interaction with the IT system in general and with the user dialogue in particular. In plain language, this deals with the last '8 cm', which equals the process from the eye registering the visual input until the input has been processed by the brain and converted into a new instruction. Thus it is closely related to and very much overlaps with the measurement of the ergonomic aspects (see under *Usability*). The focus below is on the cognitive aspects that are not covered by the concept of usability.

This type of test is task-oriented – that is, the user simulates (or even tries) to complete an actual departmental work process by means of the IT system. All these tests are recorded on video (because there is no time to digest the information during the session). Kushniruk and Patel (2004) provide a review of methods in this respect.

One of the methods used for analyzing videorecordings is a diagram of the procedure (Beuscart-Zéphir, personal communication), where the course of the dialog with the IT system is noted down in symbolic form as shown in the figure below. The example could illustrate a doctor trying to make notes in the electronic patient record while talking to the patient.

example

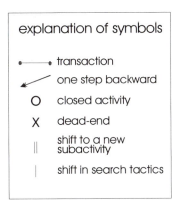

explanation of symbols	
•——•	transaction
╱	one step backward
O	closed activity
X	dead-end
‖	shift to a new subactivity
		shift in search tactics

Symbols could, for instance, be designed for the following aspects of the dialogue:

- How often did the user search in vain for information or for actual data fields where they believed them to be?
- How often was data input rejected simply because the user had misunderstood how the data had to be presented or what the field should be used for?
- How often did the user have to ask or to rack his or her brain to find out what to do? And how quickly did they find out, once they had tried it once or twice?

In an analogous approach, building on analytical constructs and techniques of Conversation Analysis, Meira and Peres (2004) suggest an evaluative approach that identifies gaps or breakdowns in user dialogues, and it maps the mismatches between user actions and software behavior.

Assumptions for Application

Assumptions for application depend entirely on what the results of the study are to be used for. It normally requires an experienced cognitive psychologist to assist in the investigation as there is still no standardized and thoroughly tested method within the current literature on IT assessment. The difficulty with the use of this method is how to find a direction of a synthesis and a conclusion on the functionality of the IT system if one does not have a cognitive psychology background. Depending on the objective of the study, a suitable person with relevant experience in the field should be engaged. It is also a prerequisite that there are detailed activity descriptions or scenarios for the user tasks within the department.

Perspectives

The difference between this method and *Cognitive Walkthrough* (below) is the approach: *Cognitive Walkthrough* starts with a technical description or a physical realization of the system and transforms this into scenarios of its use, whereas *Cognitive Assessment* starts by using the users' practical everyday tasks to develop scenarios to test the IT-based system.

During interaction with an IT system, an understanding of what goes on in the system is important for user friendliness and user satisfaction, and for the user to know what he or she has to do next or where he or she can find the relevant information. The cognitive aspect is not only of great importance when learning the system, but it is indeed of particular importance for the quantity of operator errors during its life cycle. This could be a reason why EHR seems to work perfectly well in general practice but less successfully in clinical departments: Once you have learned to use the system and you use it a great deal every day, it becomes very easy, even though the system might be a bit clumsy. However, when there are competing activities for the many and varying staff, who only use the systems for short periods of time, cognitive aspects demand much more attention.

The shortage of this type of assessment means that operational requirements, criteria, or recommendations have yet to be established. There is also a lack of established practice for incorporating the cognitive aspects into a requirements specification. Hence, cognitive aspects do not normally form an explicit part of a frame of reference in a traditional agreement with a vendor.

Frame of Reference for Interpretation

This method is normally used for explorative studies – that is, for studies intended to give a picture of a situation. Thus, there is no frame of reference in the normal sense.

However, there is a need for detailed descriptions of activities or scenarios of user activities in a department. What is an activity –in other words, what is its objective? What is its premise? What decision elements does it entail? And in what context (physically, socially, mentally) does it take place? Who performs the activity? What is the consequence of inadequate or delayed completion of the activity? This information is then used as a basis for comparison for the assessment of the cognitive aspects of an IT system. An example is the preoperative patient record taking by an anaesthesiologist (see Beuscart-Zéphir et al. 1997) – for example, where are the records physically kept during the operation (during the study in question, the paper-based record used to be placed on the patient's stomach)? And how does the doctor quickly find the information he or she needs during a crisis?

Perils and Pitfalls

Studies within this area require specialist knowledge. However, the experience and level of expertise of the user is a pitfall that even the experienced performer can fall into. There is a difference in how novices and experts work and think (see, for instance, Dreyfus 1997 and Beuscart-Zéphir et al. 2000), and experts can hardly discern between what they themselves say they do and what they actually *do* do (Beuscart-Zéphir et al. 1997; Kushniruk et al. 1997). See also the discussion in (Brender 1997a and 1999) and Part III in this handbook.

Advice and Comments

The questions raised in Description (above) can – initially – assist in finding out whether a system has serious cognitive problems, as can the analysis of operational errors in *Functionality Analysis* or the *Usability* methods.

References

Beuscart-Zéphir MC. Personal communication; 1997.

Beuscart-Zéphir MC, Anceaux F, Renard JM. Integrating users' activity analysis in the design and assessment of medical software applications: the example of anesthesia. In: Hasman A, Blobel B, Dudeck J, Gell G, Prokosch H-U, editors. Medical Infobahn Europe. Amsterdam: IOS Press. Stud Health Technol Inform 2000;77:234-8.

Beuscart-Zéphir MC, Brender J, Beuscart R, Ménager-Depriester I. Cognitive Evaluation: How to assess the usability of information technology in healthcare. Comput Methods Programs Biomed 1997;54(1-2):19-28.

Brender J. Methodology for assessment of medical IT-based systems – in an organisational context. Amsterdam: IOS Press, Stud Health Technol Inform 1997;42.

Brender J. Methodology for constructive assessment of IT-based systems in an organisational context. Int J Med Inform 1999;56:67-86.
This is a shortened version of the previous reference and more accessible regarding those aspects referred to in the text.

Dreyfus HL. Intuitive, deliberative and calculative models of expert performance. In: Zsambok CE, Klein G, editors. Naturalistic Decision Making. Mahwah: Lawrence Erlbaum Associates, Publishers; 1997. p. 17-28.

Kushniruk AW, Patel VL. Cognitive and usability engineering methods for the evaluation of clinical information systems. J Biomed Inform 2004;37:56-76.

Kushniruk AW, Patel VL, Cimino JJ. Usability testing in medical informatics: cognitive approaches to evaluation of information systems and user interfaces. Proc AMIA Annu Fall Symp 1997:218-22.
The article clearly illustrates the difference between the users' subjective understanding and the objective measure of the same.

Meira L, Peres F. A dialogue-based approach for evaluating educational software. Interacting Comput 2004;16(4):615-33.

Supplementary Reading

Carroll JM, editor. Scenario-based design, envisioning work and technology in system development. New York: John Wiley & Sons, Inc.; 1995.
This book contains a number of articles written by professionals in system development. It can therefore be on the heavy side, but there is a lot of inspiration to be had regarding scenarios. The different articles deal with different forms of scenarios, their use, as well as a discussion of advantages, disadvantages, and assumptions.

Demeester M, Gruselle M, Beuscart R, Dorangeville L, Souf A, Ménager-Depriester, et al. Common evaluation methodology. Brussels: ISAR-T (HC 1027) Health Care Telematics Project; 1997. Report No.: Deliverable 5.1.
This publicly available technical report can be obtained by

*contacting the author. It describes all the assessment methods of
the project including the ergonomic and cognitive assessments.*

Jaspers MWM, Steen T, van den Bos C, Genen M. The think aloud
method: a guide to user interface design. Inf J Med Inform
2005;73:781-95.

*The Think Aloud method combined with video recording was used
as a means to guide the design of a user interface in order to
combat the traditional problems with usability.*

Kushniruk A, Patel V, Cimino JJ, Barrows RA. Cognitive evaluation of
the user interface and vocabulary of an outpatient information system.
Proc AMIA Annu Fall Symp 1996:22-6.

Kushniruk AW, Patel VL. Cognitive computer-based video analysis: its
application in assessing the usability of medical systems. In: Greenes
RA, Peterson HE, Protti DJ, editors. Medinfo'95. Proceedings of the
Eighth World Congress on Medical Informatics; 1995 Jul; Vancouver,
Canada. Edmonton: Healthcare Computing & Communications Canada
Inc; 1995. p. 1566-9.

Kushniruk AW, Patel VL. Cognitive evaluation of decision making
processes and assessment of information technology in medicine. Int J
Med Inform 1998;51:83-90.

*Keep these two authors in mind with regard to studies of cognitive
aspects. Although some of their articles are conference
proceedings, they contain many good details.*

Patel VL, Kushniruk AW. Understanding, navigating and
communicating knowledge: issues and challenges. Methods Inf Med
1998;37:460-70.

*Describes how they carry out assessments using video recordings
and think-aloud techniques.*

Cognitive Walkthrough

Areas of Application

Assessment of user 'friendliness' on the basis of a system design, from specification, to muck-ups and early prototypes of the system, aimed at judging how well the system complies with the users' way of thinking, for instance:

- Identification of where and why operational errors occur
- Identification of causes behind problems with respect to user friendliness and consequently identification of areas for improvement

(Patel et al. 1995)

. . . and thereby also

- The assessment of a demo IT system as a step in the process of choosing a system in a bid situation

The advantage of this method compared to many others is that it can be carried out at an early stage and with just a system specification as a basis. Therefore, the method can also be used to assess immature prototypes (Beuscart-Zéphir et al. 2002).

See also under *Cognitive Assessment.*

Description

Every single task or activity in an organization requires a combination of cognitive (i.e., intellectual) functions and physical actions. *Cognitive Walkthrough* is an analytical method designed to evaluate usability. The method addresses the question of whether a user with a certain degree of system and domain knowledge can perform a task that the system is designed to support. See (Horsky et al. 2003), which provides an overview of theories and approaches used for studying usability aspects as well as a case study. It focuses on the cooperation between the cognitive functions and the parallel physical actions, while the ergonomic aspects are closely related to the organization of, and the interaction with, each of the individual fields on the screen images. There is a gentle graduation and quite an overlap between cognitive and ergonomic aspects (see *Usability* and *Cognitive Assessment*) of the user interface of an IT system.

Cognitive Walkthrough is a review method for which a group of experts prepare task scenarios either from specifications or from earlier prototypes (could be video-based) (Kushniruk et al. 1996). The experts investigate the scenarios either on their own or together with a user. The one acting as a typical user goes through the tasks with the aid of the interface of the scenario – "walking through the interface", as they pretend that the interface actually exists and works. Each step of the process is analyzed as seen from the point of the objective of the task with the intention of identifying obstacles in the interface that make it either impossible or difficult to complete the task. Complicated or roundabout ways through the system's functions indicate that the interface needs a new function or simplification of the existing one.

Assumptions for Application

The method is designed to systematically go through all the user's possibilities of interaction with every screen of the IT system. The analyst is required to perform a manual simulation of the cognitive processes that form part of the successful execution of a task. In practice it could, however, be impossible to carry out a systematic cognitive walkthrough if the system is very complex.

It is necessary to know how the user interface will look; therefore, the description of the system needs to meet a certain level of detail.

It is a prerequisite that there is a task and activity analysis. See, for instance, under *Analysis of Work Procedures*, and see (Beuscart-Zéphir et al. 2002).

Normally users of a (future) IT system do not have the experience to prospectively and methodically assess the cognitive aspects themselves, as to analyze one's own activities from a different point of view requires special awareness and some lateral thinking.

Perspectives

The difference between this method and *Cognitive Assessment* is the point of view. As a starting point *Cognitive Walkthrough* uses a technical description, or a physical realization of it, and transforms it into scenarios of its use, while *Cognitive Assessment* starts by using the practical daily tasks of the user to prepare scenarios to test the IT-based system.

A character-based system can have excellent cognitive qualities, and systems with a graphical interface can have terrible cognitive qualities, so one should get rid of a priori prejudices. What is important is whether the system and the way the user thinks work together – not whether the interface is esthetically pretty to look at. A person who knows the system can easily circumvent cognitive problems because one can learn how to navigate. Thus, thorough training can compensate for cognitive and ergonomic problems in IT-based systems.

Ordinary users and user organizations will typically experience and notice cognitive errors as operational errors with inadequacies in specific details or in the interaction between the IT system and the work-processes of the organization.

The method's systematic approach is based on the assumption that all screen actions bring discrete changes between states of the system.

Frame of Reference for Interpretation

The frame of reference is purely based on the experience of what will normally cause problems in terms of gaps in the understanding and breakdowns in actions.

Perils and Pitfalls

Development of user scenarios based on specifications or on an early prototype cannot become more complete and correct than the base upon which it has been developed. In other words, if this material is wanting, then the assessment will also be wanting, but this does not preclude that the method can be quite a valuable (constructive) assessment tool during the early development phase.

Advice and Comments

The method is suited for use, for example, during a demo of an existing system, although it is easier if you get to the keyboard yourself. Alternatively, one can stipulate that the vendor or bidder goes through one or more actual scenarios.

References

Beuscart-Zéphir MC, Watbled L, Carpentier AM, Degroisse M, Alao O. A rapid usability assessment methodology to support the choice of clinical information systems: a case study. In: Kohane I, editor. Proc AMIA 2002 Symp on Bio*medical Informatics: One Discipline; 2002

Nov; San Antonio, Texas; 2002. p. 46-50.

Horsky J, Kaufman DR, Oppenheim Mereon Institute, Patel VL. A framework for analyzing the cognitive complexity of computer-assisted clinical ordering. J Biomed Inform 2003;36:4-22.

Kushniruk AW, Kaufman DR, Patel VL, Lévescque Y, Lottin P. Assessment of a computerized patient record system: a cognitive approach to evaluating medical technology. MD Comput 1996;13(5):406-15.

Patel VL, Kaufman DR, Arocha JA, Kushniruk AW. Bridging theory and practice: cognitive science and medical informatics. In: Greenes RA, Peterson HE, Protti DJ, editors. Medinfo'95. Proceedings of the Eighth World Congress on Medical Informatics; 1995 Jul; Vancouver, Canada. Edmonton: Healthcare Computing & Communications Canada Inc; 1995. p. 1278-82.

Supplementary Reading

Carroll JM, editor. Scenario-based design, envisioning work and technology in system development. New York: John Wiley & Sons, Inc.; 1995.
> *This book contains a number of articles written by system development professionals, so it can be somewhat heavy to read, but there is a lot of inspiration regarding scenarios. The different articles deal with various forms of scenarios, their use, as well as a discussion of advantages, disadvantages, and assumptions.*

Huart J, Kolski C, Sagar M. Evaluation of multimedia applications using inspection methods: the Cognitive Walkthrough case. Interacting Comput 2004;16:183-215.
> *An exhaustive case study that also reviews usability methods.*

Kushniruk AW, Patel VL. Cognitive and usability engineering methods for the evaluation of clinical information systems. J Biomed Inform 2004;37:56-76.
> *A thorough description of a number of usability inspection methods, including the walkthrough method.*

http://jthom.best.vwh.net/usability/
> *Contains many method overviews with links and references. (Last visited 31.05.2005)*

Delphi

Areas of Application

- (Qualitative) assessment of an effect – for instance, where the solution space is otherwise too big to handle
- Elucidation of a problem area – for instance, prior to strategic planning
- Exploration of development trends

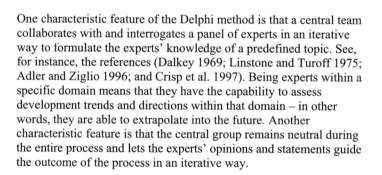

Description

The Delphi method is a consensus method for the prediction of the future (Dalkey 1969) developed by the Rand Corporation for the American military in the 1950s.

One characteristic feature of the Delphi method is that a central team collaborates with and interrogates a panel of experts in an iterative way to formulate the experts' knowledge of a predefined topic. See, for instance, the references (Dalkey 1969; Linstone and Turoff 1975; Adler and Ziglio 1996; and Crisp et al. 1997). Being experts within a specific domain means that they have the capability to assess development trends and directions within that domain – in other words, they are able to extrapolate into the future. Another characteristic feature is that the central group remains neutral during the entire process and lets the experts' opinions and statements guide the outcome of the process in an iterative way.

The approach depends on the topic, as the basis for interrogation may be predefined (for instance, some quantitative investigations) or may be the result of an open opening question (for instance, in certain qualitative investigations). An example of the latter is seen within (Brender et al. 2000):

1. Brainstorming phase based on an open question of what is relevant to address the problem area with.
2. Evaluation phase, where the individual experts comment on (prioritize, elaborate, refine) each others' contributions from the first phase.
3. Feed-back to the authors on their fellow experts' commented,

providing an opportunity for them to refine their original intention. Following this refinement, the topics are fixed.

4. Preparation of a questionnaire from previous material.
5. Collection and analysis of the expert panel's rating of the individual topic.

Assumptions for Application

The method is medium of difficulty, primarily because it assumes experience and cautiousness with the synthesis and with the preparation of a questionnaire, including the perils and pitfalls associated with a *Questionnaire* approach (see this elsewhere).

It is an assumption for a reliable outcome that the core team remains neutral toward the material and in dealing with the outcome.

Perspectives

The professional perspective behind the design of this method is that a collection of experts is capable of inspiring and correcting each other to predict the future or the nature of something, which none of them are able to judge accurately on their own. Cooperation makes them adjust and compensate for each other's weak points in an iterative process controlled by the core team so that the end results become fairly accurate. Thereby, a topic may be exhaustively investigated, while inaccuracy, nonsense, hidden agendas, and hobby horses vanish in the iterative process. It is difficult to predict anything about the future, but experience shows a fair amount of success by using the Delphi method.

Frame of Reference for Interpretation

(Not applicable)

Perils and Pitfalls

When the experts know each other, there is a risk that they become emotional or stick to the official view of the topic rather than responding according to their best convictions. Therefore, it is best to keep the contributions anonymous. This sometimes also includes the composition of experts within the panel, at least as long as the process is ongoing.

Advice and Comments

Depending on the need for precision in the outcome, one may continue iterating the last phases until the results no longer converge, indicating that the maximum level of accuracy and precision has been reached for that specific combination of experts.

References

Adler M, Ziglio E. Gazing into the oracle – the Delphi method and its application to social policy and public health. London: Jessical Kingsley Publishers; 1996.

Brender J, McNair P, Nøhr C. Research needs and priorities in health informatics. Int J Med Inform 2000;58-9(1):257-89.

Crisp J, Pelletier D, Duffield C, Adams A, Nagy S. The Delphi method? Nurs Res 1997;46(2):116-8.

Dalkey NC. The Delphi method: an experimental study of group opinion – prepared for United States Air Force project. Santa Monica (CA): Rand; 1969.

Linstone HA, Turoff M. The Delphi method, techniques and applications. Reading, MA: Addison-Wesley Publishing Company; 1975.

Supplementary Reading

Kors JA, Sittig AC, van Bemmel JH. The Delphi method to validate diagnostic knowledge in computerized ECG interpretation. Methods Inf Med 1990;29:44-50.
> *A case study using the Delphi method for validating diagnostic performance.*

O'Loughlin R, Kelly A. Equity in resource allocation in the Irish health service, a policy Delphi study. Health Policy 2004;67:271-80.
> *A case study using the Delphi method to explore policy issues in resource allocation.*

Snyder-Halpern R. Indicators of organizational readiness for clinical information technology/systems innovation: a Delphi study. Int J Med Informatics. 2001;63:179-204. Erratum in Int J Med Inform 2002;65(3):243.
> *A case study using the Delphi method for a specific evaluation purpose.*

Equity Implementation Model

Areas of Application

Examine users' reaction to the implementation of a new system, focusing on the impact of the changes such a system brings about for the users.

Description

The Equity Implementation Model is used to retrospectively investigate and understand user reactions to the implementation of an IT-based system, based on incidents in an organization. The focus of this method that originates in social science is the effect of the changes that such a system brings about (Lauer et al. 2000).

The method consists of three steps (Lauer et al. 2000):

1. Deals with the changes from the perspective of a user to identify possible stresses and benefits that may be affected by the new IT system, both of which may be positive or negative in a picture of the 'perceived benefit'

2. Examines the fairness in relation to the employer in sharing the gains or losses brought about by the change, thereby comparing the perceived benefits of the two parties

3. Compares changes perceived by individual users with that of other users or user groups

Assumptions for Application

There is a need for insight into behavioral aspects and social science to avoid the pitfalls in studying humans.

Perspectives

Implementation of an IT-based solution implies organizational change. Many attempts at implementing IT-based systems in organizations have resulted in failures, of which only a fraction are on account of technical problems, and many researchers have demonstrated that critical issues in the implementation of such systems reside with the soft human aspects of an organizational.

The method provides a means for explanation of system implementation events, leading to an understanding of user resistance or acceptance of the new technology. It is based on the perspective that there is no fundamental or irrational resistance to change (Lauer et al. 2000): Each change is evaluated as being favorable or unfavorable by each individual affected by it.

Further, the method emphasizes that it is important to pay attention to the fairness concerns of all users, a viewpoint that is highly culturally dependent.

Frame of Reference for Interpretation
(Not applicable)

Perils and Pitfalls
The sources of bias come from the method's origin in social science, and hence it is concerned with the pitfalls in observing and interrogating humans (see Part III in general).

Advice and Comments
Although the objective of Lauer et al. (2000) is that of research, it may certainly in some situations be useful for more down-to-earth investigations as well, particularly in cases of special user-satisfaction problems.

As the method in general deals with equity, it may be applied as a measuring instrument to provide the decision-making basis relation to policy planning and priority setting, as well as for examination of barriers and drivers at the implementation of change. The method may also prospectively provide a means for pointing out other problem areas that may subsequently be addressed by preventive initiatives through its focus on equity.

References

Lauer TW, Joshi K, Browdy T. Use of the Equity Implementation Model to review clinical system implementation effort, a case report. JAMIA 2000;7:91-102.

Field Study

(In the sense of observational studies)

Areas of Application

Observation of an organization to identify its practices and to elucidate mechanisms that control change.

Description

In short, observational studies are used to diagnose various conditions in an organization (Harrison 1994). This method is widely used in psychology, sociology, anthropology, and so on – that is, in professions that deal with different perspectives of human factors – to identify what goes on and how. The studies encompass all sorts of elements from social interaction and the influence of specialist cultures on work practices, through to work process analysis, as seen in the informatics part of the organizational spectrum observed. The studies can be transverse or in depth, exploring or verifying.

Assumptions for Application

This type of study normally requires professional psychological, sociological, or specialist knowledge of organizational theory.

Perspectives

It is an important aspect of field studies to understand that the reality of the actors is a determining frame for acting and maneuvering. Therefore, the outcome of the study depends on prior knowledge of the users' conditions and an understanding of their way of thinking in different contexts. The specialist culture is an acquired one.

One of the reasons why this type of study has to be performed by specialists is that the observer must be able to free himself from his perspectives and thereby from his prejudices, expectations, and assumptions, as well as from established principles and understanding. Any kind of preconception will influence the process of observation and introduce bias. Professionals in the healthcare sector including IT users are subconsciously trained to think in a specific way (a profession-oriented culture and politics) to such a degree that it is difficult for them to disregard their own way of thinking. Informatics specialists are trained to observe the movements of information units and processes of change in an organization, but not to observe (profession-oriented) cultural, social, and psychological phenomena, so even informatics specialists fall short.

There are two basic models behind field studies: Reductionist ('diffusion model') and holistic ('translation model').

The reductionistic understanding presupposes that things can be taken apart and individual items be observed in isolation, after which they are put back together as an entirety where the conclusion equals the sum of the component items. It is also an assumption in this perspective that the results from one organization will work in the same way in other organizations and that the organization(s) can be more or less suited but can adapt to the technology. Specialists of informatics, natural sciences, or technically trained people are trained to work with the reductionistic model, while there is a tendency evolving to try to incorporate holistic aspects when developing new methodologies in order to compensate for known deficiencies.

The holistic view is based on the understanding that an organization or a person comprises many different factors and units that work in complex unity and that any external influence will cause them to mutually affect each other. Specialists with a background in the humanities use a holistic view to a far greater extent than informatics specialists. However, they often have to draw very strict limitations as the totality otherwise becomes too large.

Frame of Reference for Interpretation

(Not applicable)

Perils and Pitfalls

Professionals from social and behavioral sciences are well aware of the many serious pitfalls and take the organizational and behavioral circumstances as their methodological and methodical starting point. This is why field studies require a specialist background.

One must be aware that it takes time for a person from outside the domain to reach a stage of observation enabling him to pose the right questions to the right people. This is because without prior knowledge of the domain, one cannot know anything about what should and shouldn't happen. Even though they are trained to observe, it takes time to get to the core of the matter.

Interview studies are often used to facilitate field studies, but as they are unable to elicit tacit knowledge, they embrace severe pitfalls, inasmuch as the users in an organization are unable to account for what or how they do things[6] (see the review in Brender 1997a and 1999). Instead they have a tendency to describe prescriptive procedures in a way that they would use to tell a colleague being trained in the department (Beuscart-Zéphir et al. 1997; and Beuscart-Zéphir, personal communication).

The Hawthorne effect may be significant in studies of this kind: For psychological reasons people tend to change behavior and performance when under observation (see Part III). This points at the need for addressing the complex dynamics of the wholeness and its mechanisms of change rather than single and specific variables before and after the process of change.

Advice and Comments

This method is very time consuming.

Before you even start to consider undertaking a field study yourself, you need to read Baklien (2000), who examines a number of aspects of field studies particularly concerned with constructive assessment purposes.

---

[6] This is a known phenomenon in the development of knowledge-based systems and has resulted in the establishment of a special profession, called knowledge-engineering with methods dedicated to the purpose. They still struggle to develop methods to elicit the users' knowledge of how they do things in real life and why. The focus is particularly aimed at expert knowledge in the area of diagnostics/therapy. But system analysts/informatics people struggle equally to develop efficient and reliable methods to elicit the entirety of relevant aspects in work processes (Brender 1999).

Svenningsen (2003) is a field study of an exploratory character. It does not, therefore, have any element of constructive assessment. However, the study is highly timely in its subject as it focuses on the clinical processes of changes relating to the introduction of EHR into the Danish healthcare system, and it encompasses a study of the activities and accounts of the causal explanations in order to identify the patterns of change.

References

Baklien B. Evalueringsforskning for og om forvaltningen. In: Foss O, Mønnesland J, editors. Evaluering av offentlig virksomhet, metoder og vurderinger. Oslo: NIBR; 2000. Report No.: NIBRs PLUSS-SERIE 4-2000. p. 53-77. (in Norwegian)

Beuscart-Zéphir M-C. Personal communication 1996.

Beuscart-Zéphir MC, Brender J, Beuscart R, Ménager-Depriester I. Cognitive evaluation: how to assess the usability of information technology in healthcare. Comput Methods Programs Biomed 1997;54(1-2):19-28.

Brender J. Methodology for assessment of medical IT-based systems – in an organisational context. Amsterdam: IOS Press, Stud Health Technol Inform 1997;42.

Brender J. Methodology for constructive assessment of IT-based systems in an organisational context. Int J Med. Inform 1999;56:67-86.
    This is a shortened version of the previous reference and more accessible with regard to this subject.

Harrison MI. Diagnosing organizations: methods, models, and processes. 2nd ed. Thousand Oaks: Sage Publications. Applied Social Research Methods Series 1994. vol. 8.
    The book discusses advantages and disadvantages of various methods, including field studies, for the analysis of a number of aspects within an organization.

Svenningsen S. Electronic patient records and medical practice – reorganization of roles, responsibilities, and risks [PhD thesis]. Copenhagen: Samfundslitteratur; 2003. Report No.: Ph.D.-Series 10.2003.
    A thorough Danish case study of processes of change in a clinic upon implementation of EHR.

Supplementary Reading

Jorgensen DL. Participant observation, a methodology for human studies. Newbury Park: Sage Publications. Applied Social Research Methods Series 1989. vol. 15.

Describes what field studies can be used for and how one can observe people in an organization. However, the book avoids discussing the pitfalls.

Kuniavsky M. Observing the user experience, a practitioner's guide to user research. San Francisco: Morgan Kaufmann Publishers; 2003.

Chapter 8 of this book is dedicated to the method of Contextual Inquiry, a data collection technique that studies a few carefully selected individuals in depth in order to arrive at an understanding of the work practice.

Focus Group Interview

Areas of Application

In principle this group interview method can be used for the same purpose as other *Interview* methods, but in practice it is most relevant for the following tasks (see, for instance, Halkier 2002 and Kuniavski 2003):

- During the early analysis phases (the Explorative Phase) – for instance, when eliciting the attitudes, perceptions, and problems of social groups, or when a model solution is being established.

- During operations – for instance, to identify a pattern in user attitudes to the system, norms, and behavior, or to identify problem areas of the system functionality or of operations in general.

Description

The method is a variation on other interview methods, with individual interviews being replaced by a group interview process; see also general aspects under *Interviews*.

Focus Group Interviews can be carried out during workshops or other dedicated meeting activities, where one of the purposes of the introductory steps is to get the group dynamics working. Depending on the topic discussed, a skilled moderator can use a variety of data-capture techniques (such as mind-maps, Post-it notes on a whiteboard, or similar brainstorming techniques) to ensure that the written output is generated as part of the whole process.

Stewart and Shamdasani (1990) and Halkier (2002) meticulously investigate the various methodical issues for each step starting with preparation, through completion of the interview, to transcription and analysis of the data. Halkier (2002) and Kuniavsky (2003) recommend that the whole procedure be videotaped, as it can be virtually impossible to take notes that are sufficiently thorough and accurate.

In contrast to interviews of individuals, where one is able to take firm control of the process while taking notes, group dynamics will invariably make the participants all eagerly speak at the same time.

This creates a lot of overlapping communication, and small, parallel groups that communicate informally may form from time to time. Thus, it becomes very difficult for the moderator to take notes and get the whole context down at the same time as moderating the process.

Assumptions for Application

It takes an experienced moderator and facilitator (Halkier 2002; Kuniavsky 2003), and practice of transcribing and analyzing this type of data.

Perspectives

When you gather a number of individuals under informal conditions, you get the opportunity to start a group dialog or debate right across the whole group. The advantages of this method over that of individual interviews are that the participants can mutually inspire as well as adjust and moderate each other during a brainstorming process, stimulating the creativity of the group and, even more importantly, kindling the individual's memory and perception.

During the process a synthesis of new knowledge will frequently occur, resulting directly from the interaction between the participants, which the interviewer could not possibly bring out due to the lack of prior contextual knowledge of the subject (Halkier 2002). At times it is easier to glean certain types of information from a group, maybe through group pressure, as it is precisely the social interaction that is the source of the data. For instance, members of a group can have insider information that the interviewer would not be able to draw from an individual. Hereby information will be revealed that often would not be communicated during an individual interview. At the same time one can iterate the process until the required or potential level of precision is reached.

However, there are – culturally defined – topics that will be difficult to discuss in a group, just as there is a tendency to put the official version forward rather than the real version of a topic.

Frame of Reference for Interpretation

The method is primarily used to explore a subject. Therefore, studies based on this method normally do not have a frame of reference.

Perils and Pitfalls

The psychological factors are prominent, as in *Interview* methods in general (see *Interview* section), but additionally there are the social factors to contend with. The interaction between delegates can have a powerful impact on the reliability of the result, as seen, for instance, from the domination of key persons (or the opposite). In other words, the result depends on social control, representativeness of stakeholders, the homogeneous and heterogeneous composition of the group, internal power structures (Stewart 1990; Harrison 1994), and confidentiality and sensitivity of topics or taboos.

This form of interview makes it difficult to get at the finer details or variances in individual practice or at atypical understandings (Stewart 1990; Halkier 2002), because the philosophy of the method is that of consensus seeking but also because it is difficult to get representativeness in the composition of the groups and the resulting group dynamic.

Advice and Comments

-

References

Halkier B. Fokusgrupper. Frederiksberg: Samfundslitteratur og Roskilde Universitetsforlag; 2002. (in Danish)

> *This is a very thorough handbook of methods dedicated to Focus Group Interviews, but it has the disadvantage that the error sources and pitfalls are only implicitly described.*

Harrison MI. Diagnosing organizations: methods, models, and processes. 2nd ed. Thousand Oaks: Sage Publications. Applied Social Research Methods Series 1994. vol. 8.

> *The book deals with the analysis of a number of aspects of an organization and describes advantages and disadvantages of different methods.*

Kuniavsky M. Observing the user experience, a practitioner's guide to user research. San Francisco: Morgan Kaufmann Publishers; 2003.

> *Chapter 9 of this book is dedicated to Focus Group Interview and outlines four different types thereof as well as describes what the method is suited for or not in Web applications.*

Stewart DW, Shamdasani PN. Focus groups: theory and practice. Newbury Park: Sage Publications. Applied Social Research Methods Series 1990. vol. 20.

> *Describes a number of aspects of group dynamics, strengths, weaknesses, and the risk of bias by application of the method, all of which are very important when using this method.*

Supplementary Reading

Robson C. Real world research, a resource for social scientists and practitioner-researchers. 2nd ed. Oxford: Blackwell Publishers Inc; 2002. p. 269-91.

> *This book gives a good description of different types of interviews, details and ideas regarding their use including the advantages and disadvantages of each of them.*

http://www.icbl.hw.ac.uk/ltdi/cookbook/focus_groups/index.html

> *The home page gives additional advice and guidelines on how to carry out the various phases of a Focus Group Interview. (Last visited 31.05.2005)*

http://jthom.best.vwh.net/usability,

> *The home page contains a lot of method overviews, links and references. Two of the better links from this page that are relevant for Focus Groups are those of George Silvermin and Thomas Greenbaum's (both last visited on 31.05.2005).*

Functionality Assessment

Areas of Application

- Validation of objectives fulfillment (realization of objectives) – as opposed to a pure verification of the requirements specification – that is, assessment of the degree of compliance between the desired effect and the solution realized
- Impact Assessment (also called effect assessment)
- Identification of problems in the relation between work procedures and the functional solution of the IT system

The method will also capture severe ergonomic and cognitive problems but is not dedicated to capture details of this type.

Description

The method is as objective as its user. It can include both qualitative and quantitative elements but is best suited to qualitative studies.

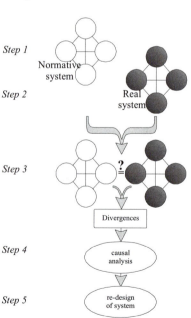

An overview of the methodological procedure is illustrated in the figure to the left (reprinted from Brender 1989 and 1997a). The 'normative system' and the 'real system' are described first (easiest when using the same modeling and descriptive techniques). The latter includes all of the IT-based solution (i.e., IT system plus the surrounding work procedures) as it works in practice, while the normative system is the planned IT-based solution. If the actual IT system of the normative system is not described, it can be replaced by the planned structure, work processes, activities of the organization, and new guidelines, for example. In step 3 all divergences between the two systems are described, indicating which of these are considered key divergences. Step 4 consists of an analysis of the causal connection. Step 5 is normally used (for development projects and constructive assessment activities) to design the new solution.

The principle behind the analysis of the causal connection is illustrated in the example given in the figure to the right: Each symptom is unwound from the end, from description of a symptom to possible causes right back to the anticipated primary source of the problem based on the philosophy in Leavitt's model for organizational changes (see under Perspectives below).

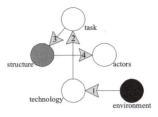

Assumptions for Application

The method is very work intensive when the complete picture of how work processes in an organization function with an IT system as an overall solution.

The degree of difficulty depends largely on the diagramming technique used (see examples under *Work Process Analysis*). However, it is most common to use the same methods of description as the ones used for analysis of the organization in earlier phases of the project, thereby also making the method accessible for a broader group of users.

The ability to be objective, persistent, and meticulous is a requirement for the causality analysis, as is in-depth knowledge of the organization in order to limit the solution space for propagating from cause to symptom in the way that best reflects the organization.

Perspectives

During a period after taking the IT system into operation – no matter how thorough you are during planning – a number of adaptations of the work processes and probably also of the IT system will take place. At the same time both the organization and the users will change; they will learn something new, giving rise to new possibilities and/or challenges. For this reason the connection between the IT system and the work processes around the system will always be sensitive to time. Thus, the method has been designed (within certain limits) to make allowances for the development of the system and changes of work procedures as a function of time when interpreting the result.

The method is based on Leavitt's model for organizational change (Leavitt 1970), so it is based on the philosophy that any change in one element of an organization will propagate to the other elements of the organization in a chain reaction until a new, steady state is reached. If problems arise within an organization, compensating reactions will thus spread to other parts of the organization, implying that the problems will be visible in terms of these changes.

At the same time, the method is based on a generalization of the philosophy of Mumford's Participatory Approach to System Design from the late 1970s (Mumford et al. 1978 and 1979). The principle is to start by identifying all variances between the IT system's or the organization's desired processes (i.e., the normative system) and the way it actually works. Mumford's system development method then focuses on finding a solution to one or more of the variances identified.

Frame of Reference for Interpretation

The method has a built-in frame of reference – namely the description of the Normative System (see above). The original method – analysis of the realization of objectives of a specific IT system – was based on a detailed Requirements Specification and a System Specification together with the user manual and minutes of meetings, and so on, as a frame of reference (the normative system) (Brender 1989), while the analysis carried out in (Beuscart et al. 1994) is based on the same method but with the needs and expectations as the frame of reference.

The difference between these two applications (see Brender 1997a) illustrates that should the normative system not explicitly be prepared prior to the introduction of the system, there is a possibility of 'making do' with the expectations of the system as a frame of reference, as, for instance, in descriptions of new work processes developed in connection with the introduction of the system.

Perils and Pitfalls

The causality analysis is the weakest point of the method because the interpretation and therefore the final conclusion is completely dependent on this analysis. It can be difficult to uncover the skeletons in an organization and to discuss the problems without hurting somebody's feelings. Alternatively, someone may try to cover up and hide the problems.

On the other hand, the method is less dependent on whether all divergences are included or whether you get the right divergences defined as key divergences because the actual causality will often manifest itself in more than just one symptom.

Advice and Comments

The method is designed to address measures according to Leavitt's model for organizational change. However, the framework addressing 'structure, process, and effect', or any other similar framework structure, can be used in the same way.

The causal analysis of this method may be supported by the *Root Causes Analysis* method (see separate section).

References

Brender J. Quality assurance and validation of large information systems – as viewed from the user perspective [Master thesis, computer science]. Copenhagen: Copenhagen University; 1989. Report No.: 89-1-22.
> *A résumé of the method and a case study can be found in (Brender 1997a). If this does not suffice, the reference can be obtained from the author.*

Brender J. Methodology for assessment of medical IT-based systems – in an organisational context. Amsterdam: IOS Press, Stud Health Technol Inform 1997;42.

Beuscart R, Bossard B, Brender J, McNair P, Talmon J, Nykänen P, Demeester M. Methodology for assessment of the integration process. Lille: ISAR (A2052) Project; 1994. Report No.: Deliverable 3.
> *This report is freely available, and contact information can be obtained from the undersigned author.*

Leavitt HJ. Applied organizational change in industry: structural, technological and humanistic approaches. In: March JG, editor. Handbook of organisations. Rand MacNally & Co: Chicago; 1970.

Mumford E, Land F, Hawgood J. A participative approach to the design of computer systems. Impact Sci Soc 1978;28 (3):235-53.

Mumford E, Henshall D. A participative approach to computer systems design, a case study of the introduction of a new computer system. London: Associated Business Press; 1979. Appendix C.

Future Workshop

Areas of Application

Evaluation and analysis of an (existing) situation with the view to
identifying focus areas for change – that is, aiming at designing future
practice.

Description

The method resembles the *Logical Framework Approach* (see
separate section) and uses the same terminology. However, the *Future
Workshop* as a method has a different focus and concentrates on
situation analysis supplemented by a follow-up and a far more
thorough interpretation of how to carry out the individual phases.
Another difference from the *Logical Framework Approach* is that in
the *Future Workshop* it is not necessary to focus on just one problem
during the implementation and process of change, but it uses a picture
of the organization and its problems as a whole.

The method is carried out through a workshop, a preparatory phase,
and a follow-up phase (Jungk and Müllert 1984; Müller 2002). The
preparatory phase of the workshop consists of a simple stakeholder
analysis and the participants getting to know each other. The purpose
of the follow-up phase is an ongoing analysis of whether the right
track is being pursued and whether it is being pursued in a satisfactory
way. The workshop itself has the following three phases:

1. The critique phase, with the purpose of identifying and discussing
   existing problems
2. The fantasy phase, with subgroups discussing problems identified
   and submitting their vision of the future (thus, the result is a
   catalogue of visions)
3. The realization phase, where means, resources, and opportunities
   to realize the visions are discussed

Assumptions for Application

Depending on the degree of accuracy and precision needed, the
person(s) in charge of the process must have sufficient experience of
group dynamics – in other words, the method requires an experienced
moderator and facilitator familiar with transcription and analysis of
this type of data. An experienced moderator may use data-capture
techniques (such as mind-maps, Post-it notes on a whiteboard, or

similar brainstorming techniques) to ensure that the written output is generated as part of the whole process. However, in some situations it might inhibit the process resulting in loss of information.

Perspectives

The Future Workshop as described is relatively neutral to political, organizational, and cultural conditions and bonds. It neither dictates nor prevents such bonds but can adapt and operate under the conditions of the organization.

There are, however, aspects of the method that makes it more suitable in certain cultures and forms of organization than in others. For instance, the proposal of a broad representation of staff as participants in the project is dependent on culture (at national and organization levels). However, there is nothing to stop you from making minor adaptations at some points, as long as you are aware of the magnitude of potential consequences and their further implications.

Frame of Reference for Interpretation

There is no frame of reference built into the method itself, but references as to whether the result is valid and applicable are the premises against which the result should be used. In other words, the frame of reference has to be the formulation of the organization's (stakeholder groups') vision, mission, and strategic initiatives, as well as other constraints within the organization and possible declared intentions for different aspects of the organization.

Perils and Pitfalls

It is a substantial pitfall in some cultures that the method description promotes broad staff participation to identify visions and objectives of the organization because there is no prior knowledge of whether management (or staff) is ready to take that step. It is the step from realizing the problem to establishing solutions and monitoring objectives that may become the point of issue. Therefore, it is important that the leader (the facilitator) of the workshop process has complete insight into, and works in accordance with, management intentions and the principles of the organization or, alternatively, that management accepts that the process of change in the organization also includes this stipulation.

Advice and Comments

The follow-up phase does not have an explicit risk monitoring in the same neat way as in *Logical Framework Approach*, but there is nothing to stop you from incorporating it.

Analogous methods that might provide further inspiration are 'Future Search' and 'Cafe-Seminar' (see http://www.futuresearch.net and www.worldcafe.dk, respectively; both last visited 31.05.2005).

References

Jungk R, Müllert N. Håndbog i fremtidsværksteder. Viborg: Politisk Revy; 1984. (in Danish)
One of the early references for this method. It encompasses a thorough investigation of the method and a case study.

Müller J. Lecture note on future workshop, design and implementation. Aalborg: Dept. of Development and Planning, Aalborg University; 2002 (a copy can be obtained from the department).

Grounded Theory

§§§

€€€

Areas of Application

Grounded Theory is a supportive analytical method for data acquisition methods that generate textual data, some open *Questionnaire* methods, and *Interviews* (individual and group interviews), for example.

Description

Grounded Theory aims at identifying and explaining phenomena in a social context through an iterative and comparative process (Cronholm 2002).

There are four steps:

1. Open coding, where single elements from the data are correlated to and named as concepts with defined characteristics, including identification of tentative categories of theoretical importance

2. Axial coding, where the named concepts are definitively defined, patterns among them identified, and are then organized into categories according to characteristics and internal relationships, including potential causal relationships

3. Selective coding, which works toward arranging the concepts according to the relationships between them, including identification of mechanisms, processes, or circumstances that may bring about the concept characteristics identified. Finally, the central category to which everything else relates is identified

4. Theoretical coding, which provides a hypothetical model (generalized relationships) based on the previous coding. The model must be able to abstract and explain the phenomena observed and their interrelationships.

Assumptions for Application
The method is considered difficult and requires special qualifications. Normally it should only be undertaken by experienced professionals.

Perspectives
The method is subjective, and it is the implementer's perceptions and evaluations that influence the outcome of the analysis. The subjectivity is somewhat compensated for by the fact that it is iterative, inasmuch as the outcome – provided you have the right end of the stick – starts out resembling chaos but converges toward a (relative) simplicity.

Frame of Reference for Interpretation
The method does not use any frame of reference.

Perils and Pitfalls
Lack of experience in the use of the method or very large amounts of data can easily result in an imprecise or inaccurate outcome.

It is necessary to be aware of the fact that the data acquisition method itself holds a pattern, precisely because an interview, a questionnaire, or literature searches, for example, are organized according to one's prior knowledge and expectations. One must therefore be careful not to restore this pattern, as the outcome as this simply creates circularity.

A bias – one that clearly must be balanced against the advantage of having prior knowledge of the application domain – lies in the risk of categorizing according to known patterns and prior experiences or attitudes, or experience reported in the literature (Goldkuhl and Cronholm 2003). This is because experiences and attitudes (often subconsciously) influence one's evaluation. Thus, preconception (but not necessarily prior knowledge) is a dangerous cocktail when executing this method, also called 'lack of neutrality' (Edwards et al. 2002). The danger is explained as the result of the analysis being driven by the user.

Another bias, as pointed out by Edwards et al. (2002), is 'personal bias' (closely related to 'hypothesis fixation' described in Part III). This appears as a risk when the researcher works on verification of a work hypothesis during observation of an actual case.

Advice and Comments

The method is difficult to apply with a reliable and reproducible result and also rather work intensive. But if you do need textual analysis, there are not many alternatives.

Edwards et al. (2002) illustrate and discuss how triangulation can be used to avoid strong elements of subjectivity during categorization. They make extensive use of feed-back from the actors of the case under study to ascertain whether it is meaningful to them. This way they get a good relationship between conceptions, attributes and categories.

Similarly, Allan (2003) and Balint (2003) give a number of ideas on how to safely manage the methodological challenges, including the coding.

References

Allan G. The use of Grounded Theory as a research method: warts & all. In: Remenyi D, Brown A, editors. Proceedings of the European Conference on Research Methodology for Business and Management Studies; 2003 Mar; Reading, UK. Reading: MCIL, 2003. p. 9-19.
> *Goes through experience of, and offers advice on, coding with Grounded Theory.*

Balint S. Grounded research methodology – a users' view. In: Remenyi D, Brown A, editors. Proceedings of the European Conference on Research Methodology for Business and Management Studies; 2003 Mar; Reading, UK. Reading: MCIL, 2003. p. 35-42.
> *Discusses how as a user one can ensure validity, quality, and stringency during its use – in other words, methodological challenges.*

Cronholm S. Grounded Theory in use – a review of experiences. In: Remenyi D, editor. Proceedings of the European Conference on Research Methodology for Business and Management Studies; 2002 Apr; Reading, UK. Reading: MCIL; 2002. p. 93-100.
> *Elaborates on the method and discusses experiences (strengths and weaknesses) of the various steps of its application, based on an analysis of the application of the method by a number of PhD students.*

Edwards M, McConnell R, Thorn K. Constructing reality through

Grounded Theory: a sport management study. In: Remenyi D, editor. Proceedings of the European Conference on Research Methodology for Business and Management Studies; 2002 Apr; Reading, UK. Reading: MCIL; 2002. p. 119-27.

Goes through a case and discusses the weaknesses of the method.

Goldkuhl G, Cronholm S. Multi-Grounded Theory – adding theoretical grounding to Grounded Theory. In: Remenyi D, Brown A, editors. Proceedings of the European Conference on Research Methodology for Business and Management Studies; 2003 Mar; Reading, UK. Reading: MCIL, 2003. p. 177-86.

Discusses certain strengths and weaknesses of the method and suggests an alternative procedure for applying the method at its weakest point.

Supplementary Reading

Proceedings from the European Conference on Research Methodology for Business and Management Studies (an annual event) can be generally recommended. There are often some good references with practical experiences of the method.

Ericsson KA, Simon HA. Protocol analysis, verbal reports as data. Cambridge (MA): The MIT Press; 1984.

This book provides a thorough review of the literature on approaches and problems in general terms at the elicitation of information about cognitive processes from verbal data.

Esteves J, Ramos I, Carvalho J. Use of Grounded Theory in information systems area: an explorative study. In: Remenyi D, editor. Proceedings of the European Conference on Research Methodology for Business and Management Studies; 2002 Apr; Reading, UK. Reading: MCIL; 2002. p. 129-36.

Discusses a number of recommendations and critical success factors for use with this method.

Jorgensen DL. Participant observation, a methodology for human studies. Newbury Park: Sage Publications. Applied Social Research Methods Series 1989. vol. 15.

Describes a number of issues with regard to observation studies and what they can be used for, including how to analyze data from the observation studies of the Grounded Theory method. Unfortunately, however, the book avoids discussing the pitfalls.

Heuristic Assessment

Areas of Application

This inspection-based method may be used when no other realizable possibilities exist – for instance, if:

- The organization does not have the necessary time or expertise
- There are no formalized methods to be applied by users
- There is not yet anything tangible to assess.

Description

Basically, this method consists of summoning experts (3-5 are recommended) from the area in question (usually the assessment of usability) and letting them make a statement – one based on experience but in a formalized way. Kushniruk and Patel (2004) and Sutcliff and Gault (2004) propose approaches and a number of heuristics.

In principle this method can be used for nearly everything, but in practice it is most commonly used for the assessment of user interfaces where few methods exist that will assist the ordinary user in carrying out his own assessment on a formal basis. The website http://jthom.best.vwh.net/usability indicates that this method can be particularly useful for the assessment of user interfaces because precisely this particular type of assessment can be difficult for the user organization itself to carry out. Therefore, it can be a really good idea to call on one or more external experts and ask their (unreserved) opinions.

Assumptions for Application

It is normally quite simple to summon experts to solve a problem. The difficulty lies in finding experts who are both professionals in the problem area and who also have an understanding of the area of application.

If you yourself have to synthesize the experts' comments into an overall conclusion afterward – for decision-making purposes, for instance, knowledge of the terminology as well as the ability and experience of assessing the consequences of the observations must be present.

Perspectives

-

Frame of Reference for Interpretation

(Not applicable)

Perils and Pitfalls

-

Advice and Comments

Although the literature states that users normally do not take part in this method, Beuscart-Zéphir et al. (2002) nevertheless show that users themselves can act as experts for certain types of IT system assessment, provided that there is suitable guidance and supervision.

References

http://jthom.best.vwh.net/usability/
This website contains a number of descriptions and links with relevant references (last visited 31.05.2005).

Beuscart-Zéphir MC, Watbled L, Carpentier AM, Degroisse M, Alao O. A rapid usability assessment methodology to support the choice of clinical information systems: a case study. In: Kohane I, editor. Proc AMIA 2002 Symp on Bio*medical Informatics: One Discipline; 2002 Nov; San Antonio, Texas; 2002. p. 46-50.

Kushniruk AW, Patel VL. Cognitive and usability engineering methods for the evaluation of clinical information systems. J Biomed Inform 2004;37:56-76.

A thorough description of a number of usability inspection methods, including the heuristic evaluation method. A number of heuristics is presented.

Sutcliff A, Gault B. Heuristics evaluation of virtual reality applications. Interacting Comput 2004;16(4):831-49.

Supplementary Reading

Graham MJ, Kubose TK, Jordan D, Zhang J, Johnson TR, Patel VL. Heuristic evaluation of infusion pumps: implications for patient safety in intensive care units. Int J Med Inform 2004;73:771-9.

A case study applying heuristic assessment for the evaluation of usability aspects to uncover design and interface deficiencies. The study is performed by a combination of specialists and a healthcare professional without prior experience of the method.

Impact Assessment

(Also called Effect Assessment)

Areas of Application

Measurement of the effect – that is, the consequence or impact in its broadest sense from degree of realization of the objective plus assessment of side effect – of an IT-based solution, with or without the original objective as a frame of reference. Hence, it includes not only the beneficial effects, but also potential adverse effects.

Description

Within the social sector, the practice has been to assess the effect of a given initiative, legislation, or project with the (political) objective as a frame of reference to obtain a measurement for assessing to what extent the objectives have been realized (also denoted 'objectives fulfillment'). However, it is worth noting, that in this sector goal-free evaluations are also gaining ground (Krogstrup 2003) – that is, the type of explorative studies aimed at reporting descriptively on a situation as seen from one or more perspectives. A goal-free evaluation has a nearly limitless solution space when the concept is interpreted in its literal meaning because it entails measurement of the impact with all its secondary effects.

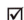

Assessment of the effect of health informatics systems can be carried out in the same way as projects and initiatives within the social sector – that is, either as assessment of objectives fulfillment or as exploratory studies. The indicators would of course have to be identified and designed for the actual purpose.

As the solution space is very large in a goal-free evaluation, you need to start by finding out what you really need to know about the effect and what the result is going to be used for in order to limit the study: For instance, is it an assessment of the gains as in the effect on the level of service or on the quality? Consequences for ways of cooperation or social interaction? Consequences on the organizational structure or culture? Legal consequences or cases derived from the system? User satisfaction? And so on and so on. The question now is whether the need is for qualitative and/or quantitative data or information. One does not necessarily exclude the other.

Depending on what you wish to know about the effect of an IT-based solution, it makes a huge difference to how you proceed. Please see the list of references with regard to additional descriptions of procedures.

Assumptions for Application

It is obvious that a measurement of fulfillment of the objective assumes that a strategic objective has been defined and can be made operational in terms of relevant and realistic measures – that is, that formulas (metrics) can be established for their measurement.

Perspectives

Few people realize the wide range of consequences an IT-based solution can have even beyond the organization normally considered as the user of the system: On implementation of a (new) IT system, it is nearly always necessary to make compromises (a bit of give and take). This is not necessarily bad, as over time many organizations develop very specific ways of doing things in a never-ending number of variations that often cannot be handled by the IT system. Some forms of rationalization will therefore typically result from the implementation of an IT system. This rationalization will impact on something or somebody, and therefore there is a risk that the changes within the user organization will reach far and wide into the surrounding organizations.

Once introduced into daily operation, the organization keeps on changing – initially as it gets accustomed to and adjusts to the system. One danger (and a pitfall) is to start measuring the effect too soon after the daily operation has started before a degree of stability has been achieved. On the other hand, after a certain period in operation staff will start using their creativity, and new ways of doing things will develop spontaneously – both appropriate ones and inappropriate ones, intentional ones and unintentional ones (as shown in van Gennip and Bakker 1995 or in Part III, Section 11.1.6.9). This phenomenon only reflects the development pattern from novice to expert: You start by following the prescribed way of doing things, but while gaining experience at a proficient level, you get to know the shortcuts (Dreyfus 1997). You could, for instance, compare the note-taking in patient records by a newly graduated physician to that of a consultant. This phenomenon may make comparisons of controlled studies and before and after studies rather difficult.

Frame of Reference for Interpretation

The strategic objective may influence all aspects of an organization, right from (partly) financially, matters of responsibility and competence, quality objectives for patient care or the overall service, overall to the number of records missing or patient and staff satisfaction. Whether there is a need for before-values (baseline data) depends on the individual study.

IT systems that do not have a written defined strategic objective could possibly have an objective defined at a lower, tactical level (for instance, in terms of the interim objectives that are expected to lead to the overall strategic objective), and this may perfectly well replace the strategic objective as a frame of reference or they can form the frame of reference together.

The frame of reference must therefore be aligned with the real objective and to the conditions of the actual study. In order to describe the conditions adequately, the objective will usually need to be covered by a whole range of indicators (measures).

Perils and Pitfalls

A consequence of the extremely dynamic situations occurring in connection with the introduction of an IT-based system could be the loss of control of what some of the effect indicators actually signify. Before-and-after assessment, as, for instance, in those recommended in (*Nytteværdi* 2002), have inbuilt pitfalls in the shape of the validity of the frame of reference. One must be sure that the concepts used are the same before *and* after in case they are directly measured and compared. It is often necessary to use different questionnaires for the before-and-after situations, as the work processes and many other aspects are different, thus making a direct comparison difficult.

It is difficult to separate the effect of different variables: For instance, what is the effect of having done anything at all? Simply focusing on an organization over a period of time, asking lots of questions about what and how things are done, has tremendous effect. How does one separate the effect arising purely from the fact that something is happening from the real (intentional) effect of the IT system or the IT solution? If the effect is caused by the first possibility, there is a strong risk that given time it will revert toward the starting point to a certain degree.

Advice and Comments

See also under the method *Functionality assessment,* which has been specifically designed with the evaluation of fulfillment of the objective of an IT-based solution in mind.

The approach in (Clements et al. 2002) of a Utility Tree with a hierarchical breakdown from overall interest areas to specific measures might be valuable for narrowing the focus of an Impact Assessment.

References

Clements P, Kazman R, Klein M. Evaluating software architectures, methods and case studies. Boston: Addison-Wesley; 2002.

Dreyfus HL. Intuitive, deliberative and calculative models of expert performance. In: Zsambok CE, Klein G, editors. Naturalistic Decision Making. Mahwah: Lawrence Erlbaum Associates, Publishers; 1997. p. 17-28.

Krogstrup HK. Evalueringsmodeller. Århus: Systime; 2003. (in Danish)
> *This little instructive book gives a good overview of applications and limitations of a couple of known assessment models. Although it originates in the social sector it is inspiring with regard to Impact Assessment and assessment of performance.*

Nytteværdi af EPJ, MTV-baseret metode til måling af nytteværdien af elektronisk journal. Roskilde: Amtssygehuset Roskilde, DSI og KMD Dialog; 2002. (in Danish)
> *This little book gives an excellent and quick overview of how to carry out an actual Impact Assessment (as in the usefulness) of an EPJ including quantitative indicators, questionnaires, and the procedure.*

van Gennip EM, Bakker AR: Assessment of effects and costs of information systems. Int J Biomed Comput 1995;39:67-72.
> *A valuable case study to learn from.*

Supplementary Reading

Bates DW, Teich JM, Lee J, Seger D, Kuperman GJ, Ma'Luf N, Boyle D, Leape L. The impact of computerized physician order entry on medication error prevention. JAMIA 1999;6(4):313-21.
> *A case study using prospective time studies to assess the effect of*

the introduction of an IT-based solution on a given activity.

Brinkerhoff RO, Dressler DE. Productivity measurement: a guide for managers and evaluators. Newbury Park: Sage Publications. Applied Social Research Methods Series 1990. vol. 19.

Measurement of productivity as a function of input and output variables (including identification of measures) is extremely important in many studies of objectives fulfillment and assessments of effect. This book is useful as inspiration for that purpose.

Collinson M. Northern province HIS evaluation, defining an evaluation framework - workshop 24 July 1998. (Available from: http://www.sghms.ac.uk/depts./phs/hceu/safrica2.htm. Last visited 31.05.2005.)

The report illustrates a fairly thorough and effective way in which to get relevant measures.

Friedman CP, Abbas UL. Is medical informatics a mature science? a review of measurement practice in outcome studies of clinical systems. Int J Med Inform 2003;69:261-72.

A thorough and critical review of studies that measure different types of effect. It includes a very useful list of earlier studies measuring effects within the healthcare sector.

Garrido T, Jamieson L, Zhou Y, Wiesenthal A, Liang L. Effect of electronic health records in ambulatory care: retrospective, serial, cross sectional study. BMJ 2005;330:581-5.

A fairly exhaustive, retrospective case study applying administrative data to assess usage and quality of care before and after implementation of an EHR.

Hagen TP. Demokrati eller effektivitet: hvad skal vi evaluere? In: Foss O, Mønnesland J, editors. Evaluering av offentlig virksomhet, metoder og vurderinger. Oslo: NIBR; 2000. Report No.: NIBRs PLUSS-SERIE 4-2000. p. 79-110. (in Norwegian)

Discusses a number of effectiveness measures, including that of "through whose 'eyes' is the organization being observed".

Hailey D, Jacobs P, Simpson J, Doze S. An assessment framework for telemedicine applications. J Telemed Telecare 1999;5:162-70.

This article outlines a list of effect measures that can be used universally, even though the design originally is for tele-medicine purposes.

Kimberly JR, Minvielle E. The quality imperative, measurement and management of quality in healthcare. London: Imperial College Press; 2000.

This anthology of quality in the healthcare sector covers many methods and problems concerned with quality measurements and many of its chapters are inspirational with regard to effect measurement.

Milholland DK. Information systems in critical care: a measure of their effectiveness. In: Greenes RA, Peterson HE, Protti DJ, editors. Medinfo'95. Proceedings of the Eighth World Congress on Medical Informatics; 1995 Jul; Vancouver, Canada. Edmonton: Healthcare Computing & Communications Canada Inc; 1995. p. 1068-70.

Development and verification of a tool to measure the effect in terms of a fulfillment of the objective of efficiency. Although it is only a proceeding, it includes valuable directions to useful statistical tools to verify the metrics and the results of the analysis.

Mitchell E, Sullivan F. A descriptive feast but an evaluative famine: systematic review of published articles on primary care computing during 1980-97. BMJ 2001;322:279-82.

One of the very few systematic reviews of the effect of IT within the primary healthcare sector. It is a supplement to (Sullivan and Michell 1995) and particularly valuable to include, as it is critical and encompasses many assessments of effect and references to studies with good case studies of this particular measurement of effect type. The authors do this without automatically keeping the non-RCT studies apart; instead they create a quality score applying a Delphi method.

Sullivan F, Mitchell E. Has general practitioner computing made a difference to patient care? a systematic review of published reports. BMJ 1995;311:848-52.

A review containing references to numerous case stories about the effect of IT on general practice. The article addresses the best studies of patient outcome effect, the effect of the consultation process, and clinical performance, respectively.

Vabo SI. Kritiske faktorer for evalueringer av kommunale reformer. In: Foss O, Mønnesland J, editors. Evaluering av offentlig virksomhet, metoder og vurderinger. Oslo: NIBR; 2000. Report No.: NIBRs PLUSS-SERIE 4-2000. p. 139-82. (in Norwegian)

Discusses specific indicators for the measurement of attitudes and behavior.

van der Loo RP, van Gennip EMSJ. Evaluation of personnel savings through PACS: a modelling approach. Int J Biomed Comput 1992;30:235-41.

Outlines a diagramming and modeling method where all divergences between before-and-after descriptions of work processes are used as a baseline for a quantitative assessment of the effect of a PACS system on staff resources.

Zoë Stavri P, Ash JS. Does failure breed success: narrative analysis of stories about computerized provider order entry. Int J Med Inform 2003;70:9-15.

Uses a narrative analysis approach to retrospectively elicit aspects of success and failure of an IT-based solution. This approach might be useful for narrowing the scope of an impact assessment through the identification of areas of interest.

Interview

(Nonstandardized interviews)

Areas of Application

This method is frequently used for qualitative studies of subjective as well as objective circumstances. Interviews are particularly suited for the elucidation of individuals' opinions, attitudes, and perceptions regarding phenomena and observations. This is especially the case when non- or semistructured techniques or group techniques are being used to promote dynamic interaction.

Description

Interviews are methods used to carry out a type of formalized conversation that can be:

- Structured at different levels (structured, semistructured, and unstructured)
- Controlled to a greater or lesser extent by the interviewer
- Conducted with individuals or in groups

The book by Fowler and Mangione (1990) (and a number of similar books) is indispensable for those who want to make an effective interview study. It describes all aspects of the method and discusses what can diminish the value (precision, accuracy) of the results and thereby the reliability of the study. It is necessary to examine thoroughly the different methodological considerations for each step from preparation (choice of theme, design) to completion of the interview, transcription and analysis of data, and verification.

An often used type of group interview is the *Focus Group Interview*, where brainstorming techniques can be useful to stimulate the dynamics and the creativity of the participants. See separate description of this variation of interviews.

Assumptions for Application

The flexibility of un- or semistructured interview methods makes it necessary to be experienced in order to achieve a reliable result from the study. The level of reliability (precision and accuracy) required is, however, the deciding factor. This is the case for both individual and group interviews.

Perspectives

The methods are based on conversation between people, but it is not a dynamic dialogue of equals between the interviewee and the interviewer. Therefore, there are a number of social and psychological factors and pitfalls that have to be taken into consideration during the interaction.

Silverman (2001) describes the different perspectives behind approaches for interviews: Positivism, emotionalism, and constructionalism. In short, positivists acknowledge that interviewers interact with the interviewees giving facts or beliefs about behavior and attitudes and demand that this interaction is defined in the protocol; emotionalists recognize that interviews are inescapably encounters between subjects, while eliciting authentic accounts of subjective experience; constructionalists see the interview as a focused interaction with its own right, while dealing with how interview participants actively and mutually create meaning.

Frame of Reference for Interpretation

In interview studies, there is normally no frame of reference in the usual sense, but it is quite possible to interview a group of people about the same subject – for instance, before-and-after the introduction of an IT-based system – and thereby get a feeling of the development or change with regard to a specific question.

Perils and Pitfalls

See (Robson 2002) and Part III in this handbook.

The influence of the interviewer(s) is a common source of errors (Rosenthal 1976; Fowler and Mangione 1990). It is significant whether or not the interviewer is known to, and respected in, the organization, whether the interviewer holds respect for the organization and its needs for privacy and anonymity, and whether the interviewer has prior knowledge of the domain. It is significant whether there are one or more interviewers, as they may not necessarily get the same result. And it is significant whether you interview staff, middle management, or executive management, as the two latter groups are used to disregarding their own personal opinions in favor of the official politics and principles of the organization.

The way the questions are posed is important for the precision of the answers, as are the procedures under which the interviews are carried out (Fowler and Mangione 1990). Questions may be seen as being threatening (Vinten 1998) or touch on (culturally based) taboos.

A potential pitfall when digging into historical information is postrationalization, see Part III.

There is also a risk of a bias in quantitative studies if the user's ability to assess assumptions and correlations is challenged (see Part III).

Last but not least, it is important to realize that users in an organization find it extremely difficult to account for how they actually carry out their activities (see the discussions in Brender 1997a and 1999).

Advice and Comments

The level of difficulty in interview methods is often underestimated, and reliability as well as internal and external validity of the outcome is correlated to the experiences as interviewer. However, this should not deter from using interview methods, but one has to get to know the methods in depth before starting and put their quality aspect up against the objective of the study. This is certainly important if the result of the research is to be published in the scientific literature. However, there is a lot of easily accessible literature about the subject.

If there is a particular need to measure the validity of one's conclusions from an interview study, triangulation of the method or of specific observations can be made, as described in Part III.

References

Brender J. Methodology for assessment of medical IT-based systems – in an organisational context. Amsterdam: IOS Press, Stud Health

Technol Inform 1997;42.

Brender J. Methodology for constructive assessment of IT-based systems in an organisational context. Int J Med Inform 1999;56:67-86.
This is a shortened version of the previous reference, so it does not go into as much depth and is more accessible.

Fowler Jr FJ, Mangione TW. Standardized survey interviewing: minimizing interviewer-related error. Newbury Park: Sage Publications. Applied Social Research Methods Series 1990. vol. 18.
This book is indispensable for those who want to make an effective interview study. It describes all aspects of the method and discusses what can diminish the value (precision, accuracy) of the results and thereby the reliability of the study.

Robson C. Real world research, a resource for social scientists and practitioner-researchers. 2nd ed. Oxford: Blackwell Publishers Inc; 2002. p. 269-91.
This book gives a good description of different types of interviews, details, and ideas regarding their use including the advantages and disadvantages of each of them.

Rosenthal R. Experimenter effects in behavioral research, enlarged edition. New York: Irvington Publishers, Inc.; 1976.
This rather unsettling book reviews the impact of the experimenters on their test objects, including biosocial attributes, psychosocial factors, and situational factors (the context of the studies).

Silverman D. Interpreting qualitative data, methods for analysing talk, text and interaction. 2nd ed. London: Sage Publications; 2001.

Vinten G. Taking the threat out of threatening questions. J Roy Soc Health 1998;118(1):10-4.

Supplementary Reading
There are a number of similar descriptions of research methodologies for research within the social sciences including interview techniques. The advice they provide is as good as the advice provided by the above references.

Ericsson KA, Simon HA. Protocol analysis, verbal reports as data. Cambridge (MA): The MIT Press; 1984.
This book provides a thorough review of the literature on approaches and problems at the elicitation of information about

cognitive processes from verbal data.

Harrison MI. Diagnosing organizations: methods, models, and processes. 2nd ed. Thousand Oaks: Sage Publications. Applied Social Research Methods Series 1994. vol. 8.

> *The book is concerned with a number of aspects of an organization, from individuals to their internal relationships (as in power structures, etc.), and discusses advantages and disadvantages of different methods in this respect, including those of interviews. It describes a number of factors with regard to individuals as well as groups in an organization.*

Leavitt F. Research methods for behavioral scientists. Dubuque: Wm. C. Brown Publishers; 1991.

> *Contains quite concrete guidelines on how to formulate questions and put them together (also in respect of questionnaires) and how to avoid the worst pitfalls (see pages 162-172).*

http://jthom.best.vwh.net/usability,

> *This contains lots of summaries of methods and references, including some inspiration regarding interview studies (last visited 31.05.2005).*

KUBI

(From Danish: "**K**valitets**U**dvikling gennem **B**ruger**I**nddragelse";
translated: Quality Development Through User Involvement)

Areas of Application

The method is used as a tool for the incremental optimization of the
outcome of a longterm development project, based on a set of user
or customer/client defined value norms and objectives.

Description

The method originates in the social sector, where it was developed
as a constructive tool to improve conditions in the healthcare and
social sectors (Krogstrup 2003). It has many points in common with
the *Balanced Scorecard* method and is applied to assess the degree
of fulfillment and subsequently to balance and re-focus on areas for
improvement. However, the KUBI method has some quite different
success indicators as its driving force for development.

The procedure follows these steps:
1. Establishment of values and criteria for the primary stakeholder
   group(s) (such as a user, customer, or client)
2. Interview phase during which selected members of the primary
   stakeholder group(s) are trained and carry out individual and
   group interviews under supervision
3. Summation of the interview data into a report that includes an
   assessment of the degree of fulfillment of user criteria
4. Preparation of plans for the areas for improvement and
   development initiatives following a discussion of the report with
   the stakeholders
5. Follow-up of the new situation with the stakeholders after about
   a year, followed by a discussion of whether the development
   plans and initiatives need revision or expansion

Assumptions for Application

-

Perspectives

The intense focus on the user-stakeholder group is somewhat unusual in IT development and implementation processes because it belongs to another world with other traditions and focal points. Nevertheless, the method has been included as it may provide inspiration in general terms. For example, one could imagine that it could be used in a slightly modified form as a hearing tool for very large IT projects, such as assessment of a regional or national strategy or implementation of an EHR where the distance from project management to the user in the field can be quite great.

Frame of Reference for Interpretation

The frame of reference is the objectives established during the first phase of the procedure.

Perils and Pitfalls

-

Advice and Comments

-

References

Krogstrup HK. Evalueringsmodeller. Århus: Systime; 2003. (in Danish)
> *Even if this reference is in Danish, the above description should enable experienced evaluators to apply the method or apply it in their own version, with benefit.*

☺☺☺
§(§)
€

Logical Framework Approach

Areas of Application

- Situation analysis either in general and at any time within a project
- Support the choice of action prior to planning of the development effort
- Incorporating risk handling within project planning

Description

Logical Framework Approach (LFA) is an objectives-oriented planning methodology. The authors call it a framework, but it serves as a methodology because it describes the overall sequence of activities for the whole process, from the start of the project to the end, and the relationships between activities and guidelines of a methodical nature.

The methodology is designed to be used for reform projects in developing countries. This in itself gives it the advantage of being intended as an incredibly simple but effective planning and implementation tool.

The methodology consists of two parts (*Handbook for objectives-oriented planning* 1992): (1) a situation analysis to identify stakeholder groups and problems and weaknesses in the existing system and (2) project design. The first part can stand alone, while the latter presupposes the first.

The philosophy of the methodology is to focus on one central problem during a change management process. The core of the process lies in producing a 'Problem Tree' where the leaves are directly converted into a 'Tree of Objectives' through a description of objectives. This is then transformed and becomes a change management tool, such as traditional activity descriptions for a project.

A. Situation Analysis

1. Stakeholder analysis: Identification of groups and subgroups in order to identify participants for the future development project.

2. Problem analysis: By means of a brainstorming technique to capture elements and symptoms in the organization, which are subsequently synthesized into a 'Problem Tree' with the trunk being the central problem and the leaves the smallest symptoms. An analysis of the causality is used as the roots of the tree in such a way that all the branches and leaves are covered and thereby accounted for.

3. Objectives Analysis: The Problem Tree is converted into a tree of corresponding solutions, the 'Objectives Tree'.

4. Analysis of the alternatives with regard to choosing the best solution for the future and the establishment of a strategy.

B. Solution Design

5. Project Elements: Define the objectives for the development (justification of the project), the resulting immediate subobjectives (which together define and limit the intended effect), and then break them down into results, activities, and resources.

6. External Factors: Identification (for each and every activity) of important risk factors.

7. Indicators: Definition of the measures for monitoring the progress of each activity.

The above approach is primarily suited for simple projects. Crawford and Bryce (2003) review other and more complex versions of the LFA and summarize the key limitations of this method, which are concerned with handling the preconditions and assumptions for the implementation work (Phase B). However, in an evaluation context it is the approach of the Situation Analysis that is of primary interest.

Assumptions for Application

There is no real precondition with regard to the educational level of the participants, precisely because its intended use is in developing countries. A very simple version of the methodology can be used. However, depending on the accuracy and precision required, it may be necessary for the leader(s) of the process to have adequate experience of group dynamics and relevant methods to supplement specific information needs. It can *not* replace traditional system development methods but may be applied to identify areas that need focused efforts and as such it may serve as a means for constructive assessment.

The methodology assumes quite a stable project plan, as it does not have any inbuilt mechanisms, such as feed-back loops, for handling modifications. However, this does not preclude changes to a project plan but requires that all elements of the plan and its methods are explicitly dealt with or taken into consideration during a possible modification.

It is clearly a prerequisite that the supporting methods and techniques are properly identified and adapted to detailed subactivities in such a way that they harmonize with the entirety and with each other. Depending on the size of project concerned with the situation analysis only – a need for supporting methods or techniques, for instance – may arise, as may a need for supporting the causal analysis. Examples of useful methods in this respect are *Stakeholder Analysis* and *Focus Group Interviews,* for example.

Perspectives

In itself the methodology is neutral to political, organizational and cultural conditions or constraints, it neither dictates nor prohibits such constraints, and it can work under their conditions. In the description there are aspects that make it more suitable in certain cultures and types of organizations than in others (as, for instance, in the suggestion for choice of project participants where the chosen procedures, principles, and criteria are clearly culture dependent). However, there is nothing to stop the use of one's own principles.

The methodology is reasonably neutral toward the methods employed and contains a number of steps for the process. As a rule it is necessary to add concrete and formalized methods or instructions (at least for large projects). As such it does not replace the stakeholder analysis method, cost-benefit analysis, impact assessments, and so on, but it has openings and rudimentary instructions where activities are prescribed and other methods therefore may supplement.

The perspective of the Problem Tree is that of focusing on just one single problem as a starting point for development. In the case of large development projects, this can often be too simplified a point of view. However, this can be resolved through a simple modification of the problem analysis. For example: 'All of the problem areas of the organization' may be defined as the trunk of the Problem Tree, instead of picking just one of the largest branches as the trunk and then disregarding the rest (Brender 1997). This will of course make the investigation into the causality more extensive or difficult, but it will also make it far more rewarding.

Frame of Reference for Interpretation

Preparation of the Problem Tree (in the Situation Analysis) is relevant as an evaluation tool in connection with an assessment of IT-based systems. But the Problem Tree does not have its own frame of reference against which to compare the outcome. The validity of the synthesized Problem Tree might be discussed with the user organization whose opinions and attitudes become a frame of reference of sorts.

Perils and Pitfalls

When eliciting the Problem Tree, one must be aware of the following sources of error (see Part III):

1. Postrationalization (may partly be redressed by brainstorming techniques through the interaction and inspiration between the stakeholders)
2. Other error sources in connection with group dynamics, as for example under *Focus Group Interview*

Advice and Comments

The methodology's principle of risk monitoring is recommended in its own right, in terms of monitoring the external factors that are incorporated in the implementation plan as explicit variables. It may be advantageous to incorporate them into other methods and strategies for ongoing monitoring (evaluation) of development trends and risk factors.

The Affinity method may be used as an aid to brainstorming and modeling of the Problem Tree or alternatively one of the other similar methods outlined on http://jthom.best.vwh.net/usability/.

References

Handbook for objectives-oriented planning. 2nd ed. Oslo: Norwegian Agency for Development Cooperation; 1992.
> *If this is not available, there is a résumé of it in the next reference. Alternatively, the reader is referred to the review in (Crawford and Bryce 2003).*

Brender J. Methodology assessment of medical IT-based systems – in an organisational context. Amsterdam: IOS Press, Stud Health Technol Inform 1997;42.

Crawford P, Bryce P. Project monitoring and evaluation: a method for enhancing the efficiency and effectiveness of aid project implementation. Int J Proj Manag 2003;21(5):363-73.

http://jthom.best.vwh.net/usability/
  Contains lots of method overviews with links and references (last visited on 31.05.2005).

Organizational Readiness

Areas of Application

Assessment of a healthcare organization's readiness to assimilate a clinical information system.

Description

A number of aspects determine the organizational readiness for change, such as organizational adaptability and flexibility, its willingness to absorb external solutions, and its ability to develop viable solutions. A potential cause of failure to innovate is the organizational inability to undergo transformation during the implementation of an information system.

The study of Snyder-Halpern (2001) briefly reviews previous attempts at determining readiness and validates a model of innovation readiness and a set of heuristics to assess organizational readiness. The method is not yet complete and has still to include the metrics of the heuristics suggested. However, the description may still serve as valuable inspiration to preventive actions through assessment at the early stages of IT systems purchase or implementation.

Assumptions for Application

-

Perspectives

-

Frame of Reference for Interpretation

(Not applicable)

Perils and Pitfalls

-

Advice and Comments

-

References

Snyder-Halpern R. Indicators of organizational readiness for clinical information technology/systems innovation: a Delphi study. Int J Med Inform 2001;63(3):179-204. Erratum in: Int J Med Inform 2002;65(3):243.

Pardizipp

Areas of Application
Preparation of future scenarios

Description
Scenarios are common-language descriptions of specific activities and of how users would normally go about executing them. They can, however, also be described diagrammatically. Pardizipp is based on the *Delphi* method. Development of scenarios, which in Pardizipp are textual, follows the six steps listed below (steps 2-4 are to be repeated jointly) (Mettler and Baumgartner 1998):

1. Definition of a general frame that will serve as the basis for group work around the creation of scenarios
2. Creation of scenarios and a thorough analysis of their consequences and assumptions
3. Quantifying and model building
4. Preparation of policies and specific actions – where a given scenario should be implemented
5. Development of a consensus scenario, which takes into account earlier scenarios developed for the same problem area
6. Preparation of recommendations for policies and actual actions

Assumptions for Application
A prerequisite for a successful result is that a good mix of stakeholder groups are represented.

It is worth noting that a centrally placed team – not the participants involved – prepares the resulting scenario(s) on the basis of the information gathered. Thus, it requires a certain degree of experience of this type of undertaking. See also under *Delphi*.

Perspectives
The philosophy behind the method is twofold: It is partly based on the philosophy built into the *Delphi* method and partly on the fact that modern technological development has a number of unfortunate effects on surrounding social and organizational conditions. This

makes the authors focus on improving the basis of decision-making and related processes, which is done by establishing a decision-making foundation built on the projections and aspirations of a broad segment of participants. In other words, they believe that the basis for decision making will improve by expanding the group preparing it. This is obviously a culturally conditioned assumption, see the discussion in the Introduction, and it has its roots in Western cultural perceptions of how things should be handled and how best to structure an organization.

Frame of Reference for Interpretation
(Not applicable)

Perils and Pitfalls
1. The principle of using scenarios gives a fragmented picture of a normally holistic entirety. Therefore, it takes some talent to organize the preparation of a combination of scenarios in such a way that together they will give an adequately holistic impression.
2. People normally find it difficult to explicitly formulate their thought about their own work situation and work procedures explicitly (see the discussions in Brender 1997a and 1999 and others). This is where the *Delphi* method shows its strength, but it cannot completely compensate in all situations.
3. One pitfall is the ethnocentricity (see Part III) – that is, lack of acknowledgement and consideration of cultural backgrounds. This may introduce a bias in the selection of participants. The authors mention principles for participation (for instance, lack of female involvement) as a caveat, but in general the method is considered to be most appropriate in cultures where there is already a tradition for participatory methods and in organizations where there is a possibility of (informal) equality among participants of different levels of competence.

Advice and Comments
Future scenarios are useful tools for the understanding of development trends and options. Methods for preparing future scenarios often have the advantage of helping the participants to fantasize – irrespective of their technological understanding. This way the participants are often able to let go of actual constraints to the technological potentials and limitations induced by many systems analysis tools.

References

Brender J. Methodology for assessment of medical IT-based systems – in an organisational context. Amsterdam: IOS Press, Stud Health Technol Inform 1997;42.

Brender J. Methodology for constructive assessment of IT-based systems in an organisational context. Int J Med Inform 1999;56:67-86.
This is a shortened version of the first reference and more easily accessible with regard to this subject.

Mettler PH, Baumgartner T. Large-scale participatory co-shaping of technological developments, first experiments with Pardizipp. Futures 1998;30(6):535-54.

Prospective Time Series

Areas of Application

Measurement of a development trend, including, for example, the effect of an intervention:

- Time series
- Before-and-after studies, where the work involved could be the introduction of an IT-based system, for instance

Description

Measurement of a number of measures over time shows how an activity or an outcome changes as a function of either time alone or as a function of different initiatives. Such studies may be either simple or controlled, depending on the level of control of experimental factors. Simple before-and-after studies address a single case before and after an intervention, while the controlled approach matches a number of cases to be studied in parallel.

Assumptions for Application

The use of time series as one's assessment design requires control over what changes take place – intentional and unintentional – within the organization during the study.

Perspectives

Time series are in principle carried out as a matched-pair design, just like traditional, controlled studies including *RCT*s. Therefore, they contain the inbuilt assumption that there is no interaction between case-specific matching characteristics and a potential intervention (Suissa 1998). The problem occurs in particular when there is just one case in the study – the simple before-and-after study – which often happens in assessment of IT-based solutions. Implementation of IT-based solutions often involves radical changes in the organization, its structure, and work processes. Consequently, when there is only one case and the intervention is the introduction of an

---

[7] The same comment is valid regarding the economy as described for *Clinical/Diagnostic Performance*.

IT-based solution, an interaction between the case and the intervention will be present. Thus, the control group (the first measurement(s) in the time series) and the intervention group are no longer identical in all aspects other than that of the intervention applied. See also Sparrow and Thompson (1999).

Frame of Reference for Interpretation

The frame of reference is generally included in the overall design – for instance, as the first point within the time series.

Perils and Pitfalls

One question to keep in mind is: Do the measures keep representing exactly the same characteristics of the system or the organization? This needs to be verified for the data collected, and it is particularly important when a time series spans the implementation of an IT system – often over several years. Evans et al. (1998) apparently elegantly handle this error source. However, they do fall into the trap of giving the decision-support system the credit for the improvements without acknowledging that, simultaneously, drastic changes to work processes take place (over and above what is needed by the system functionality).

As always, one has to ascertain that the conditions for the use of ones metrics (calculation techniques) are fulfilled, and if one does performs statistical calculations on successive steps in a series of measures, it is a requirement for the use of concrete techniques that the measures are independent ('carryover effects' and 'conditional independence on the subject'). See details in (Suissa 1998).

In cohort studies with the follow-up of cases over time, biases may occur as a consequence of cases that drop out along the way (see Pennefather et al. 1999). In principle this corresponds to cases with missing data for the later points of the time series. This bias may be caused by lack of representativeness for the drop-out group compared to the study group as a whole. An important example is successive questionnaire studies. Another example is the representativeness of the users involved around the IT system. Therefore, in the final conclusion it is important to explain the causality in connection with these missing data.

Advice and Comments

-

References

Evans RS, Pestotnik SL, Classen DC, Clemmer TP, Weaver LK, Orme JF, Lloyd JF, Burke JP. A computer-assisted management program for antibiotics and other antiinfective agents. New Engl J Med 1998;338(4):232-8.

Pennefather PM, Tin W, Clarke MP, Fritz S, Hey EN. Bias due to incomplete follow-up in a cohort study. Br J Ophthalmol 1999;83:643-5.

Sparrow JM, Thompson JR. Bias: adding to the uncertainty, editorial. Br J Ophthalmol 1999;83:637-8.

Suissa S. The case-time-control-design: further assumptions and conditions. Epidemiol 1998;9(4):441-5.

Supplementary Reading

Ammenwerth E, Kutscha A, Eichstädter R, Haux R. Systematic evaluation of computer-based nursing documentation. In: Patel V, Roger R, Haux R, editors. Proceedings of the 10th World Congress on Medical Informatics; 2001 Sep; London, UK. Amsterdam: IOS Press; 2001. p. 1102-6.

> *A good before-and-after case study of the quality of nursing documentation records and user satisfaction based on a combination of many methods (a multimethod design).*

Bates DW, Teich JM, Lee J, Seger D, Kuperman GJ, Ma'Luf N, Boyle D, Leape L. The impact of computerized physician order entry on medication error prevention. JAMIA 1999;6(4):313-21.

> *A case study using prospective time studies to assess the impact of the introduction of an IT-based solution on a concrete activity.*

Brown SH, Coney RD. Changes in physicians' computer anxiety and attitudes related to clinical information system use. JAMIA 1994;1(5):381-94.

> *In a case study the authors investigate physicians' fear of new IT technology in a before-and-after study.*

Kelly JR, McGrath JE. On time and method. Newbury Park: Sage Publications. Applied Social Research Methods Series 1988. vol. 13.

> *The book thoroughly and stringently (and with a philosophical background) discusses a number of aspects concerning time and the influence of time on experimental studies. Further, beyond the*

problems and pitfalls of time studies, it discusses, for instance, changes in the observer and problems at causal analysis of phenomena of a cyclic nature.

Murphy CA, Maynard M, Morgan G. Pretest and post-test attitudes of nursing personnel toward a patient care information system. Comput Nurs 1994;12:239-44.

A very good case study with questionnaires in a before-and-after study. Recommended for studying because they make a real effort to verify the internal validity of the elements in the questionnaire.

Ruland CM, Ravn IH. An information system to improve financial management resource allocation and activity planning: evaluation results. In: Patel V, Roger R, Haux R, editors. Proceedings of the 10th World Congress on Medical Informatics; 2001 Sep; London, UK. Amsterdam: IOS Press; 2001. p. 1203-6.

A before-and-after study of a decision-support system for nurses with the primary focus on investigating financial aspects (which in this case corresponds to evaluation of the objectives fulfillment) and user satisfaction. But, unfortunately, the study suffers (possibly) from a number of biases, typical of controlled studies (see Part III of this handbook).

Wyatt JC, Wyatt SM. When and how to evaluate health information systems? Int J Med Inform 2003;69:251-9.

Outlines the differences between the simple before-and-after and the controlled before-and-after studies as opposed to the RCTs.

Yamaguchi K. Event history analysis. Newbury Park: Sage Publications. Applied Social Research Methods Series 1991. vol. 28.

A book for those who want to conduct studies over time in an organization.

Questionnaire

(Nonstandardized questionnaires)

Areas of Application

Imagination is the only real limit to what questionnaires can, and have, been used for, but for investigations requiring a high level of accuracy their main area of application is (qualitative) studies of subjective aspects.

Note: *There is a sharp distinction between custom-made questionnaires and standardized, validated questionnaires, available from the literature or as commercial tools. The section below deals with the former. However, even if a standard questionnaire is chosen, one must still investigate the degree to which the assumptions and pitfalls and the quality meets one's needs.*

Description

The advantage of questionnaires – and probably the reason why they are so widely used – is that most people can manage to put a questionnaire together to investigate virtually any subject of one's choice.

There are a number of ways in which to ask questions, and they do not necessarily eliminate each other. However, by using a combination of them there is a risk of making the analysis (the mathematical and statistical analysis) more difficult:

- Open questions, where the respondent answers (the individual questions) the questionnaire in ordinary text
- Checklist questions, which normally consist of three boxes: "Yes", "no", and "don't know"
- The Likert scale consisting of a bar with fields to tick on a scale from "agree completely", "agree", through a neutral to "disagree" and "completely disagree"
- Multipoint scale, where the respondent indicates his or her assessment on a continuous scale indicating the two extremes with opposing rankings "agree completely" to "completely disagree"
- Semantic differential scale, which in tabular form uses columns with a value scale (for instance, "extremely", "very",

"somewhat", "neutral", "a little", "somewhat", "very", "extremely") and where the rows of the table indicate the properties that should be evaluated by means of the two extremes on the scale (for example, "easy" . . . "difficult" . . . "fun" . . . "boring"), and so on.

- Categorical scale, where the tick options (which may mutually preclude each other) are completely separated – for example, questions about sex, age, or profession.

Note: *No specific questionnaires are indicated here, as they are normally formulated for each specific case, but in the literature there are a number of more or less 'standardized' questionnaires for measuring user satisfaction, which can be used as they are or with some adaptations. These are indicated below under References.*

Assumptions for Application

Questionnaires are tools, and tools need verification with respect to construct and content validity before application. It is important that questionnaires – and all elements in them – have been tested (validated) to increase the likelihood that the questionnaire will serve its purpose as it is supposed to. It is very important that questionnaire studies are of a suitably high standard qualitatively. This concerns the preparation establishing objectives for the studies, accurate wording of hypothesizes and theories, qualitatively satisfactory questionnaires (which is probably the most difficult), clearly formulated rules of analysis, and requirements for reporting (opportunities and limitations) of the results.

Further, it is obvious that there must be a reasonable relationship between the resources required to prepare the questionnaire and the purpose of the study. Far from all studies need thorough scientific validation of the questionnaire in order to provide results leading to optimal action.

The use of concrete statistical tools normally implies assumptions, and one of the assumptions for the use of standard deviations and student's t-test is that the data come from a continuous scale (a scale with real numbers). Consequently, these statistical methods *cannot* be used for the analysis of data obtained on a categorical scale such as the Likert scale(!) but may be used for a multipoint scale, for instance.

Perspectives

The perspective of the person formulating the questionnaire depends very much on his or her level of experience. The inexperienced seem to think that it is easy to write a questionnaire and that this will produce answers and provide the truth about the questions asked. This rather naive understanding is based on the fact that we are all used to formulating lots of questions and to getting sensible answers every day. The difference is, however, that when we formulate everyday questions between us, these questions form part of a joint context in relation to the present and possibly also to a mutual past, which explains a lot about the background and what it refers to, implicitly and explicitly. If you don't get the right answer the first time around during the conversation, you repeat it once or twice without thinking about it. This type of reiteration cannot take place in questionnaires, and the creation of a mutual understanding is exactly what makes the formulation of a valid questionnaire so difficult.

Frame of Reference for Interpretation

The frame of reference depends on the purpose of the study. One may formulate before-and-after questionnaires, where the response to the first questionnaire becomes the frame of reference for the second one. A strategic objective could also be a frame of reference in a particular study. Furthermore, earlier studies from the organization, for instance, or studies described in the literature may also be used as a basis for comparison.

However, usually there is no frame of reference for the analysis or the conclusion of a questionnaire study.

Perils and Pitfalls

There is a whole range of pitfalls in questionnaires, such as the following:

- The internal validity of the questions: Does the respondent read/understand the same as the author? Do all the respondents read/understand exactly the same thing?
- The problem of postrationalization (see Part III) is a risk in studies using questionnaires presented sometime after the events addressed (Kushniruk and Patel 2004).
- Each respondent will always answer the questionnaire in his or her own context including emotional factors and the actual response will therefore vary from one day to the next.
- For psychological reasons people have problems assessing

probabilities correctly. Therefore, questions such as "how often . . .?" should be avoided.

- Certain questions may be taboos, or they may be perceived as threatening – particularly in the case of nonanonymous studies (Vinten 1998).
- When using a questionnaire from foreign literature, be aware that it needs adapting in case of national, organizational, linguistic, or cultural differences. It is not valid per se to apply a questionnaire in a foreign language, and it is not easy to translate a questionnaire while preserving the meaning, in case one wants to make a multinational survey.
- It is rare that the target group of a questionnaire study is so well grounded in a foreign language that one can expect a reliable answer should the questionnaire be used in its original language.
- Do not underestimate the pitfall that may be introduced when translating a questionnaire from one language (and culture) to another. This is by no means insignificant.
- It makes a difference who in the organization is being interviewed, because top and middle management have more training in promoting the official line at the expense of their own personal opinion without even thinking about it. The same is the case in certain cultures, such as in Asia and in the former Soviet republics. The fact that these cultures belong to countries a great distance away from your own does not automatically preclude that these same attitudes and manners exist in your country or in the subculture of your society – because they do.

Although there are many pitfalls and difficulties, one should not give up because it *is* to allay the problems. Depending on the intended use of the study result and how accurate it needs to be, the list above illustrates that the task of formulating a questionnaires often is one to be carried out by people with this expertise.

Advice and Comments
Do look for guidelines to qualitative evaluation studies, as they give lots of tangible advice on the wording of questionnaires and examples of these.

References like (Ives et al. 1983; Murphy et al. 1994; Jacoby et al. 1999; and Paré and Sicotte 2001) are examples of how to verify and adapt a questionnaire for, for instance, reliability, predictive validity, accuracy, content validity, and internal validity.

References

Ives B, Olson MH, Baroudi JJ. The measurement of user information satisfaction. Communications of the ACM 1983;26(19):785-93.

> *Brilliant little article with advice and guidelines regarding the measurement and adaptation of different quality measures for a questionnaire.*

Jacoby A, Lecouturier J, Bradshaw C, Lovel T, Eccles M. Feasibility of using postal questionnaires to examine career satisfaction with palliative care: a methodological assessment. Palliat Med 1999;13:285-98.

Kushniruk AW, Patel VL. Cognitive and usability engineering methods for the evaluation of clinical information systems. J Biomed Inform 2004;37:56-76.

Murphy CA, Maynard M, Morgan G. Pretest and post-test attitudes of nursing personnel toward a patient care information system. Comput Nurs 1994;12:239-44.

> *Recommended for studying, precisely because it makes a real effort to verify the internal validity of the elements of the questionnaire and explains how one can use questionnaires in a before-and-after study.*

Paré G, Sicotte C. Information technology sophistication in health care: an instrument validation study among Canadian hospitals. Int J Med Inform 2001;63:205-23.

Vinten G. Taking the threat out of threatening questions. J Roy Soc Health 1998;118(1):10-4.

References to Standard Questionnaires

Aydin CE. Survey methods for assessing social impacts of computers in health care organizations. In: Anderson JG, Aydin CE, Jay SJ, editors. Evaluating health care information systems, methods and applications. Thousand Oaks: Sage Publications, 1994, pp. 69-115.

> *The chapter refers to a number of questionnaires used in the literature and contains a couple of actual examples in the Appendix.*

Harrison MI. Diagnosing organizations: methods, models, and processes. 2nd ed. Thousand Oaks: Sage Publications. Applied Social

Research Methods Series 1994. vol. 8.

Appendix B of the book contains a number of references to standard questionnaires for (nearly) every purpose regarding conditions in an organization.

Supplementary Reading, Including Case Studies

Ammenwerth E, Kaiser F, Buerkly T, Gräber S, Herrmann G, Wilhelmy I. Evaluation of user acceptance of data management systems in hospitals – feasibility and usability. In: Brown A, Remenyi D, editors. Ninth European Conference on Information Technology Evaluation; 2002 Jul; Paris, France. Reading: MCIL; 2002:31-38. ISBN 0-9540488-5-7.

This reference and the next deal with the same case study, but at different phases of the assessment.

Ammenwerth E, Kaiser F, Wilhelmy I, Höfer S. Evaluation of user acceptance of information systems in health care – the value of questionnaires. In: Baud R, Fieschi M, Le Beux P, Ruch P, editors. The new navigators: from professionals to patients. Proceedings of MIE2003; 2003 May; St. Malo, France. Amsterdam: IOS Press. Stud Health Technol Inform 2003;95:643-8.

A case study of user satisfaction, which also assesses the quality aspects (reliability and validity) of the questionnaire used.

Andersen I, Enderud H. Udformning og brug af spørgeskemaer og interviewguides. In: Andersen I (Ed.). Valg af organisations-sociologiske metoder – et kombinationsperspektiv. Copenhagen: Samfundslitteratur; 1990. p. 261-81. (in Danish)

This reference contains some advice on how (not) to do things.

Bowman GS, Thompson DR, Sutton TW. Nurses' attitudes towards the nursing process. J Adv Nurs 1983; 8(2):125-9.

Concerns (measurement of) user attitudes to the nursing process.

Chin JP. Development of a tool measuring user satisfaction of the human-computer interface. In: Proceedings of the Chi'88 Conf. on Human factors in Computing. New York: Association for Computing Machinery; 1988. p. 213-8.

Addresses user attitudes toward specific characteristics of nursing documentation.

Hicks LL, Hudson ST, Koening S, Madsen R, Kling B, Tracy J, Mitchell J, Webb W. An evaluation of satisfaction with telemedicine among health-care professionals. J Telemed Telecare 2000;6:209-15.

A user satisfaction case study.

Leavitt F. Research methods for behavioral scientists. Dubuque: Wm. C. Brown Publishers. 1991.

Contains quite tangible instructions on how to formulate and put questions together (also for interviews) and avoids the worst pitfalls, see pages 162-72.

Lowry CH. Nurses' attitudes toward computerised care plans in intensive care. Part 2. Nurs Crit Care 1994; 10:2-11.

Deals with attitudes toward the use of computers in nursing, particularly in connections with documentation.

Lærum H. Evaluation of electronic medical records, a clinical perspective [Doctoral dissertation]. Faculty of Medicine, Norwegian University of Science and Technology, Trondheim: NTNU; 2004. Report No.: 237. ISBN-82-471-6280-6.

This doctoral dissertation is a multimethod evaluation study, including an extensively validated questionnaire.

Murff HJ, Kannry J. Physician satisfaction with two order entry systems. J Am Med Inform Assoc 2001;8:499-509.

A very well-planned case study when it comes to the comparison of two systems, as the users are the same for both systems. They also seem to have the statistics under control.

Nickell GS, Pinto JN. The computer attitude scale. Comput Human Behav 1986;2:301-6.

Deals with user attitudes toward computers in general (for everyday use).

Ruland CM. A survey about the usefulness of computerized systems to support illness management in clinical practice. Int J Med Inform 2004;73:797-805.

A case study applying a questionnaire to survey clinical usefulness.

Rådgivende Sociologer. Manual om spørgeskemaer for Hovedstadens Sygehusfællesskab.Rådgivende Sociologer; 2001. Report No.: manual om spørgeskemaer for H:S. (Available from: www.mtve.dk under 'publications'. Last visited 31.05.2005.) (in Danish)

This is a very useful reference for formulating a questionnaire study. It contains both instructions and actual finished questionnaires for different purposes within the healthcare sector.

Shubart JR, Einbinder JS. Evaluation of a data warehouse in an academic health sciences center. Int J Med Inform 2000;60:319-33.

Is a structured, hypothesis driven case study with verification and validation of the questionnaire and explicit validation of the results.

Sleutel M, Guinn M. As good as it gets? going online with a clinical information system. Comput Nurs 1999;17(4):181-5.

A good case study to learn from because they are aware of an analysis of the internal validity of the questionnaire and because they dig down and investigate unexpected observations. However, the drawback is that they do not mention the formal requirements for the use of their statistical tools.

Terazzi A, Giordano A, Minuco G. How can usability measurement affect the re-engineering process of clinical software procedures? Int J Med Inform 1998;52:229-34.

Addresses 'perceived usability' –that is, the user's subjective understanding of usability, using standard questionnaires for this purpose.

Weir R, Stewart L, Browne G, Roberts J, Gafni A, Easton S, Seymour L. The efficacy and effectiveness of process consultation in improving staff morale and absenteeism. Med Care 1997;35(4):334-53.

A well-executed case study applying the RCT method based on existing, validated questionnaires covering subjects such as job satisfaction, attitudes, and personalities. Unfortunately, they have problems with the differences in the intervention between the two groups compared.

See also:

http://jthom.best.vwh.net/usability

Contains lots of method overviews with links and references (last visited 31.05.2005).

Goldfield GS, Epstein LH, Davidson M, Saad F. Validation of a questionnaire measure of the relative reinforcing value of food. Eat Behav 2005;6:283-92.

The advantage of this reference is the suggestions for statistical analysis methods taking into account the nature of the investigation data.

McLinden DJ, Jinkerson DL. Picture this! multivariate analysis in

organisational development. Evaluation Program Planning
1994;17(1):19-24.

> *This little article can be inspirational in how to treat and present
> data in a different way.*

http://qpool.umit.at

> *This website is still under construction, but it will eventually
> include a list of more or less validated questionnaires from the
> literature (last visited 31.05.2005).*

RCT, Randomized Controlled Trial

☺

§§§

€€€

Areas of Application

The purpose of this type of study is verification of efficacy[8] (Wall 1991; Goodman 1992) – that is, that the IT system – under ideal conditions – makes a difference to patient care.

RCT is used to identify marginal differences between two or more types of treatment. This method has been particular useful in assessment studies of IT-based solutions for decision-support systems and expert systems, only to a limited degree for other types of systems.

Description

Randomization is used to avoid bias in allocation or choice of cases and actors. In clinical studies randomization is used in relation to selection of clinical personnel or patient treatment groups, respectively, while in the assessment of IT-based solutions, for instance, it may be used to select study organization(s) or users.

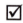

The concept 'controlled' is used in relation to studies with a minimum of two groups, one of which is a reference group (control group, treated in the traditional way). The control group is used for comparison of whether there is an effect on the intervention group – that is, as the frame of reference. The principle being that the control group and the intervention group are treated in exactly the same way (except for the intervention), thereby making it possible to measure differences in the effect of the intervention. The problem with RCT for IT-based solutions is to secure and achieve identical treatments between the two or more groups.

Assumptions for Application

Use of RCT in medicine is fairly standard, and the method is therefore known to many. However, it is not possible to transpose the method directly to assessment of IT-based solutions, as it is by no means trivial to handle the assumptions on randomization and to

---

[8] "'[E]fficacy' addresses the performance of the application under ideal circumstances, while 'effectiveness' is related to application under real circumstances (the capability of bringing about the result intended – i.e., doing the right things); and 'efficiency' is related to a measure of the capability of doing the things right." (from Brender 1997a)

obtain comparable groups. One of the challenges is to identify criteria to select the study objects and thereby the population (cases, users, and patients) with consideration to the size of the population and the generalization of a later conclusion. See below regarding the many pitfalls.

Perspectives

RCT is widely used for testing clinical procedures and pharmaceutical products. One argument in favor of RCT is that this procedure is so well established that a number of biases can be avoided. It is a characteristic of medical and pharmaceutical tests that the effect is often marginal in comparison to existing pharmaceuticals and procedures. Thus, it is necessary to be extremely careful about as many types of bias as possible in order to document that the new product makes a difference at all. This is not necessarily the case with similar studies of IT systems. Neither is it a forgone conclusion that such a study would conclude to the IT system's advantage if impact parameters were viewed unilaterally. The reward might be found in quite a different place that is not addressed by an RCT – for example, in the soft human aspects of the system, in the system's feasibility to support change management in the organization, or, in the longer term, to other profession-oriented or management aspects of the system.

RCT is carried out under ideal conditions, and it is focus driven. But who is to say that day-to-day reality is ideal?

Some people promote the viewpoint that RCT can be carried out very cheaply because the existing infrastructure, service function, and resources of a hospital or a department can be used free of charge and therefore only needs compensation for extraordinary expenses such as analysis of statistics. No doubt, this is feasible in many cases today. In principle this is also the case for RCT of IT-based systems, but it is naive to believe that real life is that simple.

Frame of Reference for Interpretation

It is possible to carry out controlled studies in several different ways, as, for instance, (1) by some patients being treated under the old system and others under the new system, or equally with regard to staff; (2) by some departments keeping the old system and other department getting the new system; or (3) by comparing similar departments in different hospitals.

Perils and Pitfalls

Quite the biggest problem is to make the groups being compared truly comparable. This includes having the groups go through the same conditions and circumstances during the process so that only relevant factors influence the outcome of the study.

Randomization depends on the feasibility of a real choice between participants to ensure that the resulting groups are comparable. It is of course possible to make a draw between two departments to find the one that gets an EHR implemented and the one that will not – in other words, which is the intervention group and which is the control group, although this in itself does not render the control group and the intervention group comparable (see the review in Part III).

- Matching control and intervention groups. It is not always enough just to have comparable cases, as in different but comparable medical departments and comparing two departments with six physicians each, for instance. For certain systems, such as EHR and decision-support systems, the categories of physicians the group is made up of makes a difference because they have different backgrounds and levels of competence, medically and in terms of IT experience.

- One must be cautious when comparing groups from different medical specialist areas. This is the case not only during planning, but also in the interpretation (or worse, in extrapolation) of the result with the purpose of later putting it into wide practical use.

- Inclusion and exclusion criteria for involving cases and users as well as patients will normally cause the conclusion to be valid for a (well-defined) fraction of the daily practice in the department or clinic.

- A demand for an RCT study will normally be to undertake comparable treatment of both groups throughout the study. For IT systems this may be achieved by carrying out the phases of requirements specification, design, and implementation – that is, the Explorative Phase and the Technical Development Phase, on both the intervention group and the control group with a delayed start in one of the departments. This way you may obtain a measure of the effect on the intervention group. However, one must still be careful and avoid other biases, such as the Hawthorne effect, for example.

Advice and Comments

It is sometimes feasible to use the balanced block design when the IT-based system includes a number of parallel applications (such as knowledge-based support for a number of medical problems). The application will then be divided in to smaller clusters, each containing a proportion of the medical problems covered by the system. Each participant is assigned to one of the clusters, while serving as a control group for the other clusters and vice versa. See this approach in (Bindels et al. 2004), for instance.

There are a number of initiatives and advocates for RCT to be used as the sole usable method for documenting the justification of a given IT system. But there are also well-argued debates, as, for instance, in (Heathfield 1998). The authors discuss the problems of using RCT for IT-based solutions and do not at all agree with those who promote the use of RCT to assess IT-based systems and solutions in the healthcare sector.

The personal view of the author is that every method should be used in the situation to which it is suited. However, in the absence of more suitable methods, or if none can be applied to the objective, one may have to compromise. This is rarely in RCT's favor in case of IT systems.

Campbell et al. (2000) give advice and guidelines on the handling of RCT studies of complex interventions. It might be of some assistance to those who may be considering an RCT for IT-based systems.

References

Bindels R, Hasman A, van Wersch LWJ, Talmon J, Winkens RAG. Evaluation of an automated test ordering and feed-back system for general practitioners in daily practice. Int J Med Inform 2004;73:705-12.

Campbell M, Fitzpatrick R, Haines A, Kinmonth AL, Sandercock P, Spiegelhalter D, Tyrer P. Framework for design and evaluation of complex interventions to improve health. BMJ 2000;321:694-6.

Goodman C. It's time to rethink health care technology assessment. Int J Technol Assess Health Care 1992;8:335-58.

Heathfield H, Pitty D, Hanka R. Evaluating information technology in health care: barriers and challenges. BMJ 1998;316:1959-61.

Wall R. Computer Rx: more harm than good? J Med Syst 1991;15:321-34.

Supplementary Inspiration and Critical Opinions in the Literature, Including a Couple of Case Studies

Altman DG, Schultz KF, Moher D, Egger M, Davidoff F, Elbourne D, Gøtzsche PC, Lang T. The revised CONSORT statement for reporting randomized trials. Ann Intern Med 2001;134(8):663-94.

> *This reference is a 'must' before getting started with putting anything about an RCT study in writing, and therefore it can also serve as an inspiration during planning of such a study.*

Ammenwerth E, Eichstädter R, Haux R, Pohl U, Rebel S, Ziegler S. A randomized evaluation of a computer-based nursing documentation system. Methods Inf Med 2001;40:61-8.

> *The authors have chosen a design using a carryover effect between the study group and the control group to get a good frame of reference for the comparison See also the discussion in Part III, Section 11.1.6.5.*

Assman SF, Pocock SJ, Enos LE, Kasten LE. Subgroup analysis and other (mis)uses of baseline data in clinical trials. Lancet 2000;355:1064-9.

Biermann E, Dietrich W, Rihl J, Standl E. Are there time and cost savings by using telemanagement for patients on intensified insulin therapy? a randomized, controlled trial. Comput Methods Programs Biomed 2002;69:137-46.

> *This case illustrates how difficult it is to design a study to obtain truly comparable groups – one with, the other without, IT support. Without comparable procedures for the control group and the study group it is not possible to express what causes the potential (lack of) effect. At the same time the article shows how difficult it is to unambiguously describe similarities and differences in the procedures of the two groups.*

Brookes ST, Whitney E, Peters TJ, Mulheran PA, Egger M, Davey Smith G. Subgroup analyses in randomized controlled trials; quantifying the risks of false-positives and false-negatives. Health Technol Assess 2001;5(33).

> *Analyzes and discusses pitfalls in subgroup analysis when using RCT.*

Chuang J-H, Hripcsak G, Jenders RA. Considering clustering: a methodological review of clinical decision support system studies. Proc Annu Symp Comput Appl Med Care. 2000:146-50.

Review of RCT studies for decision-support systems and expert systems.

Friedman CP, Wyatt JC. Evaluation methods in medical informatics. New York: Springer-Verlag; 1996.

A good book that also discusses the role of different approaches to evaluation.

Gluud LL. Bias in intervention research, methodological studies of systematic errors in randomized trial and observational studies [Doctoral dissertation]. Faculty of Health Sciences, University of Copenhagen; 2005. (ISBN 87-990924-0-9)

A valuable discussion of different types of biases and their implication in RCTs and other intervention approaches.

Hetlevik I, Holmen J, Krüger Ø, Kristensen P, Iversen H, Furuseth K. Implementing clinical guidelines in the treatment of diabetes mellitus in general practice; evaluation of effort, process, and patient outcome related to implementation of a computer-based decision support system. Int J Technol Assess Health Care 2000;16(1):210-27.

A thorough case study, randomizing the practices involved, but note that with their procedure the control group remains completely untreated, while along the way, the intervention group gets an IT system, training, and follow-up in several different ways. In other words, it is not just the impact of the decision-support system that is measured.

Kuperman GJ, Teich JM, Tanasjevic MJ, Ma'luf N, Rittenberg E, Jha A, Fiskio J, Winkelman J, Bates DW. Improving response to critical laboratory results with automation: results of a randomised controlled trial. JAMIA 1999;6(6):512-22.

The same team and just as good a study as in (Shojania et al. 1998), but in this study the authors do not have the same co-intervention problem.

Marcelo A, Fontelo P, Farolan M, Cualing H. Effect of image compression on telepathology, a randomized clinical trial. In: Haux R, Kulikowski C, editors. Yearbook of Medical Informatics 2002:410-3.

A double-blind RCT case study.

Rotman BL, Sullivan AN, McDonald T, Brown BW, DeSmedt P, Goodnature D, Higgins M, Suermondt HJ, Young YC, Owens DK. A randomized evaluation of a computer-based physician's workstation: design considerations and baseline results. In: Gardner RM, editor. Proc

Ann Symp Comput Appl Med Care 1995:693-7.
(See under the next reference.)

Rotman BL, Sullivan AN, McDonald TW, Brown BW, DeSmedt P, Goodnature D, Higgins MC, Suermondt HJ, Young C, Owens DK. A randomized controlled trial of a computer-based physician workstation in an outpatient setting: implementation barriers to outcome evaluation. JAMIA 1996;3:340-8.

> *An RCT combined with a before-and-after design to measure user satisfaction and costs of medication as well as compliance to the recommendations concerning drug substitution. The two studies referenced from this group show the design considerations and the execution of an RCT, respectively.*

See Tai S, Nazareth I, Donegan C, Haines A. Evaluation of general practice computer templates, lessons from a pilot randomized controlled trial. Methods Inf Med 1999;38:177-81.

> *The study uses an elegant way to handle control group problems. See also the discussion in Part III, Section 11.1.6.1.*

Shea S, DuMouchel W, Bahamonde L. A meta-analysis of 16 randomized controlled trial to evaluate computer-based clinical reminder systems for preventive care in the ambulatory setting. JAMIA 1996;3(6):399-409.

> *The article contains a meta-analysis of RCT, and thus it can also be used to identify a number of case studies for inspiration.*

Shojania KG, Yokoe D, Platt R, Fiskio J, Ma'luf N, Bates DW. Reducing Vancomycin use utilizing a computer guideline: results of a randomized controlled trial. JAMIA 1998;5(6):554-62.

> *Shows a well-executed RCT case study despite having a problem with co-intervention (see Part III, Section 11.1.6.3).*

Tierney WM, Miller ME, Overhage JM, McDonald CJ. Physician inpatient order writing on microcomputer workstations. JAMA 1993;269:379-83 (reprinted in: Yearbook of Medical Informatics 1994;1994:208-12).

> *A thorough case study, but with the usual problem of making the control group and the intervention group comparable.*

Weir R, Stewart L, Browne G, Roberts J, Gafni A, Easton S, Seymour L. The efficacy and effectiveness of process consultation in improving staff morale and absenteeism. Med Care 1997;35(4):334-53.

> *Another well-executed RCT case study with existing, validated questionnaires. But this also has problems with differences between the two groups.*

van Wijk MAM, van der Lei J, Mosseveld M, Bohnen AM, van Bemmel JH. Assessment of decision support for blood test ordering in primary care, a randomized trial. Ann Intern Med 2001;134:274-81.

A case study.

Wyatt JC, Wyatt SM. When and how to evaluate health information systems? Int J Med Inform 2003;69:251-9.

Outlines the differences between the simple before-and-after and the controlled before-and-after studies as opposed to the RCTs.

Requirements Assessment

$§(§)$

$€$

Areas of Application

Within the European culture the User Requirements Specification forms the basis for the choice and purchase of an IT-based solution or for entering into a development project. Consequently, the User Requirements Specification is a highly significant legal document, which needs thorough assessment.

Description

When assessing a requirements specification, it is important that it includes a description of (see Brender 1997a and 1999):

1. The user organization's needs
2. The conditions under which the organization functions (including its mandate, limitations, and organizational culture)
3. The strategic objective of the organization
4. The value norms of future organizational development
5. Whether the functionality can be made to adapt to the work procedures in the organization or the reverse

Furthermore, there are some overriding general issues of importance:

- *Relevance*: Assessment of whether the solution in question or a combination of solutions is at all able to solve the current problems and meet the demands and requirements of the organization.
- *Problem Areas*: Where are the weaknesses and the elements of risk in the model solution? For instance, an off-the-shelf product may have to be chosen because the old IT system is so unreliable that it is not possible to wait for a development project to be carried out. Or plans may be based on a given operational situation albeit a lack of know-how would occur should certain employees give notice.
- *Feasibility*: Does the organization have the resources needed to implement the chosen solution (structurally in the organization, in terms of competence and financially, for example), as well as the support of management, staff, and politicians?
- *Completeness and Consistency*: Is the solution a coherent entity that is neither over- nor undersized?
- *Verifiability (or Testability)*: One must consider how to check

that every small requirement and function in the model solution have been fulfilled once the complete system is implemented and ready to be put to use.

- *Elements of Risk*: Are there any external conditions outside organizational control that will involve a substantial risk to the project should it/they occur? This could, for instance, be dependence on a technology that is not yet fully developed, or dependence on (establishment or functional level of) of the parent organization's technical or organizational infrastructure that has to fall into place first, or dependence on coordination and integration with other projects. See also *Risk Assessment.*

There are at least as many ways in which to assess a requirements specification as there are methods to produce it, and its flexibility is nearly as broad as its formalism is limited. Formal methods of formulating requirements specifications are primarily the ones that have the formal methods of verification. Apart from that, assessment of a requirements specification is usually carried out informally but covering the aspects mentioned above.

A couple of formal methods are:

1. Formal specification methods have their own tools to formulate the requirements specification, often IT-based, and they have their own verification techniques, such as consistency control. These methods are mainly used to specify technical systems and are only occasionally suited for application by the users themselves.
2. Prototyping methods are based on repeated assessment workshops with user scenarios from real life; see, for example, the study in (Nowlan 1994). The scenarios are tested on a prototype, which gradually evolves from one workshop to the next (spiral development).

Instead, a number of standards contain recommendations on how to prepare a requirements specification and what it should include as a minimum as well as what should be taken into consideration. These standards are therefore valuable sources of inspiration or checklists to assess a requirements specification. See under *Standards.*

Assumptions for Application

Assessment methods for requirements specifications depend entirely on the method used to prepare the specification.

Perspectives

It is necessary to be quite clear about where in the organization the most serious problems occur (1) because you cannot solve a problem simply by introducing a new IT system, and (2) such weaknesses can be quite disastrous for the implementation work or for achieving the intended benefit.

It is the author's opinion that (1) ordinary users in the healthcare sector do not normally have a background enabling them to use the formal methods to produce a requirements specification, because they cannot separate the details from the entirety and the entirety from the details, and neither do they have experience of formulating the complexity. (2) It is not always enough to have IT consultants to assist in this particular task, and, therefore, (3) the users should apply their own premises and express themselves in their own language (Brender 1989). The case analyzed dealt with the development of the first large IT-based solution for the organization. The longer an organization has had IT, the better able it will be to participate on technological premises – that is, use slightly more formal methods to formulate requirements specifications because its existing IT solution can be used as a kind of checklist.

Frame of Reference for Interpretation

The frame of reference for assessing a requirements specification is the whole of the organization (structure, technology, actors, work procedures, . . .), and its needs and premises, including conditions and objectives for acquiring an IT-based solution.

Perils and Pitfalls

The pitfalls for assessing requirements specifications, which have been developed incrementally as a prototype (see under number 2 above), are used to illustrate where things may go wrong, such as:

- Representativeness of real operational details. Are all the exceptions included, or can they be dispensed with? If you work with prototyping, you risk that a number of details are not included until the end.
- Representativeness of real operational variations. The way the organization has prescribed rules and procedures are different from how they are carried out in daily practice – during the process of formulating the requirements specification the users run the risk, subconsciously, of switching between the prescribed procedures and the actual ones.

- Representativeness of the context of operations. There are differences between how an activity is carried out when you have peace and quiet and nothing else to do and, for instance, when in clinical practice your activities are constantly being interrupted, and you are forced to leave a problem and return to it at a later stage. This and similar domain circumstances need to be taken into consideration in a requirements specification.
- Representativeness of all the stakeholder groups that are actually involved in the assessment activities. This is particularly difficult (or rather costly) in an organization with a high degree of specialization.

Advice and Comments

See also under *Standards*.

References

Brender J. Quality assurance and validation of large information systems – as viewed from the user perspective [Master thesis, computer science]. Copenhagen: Copenhagen University; 1989. Report No.: 89-1-22.

> *A résumé of the method can be found in (Brender 1997a), or it can be obtained from the author.*

Brender J. Methodology for assessment of medical IT-based systems – in an organisational context. Amsterdam: IOS Press, Stud Health Technol Inform 1997;42.

Brender J. Methodology for constructive assessment of IT-based systems in an organisational context. Int J Med Inform 1999;56:67-86.

> *This is a shortened version of the previous reference and more accessible with regard to this subject.*

Nowlan WA. Clinical workstations: identifying clinical requirements and understanding clinical information. Int J Biomed Comput 1994;34:85-94.

Supplementary Reading

Bevan N. Cost effective user centred design. London: Serco Ltd. 2000. *(Available from: http://www.usability.serco.com/trump/. The website was last visited on 31.05.2005.)*

> *This report, originating from a large EU telematics project, contains advice and guidelines for the formulation of requirements, measurement of usability, and so forth, in relation to Usability.*

This little technical report also contains a lot of literature references and links to websites on the subject of Usability.

Risk Assessment

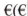

Areas of Application

Identification and subsequent monitoring of risk factors in a development or assessment project to make it possible to take preemptive action.

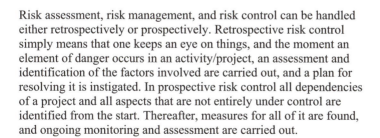

Description

Risk is defined as the *"the possibility of loss"* (Hall 1998), and a risk factor is a variable controlling the likelihood of such a loss. In other words, a risk is an aspect of a development, assessment, or operational project, which in case it is brought to bear, will lead to an undesirable condition. There must, however, be a reasonable likelihood for such a condition to occur before it is called a risk. Therefore, risk assessment together with the matching risk control is a constructive project management tool.

⇔

Risk assessment, risk management, and risk control can be handled either retrospectively or prospectively. Retrospective risk control simply means that one keeps an eye on things, and the moment an element of danger occurs in an activity/project, an assessment and identification of the factors involved are carried out, and a plan for resolving it is instigated. In prospective risk control all dependencies of a project and all aspects that are not entirely under control are identified from the start. Thereafter, measures for all of it are found, and ongoing monitoring and assessment are carried out.

Risk assessment can be carried out either ad hoc or formally – the latter certainly giving the better result. But even formal techniques may not require a large methodical foundation and may be carried out by means of consequence analysis supplemented by weighting principles – for instance, based on probability, implications of actual occurrences (such as 'medical' side effects), chance of timely realization, resources needed to compensate or rectify the unwanted situation should it actually occur, and so on. If this semiformal level is insufficient, help should be searched for in the original literature.

Assumptions for Application

Special experience is only required for strictly formal risk assessments of large or complex projects.

Perspectives

Risks will typically occur – but not solely – at the interfaces between persons, organizations, and activities and will usually arise in their input/output relationships. This also includes the time aspects, particularly within the political and administrative decision process. This is because external parties do not have the same commitment and motivation and because they do not depend on a given decision or product and thus do not have the same impetus for a solution (a timely one), as does the project itself.

Frame of Reference for Interpretation

The frame of reference for a development project is its objective, including its future plans for progress and resource requirement.

Perils and Pitfalls

A bias occurs where there is unease in revealing specific risk factors long before these have been realized. There might, for instance, be political, psychological, or other tactical reasons to omit monitoring specific circumstances.

Advice and Comments

Integration of a prospective risk, if required, can be done by establishing monitoring points in terms of indicators (measures) of the risk factors and if possible by defining milestones and deadlines in a project's contractual basis. One way of handling this is described in *Logical Framework Approach* (see relevant section), where risks are explicitly handled by means of the concept of external factors and corresponding measures that are identified and evaluated for all planned activities prior to the commencement of the project.

There is a lot of literature about this area, also concerning IT projects, so just go ahead and search for precisely that, which suits you the best.

References

Hall EM. Managing Risk: Methods for software systems development. Reading: Addison-Wesley; 1998.

Root Causes Analysis

Areas of Application

Exploration of what, how, and why a given incident occurred to identify the root causes of undesirable events.

Description

Root Causes Analysis is a family of methods, applying a sequence of component methods: (1) schematic representation of the incident sequence and its contributing conditions, (2) identification of critical events or active failures or conditions in the incident sequence, and (3) systematic investigation of the management and organizational factors that allowed the active failures to occur (Livingston et al. 2001). The reference mentioned provides an exhaustive review of the literature and case studies applying Root Causes Analysis.

Assumptions for Application

-

Perspectives

The highly structured and prescriptive approach will aid domain people to perform the investigation themselves, which is necessary given the need for domain insight to get hold of the propagation of root causes in an organization.

Frame of Reference for Interpretation

(Not applicable)

Perils and Pitfalls

The issue is to get to the root of the cause of a problem rather than to obtain a plausible explanation. The point being that in order to be able to prevent similar incidents in the future one has to get hold of the root cause before proper action can be taken; otherwise the incident will reoccur.

Advice and Comments

This method may be valuable in combination with Continuous Quality Improvement strategy for quality management.

References

Livingston AD, Jackson G, Priestly K. Root causes analysis: literature review. Health & Safety Executive Contract Research Report 325/2001. *(Available from: www.hse.gov.uk/research/crr_pdf/2001/CRR01325.pdf. Last visited 15.05.2005.)*

Social Networks Analysis

Areas of Application

Assessment of relationships between elements within an organization (such as individuals, professions, departments, or other organizations), which influence the acceptance and use of an IT-based solution. This could be used to identify key persons for success and opinion makers in an organization.

Description

Social network analysis is carried out by means of diagramming techniques, which do vary a little depending on the actual study (Rice and Anderson 1994; Anderson 2002): They are all described as networks with the knots being the actors (for instance, an individual, a profession, a department or a project, ...) and the relationships being described as named arrows between the knots. The type of relationships could, for instance, be that of communication, state of competence, or economy. The relationships are described by a number of characteristics such as frequency, type of relationship, level or strength of the interaction, and so on. Finally, the data collected are analyzed by means of several techniques that illustrate the relationships.

Assumptions for Application

Some experience of the techniques used is needed.

Perspectives

Attitudes toward information technology and its use are strongly influenced by the relationship between the individuals that form part of an organization (Rice and Anderson 1994; Anderson 2002).

Frame of Reference for Interpretation

(Not applicable)

Perils and Pitfalls

Pitfalls, the same as under diagramming techniques in general (see under Work Procedure Analysis), are that one must judge the suitability of the specific modeling technique to answer one's information needs and to which degree variations (and exceptions) can/should be included.

Advice and Comments

This method may be used to carry out stakeholder analysis, but it may also be used as a basis to uncover what and why things happen in an organization and to identify individual or professional interfaces within or between different activities in a work procedure (Rice and Anderson 1994). This is particularly important, as both internal and external interfaces in an organization constitute points of risk where, for instance, the execution or transfer of a task may fail.

The reference (Rice and Anderson 1994) contains a vast number of references to description of methods and their use.

References

Anderson JG. Evaluation in health informatics: social network analysis. Comput Biol Med 2002;32:179-93.

Rice RE, Anderson JG. Social networks and health care informations systems, a structural approach to evaluation. In: Anderson JG, Aydin CE, Jay SJ, editors. Evaluating health care information systems, methods and applications. Thousand Oaks: Sage Publications; 1994. p. 135-63.

Stakeholder Analysis

Areas of Application

Assessment of stakeholder features and their inner dynamics, aiming to identify participants for the completion of a given task, a problem-solving activity or a project.

Description

An in-depth stakeholder analysis covers a whole range of considerations, including:

1. Analysis of the rationale behind undertaking a stakeholder analysis: What are the value norms or the motivation behind a stakeholder analysis (legislative, moral, ethic, or labor-related, etc.)? What difference would it make if one stakeholder group were not involved? And what potential risks will it entail if they do not get involved?

2. Analysis of what definitive characteristics of a stakeholder group determine its influence on the decision makers, including the elucidation of the stakeholders' own expectations.

3. Observation of the stakeholder group's internal and mutual dynamics (including organizational culture, power structure, control mechanisms, etc.) and their influence on the decision-making processes as a function of internal and external factors.

4. Selection of participants and participating stakeholder groups by optimizing factors ('performance management indicators') that fulfill the policy of the organization – that is, beyond those of legal consideration as, for instance, the principles of user involvement, democracy or other principles of justice, motivational principles, know-how principles, minimizing risks by involving leading figures and spokespersons, and so on.

Assumptions for Application

The task of formal stakeholder analysis is not something that just anybody can undertake, as it requires some prior knowledge of organizational theories and administrative law. In some situations an intuitive analysis, or one with the aforementioned aspects in mind, may suffice. In other words, unless it is quite a new type of task or a very large investigation involving several organizations (particularly if they are not known beforehand) or if there is a risk of resistance severely compromising the course of the project or its outcome, there is no reason for the investigation to be as explicit and thorough as indicated in the description. If that is the case, most people can carry out a stakeholder analysis.

Perspectives

A frequently quoted definition of a stakeholder within the discipline of stakeholder analysis is Friedman's (quoted in Simmonds and Lovegrove 2002): *"any group or individual who can affect or is affected by the achievement of the organization's objectives"*. From this the perspective is derived that anybody who is influenced by a concrete solution should also be involved in the preparation of the solution model.

As often as not a number of conditions to make allowances for the different stakeholder interests are normally implicitly or explicitly incorporated into the organizational culture. This means that precedents from earlier projects and circulars and so on will implicitly make allowances for who is (officially) accepted as a stakeholder.

Principles of involvement of stakeholders in a problem-solving context are highly dependent on the culture (see the discussion on the concept of perspective in the introductory part, Section 2.4). One of the differences is to be found in the interpretation of the two English notions of 'decision maker' and 'decision taker', as seen in their extremes: 'Decision making' reflects that there is a process between the stakeholders involved in various ways, whereby a basis for a decision is created and a decision made. Conversely 'decision taking' represents the attitude that somebody has the competence to make decisions singlehandedly. In some cultures (like the Asian culture, for instance) there is no discussion about it being the leader who decides – and he or she is presumed to be knowledgeable about issues of relevance to the decision. Consequently, a stakeholder analysis will be superfluous to these cultures, and it should be noted that before using the Stakeholder Analysis method it must be adapted to the organization's own perspective of stakeholder participation in a given problem-solving context.

Frame of Reference for Interpretation
(Not applicable)

Perils and Pitfalls
See the discussion under Perspectives: If the wrong perspective is used in an actual stakeholder analysis you run the risk of taking account of the wrong factors for solving the problem or for organizing the project, and if the worst is brought to bear, internal strife in the organization or an incomplete decision-making foundation will result.

Advice and Comments
Logical Framework Approach or *Social Network Analysis* can be inspirational when a formal analysis is not required.

Also see the Stakeholder Assessment method in (Krogstrup 2003), where all stakeholder groups get involved in a given assessment activity, and the result is subsequently summarized and negotiated. The same reference summarizes the Deliberative Democratic Assessment method, which also involves all the stakeholder groups. The latter focuses on identification of value norms, and the questions asked are extremely relevant in deciding who should be involved in an assessment activity (or any sort of task) when not everybody can take part.

References

Krogstrup HK. Evalueringsmodeller. Århus: Systime; 2003. (in Danish)
> *This little informative book from the social sector gives quite a good overview of possibilities and limitations of a couple of known assessment models.*

Simmonds J, Lovegrove I. Negotiating a research method's 'conceptual terrain': lessons from a stakeholder analysis perspective on performance appraisal in universities and colleges. In: Remenyi D, editor. Proceedings of the European Conference on Research Methodology for Business and Management Studies; 2002 Apr; Reading, UK. Reading: MCIL; 2002. p. 363-73.
> *The article is a theoretical debate and review, making it difficult to grasp.*

Supplementary Reading

Eason K, Olphert W. Early evaluation of the organisational
implications of CSCW systems. In: Thomas P, editor. CSCW
requirements and evaluation. London: Springer; 1996. p. 75-89.

> *Provides an arbitrary rating approach to assess cost and benefit
> for the different user groups and stakeholders.*

SWOT

Areas of Application

- Situation analysis: The SWOT method is intended for establishing a holistic view of a situation or a model solution as objectively as is feasible.

This method was originally developed to evaluate business proposals and process re-engineering effects to assist in identifying strategic issues to assist in the formulation of a strategy.

Description

SWOT is an acronym for "**S**trengths, **W**eaknesses, **O**pportunities, and **T**hreats". For most purposes these four concepts can be used in their common sense: 'Weaknesses' are characteristics of the object of the study, usually ongoing and internal, and which will hinder development in the desired direction. 'Threats' are risks that lurk but do not necessarily happen and over which you do not have any control; there should be a certain probability that they may happen before you choose to include them. They are usually to be found in the internal or external interfaces of the organization (see also under *Risk Assessment*). 'Strengths' are to be interpreted similarly as having the same characteristics as internal assets, while 'Opportunities' are assumptions of possibilities or options, which might alleviate some of the problems arising during implementation of the actual model solution.

The SWOT method is intended to identify and analyze the four aspects mentioned for an object of study, based on a combination of facts, assumptions, and opinions (the description should indicate what information and of which type). The object of the study could, for instance, be a decision-making situation, where the choice between alternative solutions has to be made or as an introduction to a discussion on problem solving in a deadlocked situation. For a review see Dyson (2004).

A SWOT analysis can be carried out in a simple way or with increasing formality depending on the size of the topic and its complexity. A detailed SWOT analysis should, for instance, include:

- The probability that the opportunities can be realized and utilized
- The possibility to eliminate weaknesses and exploit strengths
- The probability that a given risk (threat) will occur and if so, what the consequences will be
- The possibility of ongoing monitoring in order to detect and identify risks in time
- The possibility to compensate for a given risk should it become threatening

Assumptions for Application

-

Perspectives

The SWOT method is an incredibly simple and yet useful tool whose primary function is that of a framework structure ensuring the preparation of an elaborate picture for any given situation.

Frame of Reference for Interpretation

(Not applicable)

Perils and Pitfalls

By nature the method is subjective. Therefore, should an organization have strongly conservative forces or groups of employees who are afraid of change, a certain aspect could move from one category to another. For example, some could perceive the introduction of IT in an organization as a threat because it could entail rationalization and redundancies, while to management it can be an opportunity to solve a bottleneck problem in the organization.

The method can be misused if it is not used in an unbiased way – hence, group work is recommended. What might happen is that the balance between the sequences of aspects included is (sub)consciously askew or that important aspects are left out.

Advice and Comments

The method is useful as a brainstorming method to elucidate and evaluate each of the aspects brought forward.

References

Dyson RG. Strategic development and SWOT analysis at the University of Warwick. Eur J Operational Res 2004;152(3):631-40.

Supplementary Reading

Balamuralikrishna R, Dugger JC. SWOT analysis: a management tool for initiating new programs in vocational schools. J Vocational Technical Education 1995;12(1). (Available from: http://scholar.lib.vt.edu/. Last visited 10.05.2004.)

An example of its use as an illustration.

Jackson SE, Joshi A, Erhardt L. Recent research on team and organizational diversity: SWOT analysis and implications. J Manag 2003;29(6):801-30.

An extensive literature appraisal applying the SWOT method for the analysis of the literature.

Technical Verification

☺☺☺

§§

€€€

Areas of Application

Verification that the agreed functions are present, work correctly, and are in compliance with the agreement.

The purpose of technical verification is to ensure that the management of the organization can/will take administrative responsibility for the operation of an IT-based system and for its impact on the quality of work in the organization. This should not be understood as the responsibility of an IT department for the *technical operation* of the IT system, but as users applying the system in their daily operations such as their clinical work. This is the case:

- In connection with acceptance tests at delivery of an IT system or a part-delivery
- Prior to taking the system into daily operation and before all subsequent changes to the IT system (releases, versions, and patches)

Description

With the exception of off-the-shelf IT products (see under perspectives below), technical verification is carried out by checking the delivery, screen by screen and field by field, interface by interface, function by function, and so on to see if everything is complete, correct, consistent, and coherent. For each of the modular functionalities agreed on the following questions are assessed:

☑

1. Re.: *Completeness* of the functionality
   - Is everything that was promised included?
   - Has it been possible to verify all aspects of the functionality supplied, thereby all/most possibilities of data input, including exceptions? Or has it been impossible due to errors or shortfalls in the product delivered?
   - To which degree has it been possible for the users to simulate normal daily activities?
   - To which degree does the functionality supplied comply with that expected functionality?
   - How well does the system's functionality fulfill the functionality described in the contract – that is, the actual

requirements in the contract?

2. Re.: *Correctness* of the functionality

- Does the system work as it should? That is, can the users work with data that have a logical similarity to normal production and function?
- And does it all happen correctly?

3. Re.: *Coherence* of the functionality

- When data depend on each other (some data are only valid when other given data have actual values): Does the system control these internal constraints and ensure that data are correct?
- Or does the user have to ensure this manually?

4. Re.: *Consistency* of the functionality

- Is the data being duplicated, running the risk of getting different instances of the same information?
- And has this actually been observed as happening? This normally only happens when several independent IT systems are put together to make up one IT-based solution.

5. Re.: *Interconnectivity* of the functionality: This means that technical (syntactic) aspects of communications between several IT-based systems, such as communication of patient data from one patient-administration system or a hospital information system to a laboratory system, and communication with systems dedicated to controlling user-access criteria.

- Is it the right (complete and correct) information that is received?

6. Re.: *Interoperability* of the functionality: The semantic aspects of the interaction between several IT-based systems. One example is that the change of a patient's hospital address or status in a patient administration system has to be communicated to other systems that depend on this information. See further details under *Measures and Metrics*. This is not necessarily updated immediately in the interconnected systems. It has a big impact on the perceived functionality in a ward, irrespective of how correctly an IT system seems to work. Coordination of updated data between various systems can easily go wrong. One reason could be that, for capacity reasons, the system developers store this type of information in a queue, which is only emptied every five minutes, for instance. This could be significant under some acute conditions.

7. Re.: *Reliability:*

- How often does the system go down, and what are the

consequences?

- How does the system handle error situations, and what interventions are necessary to re-create data or reestablish operations when this happens?
  - What happens when an error situation is created on purpose – during simulated breakdowns of parts of the network, for instance?
  - What happens at monkey tests or at a database locking?
8. Re.: *Performance*: Response time and throughput time for transactions on the system, as well as capacity. See also under *Measures and Metrics*.

What types of problems are users likely to run into? And how do they relate to the contract?

See also many of the concepts under *Measures and Metrics*.

Assumptions for Application

It is a prerequisite that each of the requirements of the contract are operational or that they can be rendered operational without problem.

It requires previous experience in planning and implementation of such investigations, as well as punctiliousness with regard to details. It is an advantage to have tried it before. Should one want an in-depth technical verification, it could be an advantage to seek help for the more complex issues – for instance, to ensure systematism in the verification of the interoperability.

Perspectives

In a contractual relationship with regard to the supply of a system, you cannot expect more than what is stipulated in the agreement between the customer and the vendor. Technical verification serves the purpose of assessing whether the contract has been fulfilled. Thus, the contract is an indispensable frame of reference for technical verification. This does not necessarily mean that the system is appropriate, even if it has been verified with a successful outcome, or that it works properly, should the contract not make sure of this. Remember, it is not easy to formulate a good requirements specification. Management then must decide whether the system is good enough for it to undertake administrative responsibility for the system in operation. If not, it is necessary to take the consequences and say "Stop", regardless of whether the fault lies with the vendor or the client, and thereafter to find out what the next step should be.

Whether the vendor of the IT-based system is internal or external makes no difference – that is, whether it is an independent company or the IT department of the hospital or the region.

Technical verification of off-the-shelf products, such as Microsoft Word for word processing, has a different purpose if the organization chooses to carry it out. For instance, this could be to get acquainted with the details of the system's functions in order to establish new and changed work processes. Whether the product is used for its intended purpose and whether management undertakes responsibility for its introduction are questions that must be addressed before its purchase.

Frame of Reference for Interpretation

The frame of reference is the contract – or a similar agreement with attachments.

Perils and Pitfalls

The most common pitfall is the lack of testing of specific conditions, which then show up during day-to-day use. The possible combinations, the aspects of capacity in its widest sense and the interoperability are particularly difficult to test – also for the vendor. Furthermore, not all vendors have sufficiently detailed insight into the application domain to be able to test from a real-life perspective, implying that the focus and efforts put into technical verification depend on the number of similar reference sites of the IT system in question. In other words, even if the vendor has carried out a thorough test, undetected errors and omissions may occur when new people examine the same system with different data.

Advice and Comments

In practice it is impossible to physically test all fields, types of data, and functions of nontrivial IT systems in all their relevant and irrelevant combinations. It is important explicitly to keep to this in an accreditation or certification situation (see separate description in Chapter 8).

References

(See under *Measures and Metrics.*)

Think Aloud

Areas of Application

An instrument for gaining insight into the cognitive processes as feed-back for the implementation and adaptation of IT-based systems.

Description

Think Aloud is a method that requires users to speak as they interact with an IT-based system to solve a problem or perform a task, thereby generating data on the ongoing thought processes during task performance (Kushniruk and Patel 2004). The user interaction data collected typically include the video recording of all displays along with the corresponding audio recording of the users' verbalizations.

The resulting verbal protocols together with the videos are transcribed and systematically analyzed to develop a model of the user's behavior while performing a task.

Assumptions for Application

Kushniruk and Patel (2004) describe carefully the recording and analysis tasks and illustrates implicitly the need for prior experience of using this method: The data constitutes raw data that require substantial analysis and interpretation to gain in-depth insight in the way subjects perform tasks.

Perspectives

Jaspers et al. (2004) outline the various types of memory systems with different storing capacities and retrieval characteristics, putting across the message that humans are only capable of verbalizing the contents of the working memory (the currently active information), not the long-term memory.

A perspective behind this method is that the user's mental model is independent of his or her level of expertise. Thus, while using the output as input for a development process, the key issue is to elicit the joint mental model across different levels of expertise, as these present themselves differently in the interaction with the IT-based system (see also the discussion under Pitfalls in *Cognitive Assessment*, as well as in Part III). This perspective is clearly opposed by Norman (1987) as being incorrect, stating that mental models are incomplete, parsimonious, and unstable; they change, and do not have firm boundaries. Nevertheless, the Think Aloud method may have its value for small and down-to-earth practical assessments, provided that the assessor knows these constraints and consequently does not overinterpret the outcome.

Frame of Reference for Interpretation
(Not applicable)

Perils and Pitfalls
-

Advice and Comments
-

References

Jaspers MWM, Steen T, van den Bos C, Genen M. The Think Aloud method: a guide to user interface design. Int J Med Inform 2004;73:781-95.

Kushniruk AW, Patel VL. Cognitive and usability engineering methods for the evaluation of clinical information systems. J Biomed Inform 2004;37:56-76.

Norman DA. Some observations on mental models. In: Baecker RM, Buxton WAS, editors. Readings in human-computer interaction: a multidisciplinary approach. Los Altos: Morgan Kaufman Publishers, Inc.; 1987. p. 241-4.

Supplementary Reading

Cho I, Park H-A. Development and evaluation of a terminology-based electronic nursing record system. J Biomed Inform 2003;36:304-12.

Use the Think Aloud *method to identify success and failure in matching a precoordinated phrase with what the user wanted to document.*

Ericsson KA, Simon HA. Protocol analysis, verbal reports as data. Cambridge (MA): The MIT Press; 1984.

This book provides a thorough review of the literature on approaches to and problems of elicitation of information about cognitive processes from verbal data.

Preece J. Part VI, Interaction design: evaluation. In: Human-computer interaction. Wokingham: Addison-Wesley Publishing Company; 1994.

Part VI of this book describes a number of conventional methods for measuring Usability, *from traditional Usability Engineering via analysis of video data, verbal protocols,* Think Aloud *protocols,* Interviews, *and* Questionnaire *studies to ethnographic studies. Even though the perspective on page 693 indicates that the methods are intended for professionals, it may still be useful for others to read these chapters.*

Usability

Areas of Application

"Usability is the quality of interaction in a context"

(Bevan and Macleod 1993)

- Assessment of user friendliness in terms of ergonomic and cognitive aspects of the interaction between an IT system and its users.

It can be used during all phases of an IT system's life cycle – for instance:

- During the analysis and design phase (the Explorative Phase)
- For assessment of bids (the Explorative Phase) – see (Beuscart-Zéphir et al. 2002 and 2005) and *Assessment of Bids*
- In connection with a delivery test (after installation at the end of the Technical Development Phase)

- As constructive assessment during the implementation process or during adjustment of the functionality, also called usability engineering. See, for instance, the reviews in (Kushniruk 2002; and Kushniruk and Patel 2004).

Description

Usability is an aspect that must be taken into account in the functionality from the very first description of the idea and the objective of introducing the system until the system functions (well) in day-to-day use and during maintenance.

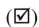

This is a very large subject area, stretching from vendors' and universities' advanced 'usability labs' with video monitoring of eye and hand movements attached to a log that tracks everything that goes on in the system. On the opposite scale you will find an assessment during hands-on use in a workplace. Somewhat dependent on the authors, the concept includes both ergonomic and cognitive aspects, as they are closely related. As already defined in a previous footnote (see *Field Studies*), this handbook distinguishes between the work procedure-related aspects (usually denoted as the functionality aspects), the dialogue-related aspects (the ergonomic aspects), and the perception-oriented aspects (the cognitive aspects).

There is definitely an overlap between them, and they are all concerned with the functionality that users are confronted with during daily use of an IT-based system.

For a review of inspection methods as well as different measurement methods ranging from formal over automatic and empirical to informal usability assessment methods, see (Huart et al. 2004).

Measurement of cognitive aspects is still at an experimental stage with regard to assessment of IT-based systems and has not yet been sufficiently addressed in the development methodologies. This is one of the reasons why only simple measurements and assessments of ergonomic aspects are included in this section, as they are easy enough to undertake by a user organization with some prior experience. Assessment of the cognitive aspects is described elsewhere (see separate sections, *Cognitive Assessment* and *Cognitive Walkthrough*).

Usability, with regard to ergonomic assessments, is concerned with characteristics of how difficult it is to carry out a user dialog with the IT system or – phrased in a positive sense – how effective an IT system is to use and how easy it is to learn to use it.

The work of ergonomic assessments is task-oriented that is, you simulate real small operational tasks. Use scenarios from every day as a base to identify suitable tasks. Correction of data is usually a good task to evaluate in this respect, although data entry and other limited activities should also be assessed. For example, how effective does the user interface work when the user uses the prototype to simulate an actual task, such as correcting a patient ID? The effectiveness can be calculated in (1) the number of shifts between screens; (2) the distance between fields on a given screen where data has to be entered or changed in other words, how many times and how far does the cursor have to be moved actively; or (3) is it necessary manually to correct data that are logical functions of each other (for instance, affiliation of staff and patients to a ward and a department) with the risk of inconsistencies?

In practice this has been made operational by a number of metrics and suggestions of things to keep an eye out for. The report (Bastien and Scapin 1993), a pioneering work in this area, goes through a number of examples of relevant aspects including recommendations and criteria gathered under a series of headings, such as:

- *Prompting*: Which tools are used to prompt the user to the next specific step of an action (a data entry field or a new action)?

- *Grouping of information and fields*: Is there a logical task-related, coherent, visual organization of the fields? This could be a topological (area) or a graphical (color, format, or similar) grouping

- *Immediate feed-back*: What is the immediate reaction of the system when the user performs something and completes it?

- *Readability*: Concerns characteristics of the readability, equivalent to the lix value (readability index) of a text. Is it readable (also for those who have early stages of age-related eyesight problems or are colorblind)?

- *Load (on the user)*: This concerns all aspect that play a part in reducing the sensual and cognitive strains on the user and the effectiveness of the dialog between the user and the system

- *Consistency*: Deals with uniformity of the design of the screens (does it show that different people have programmed it?)

- *Handling of errors*: Deals with tools to handle errors and ways to prevent them

- *Flexibility*: Deals with the overall flexibility of the system

Assumptions for Application

Experience is a prerequisite to really be able to employ the usability method and to profit from it as constructive feed-back tool during a development process. However, a usability assessment requires special professional background to have any deep impact.

Perspectives

Bastien and Scapin's report builds on an anthropocentric perspective that is, the users are not robots that have to learn and adapt to the system and that the best overall function is achieved when the user understands what goes on and is in charge of what happens and what needs to be done (see Bastien and Scapin 1993).

Usability is not just a fashion fad, but it has a decisive influence on user satisfaction, learning and training needs, and the strain of screen work, so it influences the frequency of operational errors and omissions. The ergonomic aspects are not only decisive for the efficiency of the operation of the system, but also when users try to avoid certain activities. For example, if the system is too cumbersome to handle, there is a risk that the user will carry out the activities in an incorrect way or maybe jot down the information on a piece of paper, put it in a pocket, and delay the inputting or even forget all about it.

Frame of Reference for Interpretation

The report (Bastien and Scapin 1993) may work as a de facto standard for what is 'good practice' – at least from the view of what a user organization is normally capable of dealing with itself.

Perils and Pitfalls

A significant source of error is the bias inherent in people's subjective evaluations (see Kieras 1997 and Part III): One has to find objective metrics and measures if the ergonomics are a point of discussion and negotiation with a development team or, even worse, with an external vendor.

Advice and Comments

You can find some good rules of thumb for evaluations and assessments on http://jthom.best.vwh.net/usability/ under "heuristic evaluation" under the reference to "Nielsen".

When assessing usability, one should be aware that the context in which measures are taken is very important and needs to simulate real life as closely as possible (i.e., ideally in actual use) (Bevan and Macleod 1993; Coolican 1999).

If the usability cannot be measured directly, it is sometimes possible to register and analyze the causes behind typical errors of operation and other unintentional events.

References

Bastien JMC, Scapin DL. Ergonomic criteria for the evaluation of human-computer interfaces. Rocquencourt (France): Institut National de Recherche en Informatique et en Automatique; 1993. Report No.: 156.

> *The report is available from the institute's website: http://www.inria.fr/publications/index.en.html. Click on 'Research Reports & Thesis', type "ergonomic criteria" in the text field of the search engine, and press 'Enter'. Find the report RT0156, mentioned under the description of 'Usability' assessment. By clicking on 'pour obtenir la version papier', you get the e-mail address of the person concerned, and you may request the report (last visited 10.12.2003).*

Beuscart-Zéphir MC, Watbled L, Carpentier AM, Degroisse M, Alao

O. A rapid usability assessment methodology to support the choice of clinical information systems: a case study. In: Kohane I, editor. Proc AMIA 2002 Symp on Bio*medical Informatics: One Discipline; 2002 Nov; San Antonio, Texas; 2002. p. 46-50.

Beuscart-Zéphir M-C, Anceaux F, Menu H, Guerlinger S, Watbled L, Evrard F. User-centred, multidimensional assessment method of clinical information systems: a case study in anaesthesiology. Int J Med Inform 2005;74(2-4):179-89.

Bevan N, Macleod M. Usability Assessment and Measurement. In: Kelly M. Management and measurement of software quality. Uxbridge: Unicom Seminars Ltd; 1993. p. 167-92.
An easily accessible opening for usability measurement.

Coolican H. Introduction to research methods and statistics in psychology. 2nd ed. London: Hodder & Stoughton; 1999.
Describes (mainly in the early chapters) problems of experimental conditions of psychological phenomena.

Huart J, Kolski C, Sagar M. Evaluation of multimedia applications using inspection methods: the Cognitive Walkthrough case. Interacting Comput 2004;16:183-215.

Kieras D. A guide to GOMS model usability evaluation using NGOMSL. In: Helander MG, Landauer TK, Prabhu PV, editors. Handbook of human computer interaction. 2nd ed. Amsterdam: Elsevier Science B.V.; 1997. p. 733-66.

Kushniruk A. Evaluation in the design of health information systems: application of approaches emerging from usability engineering. Comput Biol Med 2002;32(3):141-9.

Kushniruk AW, Patel VL. Cognitive and usability engineering methods for the evaluation of clinical information systems. J Biomed Inform 2004;37:56-76.

http://jthom.best.vwh.net/usability
The page contains numerous links to method descriptions and references, including, for instance, Jacob Nielsen's ten recommended aspects (last visited 15.05.2005).

Supplementary Reading

Baecker RM, Buxton WAS. Readings in human-computer interaction:

a multidisciplinary approach. Los Altos: Morgan Kaufman Publishers, Inc.; 1987.

Chapter four of this book contains a brilliant little review of methods for assessing user interfaces and is thus an easy opening for those thinking of getting started with this subject.

Bastien JMC, Scapin DL, Leulier C. The ergonomic criteria and the ISO 9241-10 dialogue principles: a comparison in an evaluation task. Interacting Comput, 1999;11(3):299-322.

Bevan N. Cost effective user centred design. London: Serco Ltd. 2000. (*Available from http://www.usability.serco.com/trump/. The website was last visited 15.06.2005.*)

This report, which originates from a large EU telematics project, contains advice and guidelines on requirement formulation, usability measures, and so forth, including lots of literature references and links to websites on Usability.

Carroll JM, editor. Scenario-based design, envisioning work and technology in system development. New York: John Wiley & Sons, Inc.; 1995.

This book contains a number of articles written by system development professionals; therefore, it may seem on the heavy side, but it is inspirational with regard to scenarios, and it is an excellent tool during preparation. The various articles deal with different types of scenarios, their use, advantages, disadvantages, and assumptions.

Graham MJ, Kubose TK, Jordan D, Zhang J, Johnson TR, Patel VL. Heuristic evaluation of infusion pumps: implications for patient safety in intensive care units. Int J Med Inform 2004;73:771-9.

A case study applying heuristic assessment for the evaluation of usability aspects.

Helander MG, Landauer TK, Prabhu PV, editors. Handbook of human computer interaction. 2nd ed. Amsterdam: Elsevier Science B.V.; 1997.

Part IV of the book consists of a selection of independent articles on Usability assessment methods, each with good lists of references to the original literature.

Jaspers MWM, Steen T, van den Bos C, Genen M. The Think Aloud method: a guide to user interface design. Inf J Med Inform 2005;73:781-95.

The Think Aloud *method combined with videorecording was used as a means to guide the design of a user interface in order to combat the traditional problems with usability.*

Karat J. User-centered software evaluation methodologies. In: Helander MG, Landauer TK, Prabhu PV, editors. Handbook of human computer interaction. 2nd ed. Amsterdam: Elsevier Science B.V.; 1997. p. 689-704.

See (Helander et al. 1997).

Kuniavsky M. Observing the user experience, a practitioner's guide to user research. San Franscisco: Morgan Kaufmann Publishers; 2003.

There are many books dealing with usability This is just one of them and is a quite practical tool. Chapter 10 of this book is dedicated to the assessment of usability of Web applications.

Kushniruk A, Patel V, Cimino JJ, Barrows RA. Cognitive evaluation of the user interface and vocabulary of an outpatient information system. Proc AMIA Annu Fall Symp 1996:22-6.

Kushniruk AW, Patel VL, Cimino JJ. Usability testing in medical informatics: cognitive approaches to evaluation of information systems and user interfaces. Proc AMIA Annu Fall Symp 1997:218-22.

Keep an eye on these two authors with regard to investigations of the cognitive aspects and usability (they do not distinguish sharply between them). Although some of the articles simply are proceedings from conferences, they do use very little space to say a lot about the methods relating to video-based studies and the measurement of usability.

Lewis C, Wharton C. Cognitive Walkthroughs. In: Helander MG, Landauer TK, Prabhu PV, editors. Handbook of human computer interaction. 2nd ed. Amsterdam: Elsevier Science B.V.; 1997. p. 717-32.

See (Helander et al. 1997).

Mayhew DJ. The usability engineering lifecycle, a practitioner's handbook for user interface design. San Francisco: Morgan Kaufmann Publishers;1999.

Pages 126-137 and Chapters 10, 13, and 16 are particularly relevant in connection with evaluations.

Preece J. Part VI, Interaction design: evaluation. In: Human-computer interaction. Wokingham: Addison-Wesley Publishing Company; 1994.

Part VI of this book describes a number of conventional methods for measuring usability, from traditional Usability Engineering via analysis of video data, verbal protocols, Think Aloud protocols, interviews, and questionnaire studies to ethnographic studies. Even though the perspective on page 693 indicates that the methods are meant for professionals, it may still be useful for others to read these chapters.

Scapin DL, Bastien JMC. Ergonomic criteria for evaluating the ergonomic quality of interactive systems. Behav Inf Technol 1997;16:220-31.

Terazzi A, Giordano A, Minuco G. How can usability measurement affect the re-engineering process of clinical software procedures? Int J Med Inform 1998;52:229-34.

> *Addresses 'perceived usability' – that is, the users' subjective impression of usability as opposed to the more objective studies based on many of the other articles, and for this purpose it uses standard questionnaires.*

Virzi RA. Usability inspection methods. In: Helander MG, Landauer TK, Prabhu PV, editors. Handbook of human computer interaction. 2nd ed. Amsterdam: Elsevier Science B.V.; 1997. p. 705-15.

> *See (Helander et al. 1997).*

Wixon D, Wilson C. The usability engineering framework for product design and evaluation. In: Helander MG, Landauer TK, Prabhu PV, editors. Handbook of human computer interaction. 2nd ed. Amsterdam: Elsevier Science B.V.; 1997. p. 653-88.

> *See (Helander et al. 1997).*

Furthermore, see the list of websites with relevant information at the end of Part III. The following are particularly relevant:

http://www.infodesign.com.au/usabilityresources/general/readinglist.asp

> *Contains a list of references to books on usability assessment (last visited 31.05.2005).*

http://web.mit.edu/is/usability/usability-guidelines.html

> *The home page contains a number of factors worth keeping in mind for an assessment (last visited 31.05.2005).*

☺(☺☺)
§(§)
€(€)

User Acceptance and Satisfaction

Areas of Application

Assessment of user opinions, attitudes, and perceptions of an IT system during daily operation.

Description
Measurement of user satisfaction is largely concerned with the assessment of user opinions, attitudes, and perceptions of phenomena and possibly with patterns of reaction in given situations. Below are a few of the most common methods.

(⇔)

1. Interview techniques (individual as well as group interviews); see under *Interviews* or *Focus-Group Interviews*.
2. Questionnaires – there are a number of more or less standardized questionnaires, see, for instance, (Harrison 1994 and Ohmann et al. 1997). See also under *Questionnaires*.
3. The Equity Implementation Model is used to investigate and understand user reactions to the implementation of an IT-based system (Lauer et al. 2000). See separate section, *Equity Implementation Model*.

Assumptions for Application
-

Perspectives
One of the more precarious issues when measuring user satisfaction (which most studies avoid discussing) is what satisfaction really is or to which measures do they correlate. This is not an easy question, and most studies circumvent it by simply defining exactly what they do measure. Or they avoid it by asking the users if, for instance, they would do without the system. See also the discussion in (Mair and Whitten 2000); although it deals with patient satisfaction, the problem is general.

Frame of Reference for Interpretation
(Not applicable)

Perils and Pitfalls
When measuring user satisfaction, it is important to involve all the right stakeholders with the study, otherwise the picture will be askew. As in (Chin and Haughton 1995) it is possible consciously to choose only to ask one specific user group, which could be the one responsible for operations. However, you need to be aware that it can be difficult to extrapolate the conclusion to cover other user groups as well.

See also under *Questionnaires*, which is the tool most commonly used when measuring user satisfaction.

Advice and Comments
It is evident how difficult it is to find generally applicable tools to measure user satisfaction by the fact that authors of so-called 'standard' user-satisfaction questionnaires often do not use these same 'standard tools' in reports from new studies of user satisfaction. This is the case with Chin and Haughton (1995), who apparently no longer use their own QUIS form, and neither do Ohmann et al. (1997) or Boy et al. (2000). This can probably be explained by variations in information needs or in the object of study leading to a demand for adaptation of the old or a completely new questionnaire.

Ives et al. (1983) show how you can verify and correct for aspects such as reliability, predictive value, accuracy and content validity, and internal validity.

References

Boy O, Ohmann C, Aust B, Eich HP, Koller M, Knode O, Nolte U. Systematische evaluierung der anwenderzufriedenheit von ärzten mit einem krankenhausinformationssystem – erste ergebnisse. In: Hasman A, Blobel B, Dudeck J, Engelbrecht R, Gell G, Prokosch H-U, editors. Medical Infobahn for Europe. Proceedings of the Sixteenth European Congress on MIE2000 and GMDS2000; Aug 2000; Hannover, Germany. Amsterdam: IOS Press. Stud Health Technol Inform 2000;77:518-22.

Chin L, Haughton DM. A study of users' perceptions on the benefits of information systems in hospitals. J Healthc Inf Manag Sys Soc 1995;9:37-46.

Harrison MI. Diagnosing organizations: methods, models, and processes. 2nd ed. Thousand Oaks: Sage Publications. Applied Social Research Methods Series 1994. vol. 8.

Appendix B of the book contains a number of references to standard questionnaires for all purposes relating to organizations.

Ives B, Olson MH, Baroudi JJ. The measurement of user information satisfaction. Communications of the ACM 1983;26(19):785-93.

Brilliant little article with advice and guidelines on measurements and corrections of different quality objectives in a questionnaire.

Lauer TW, Joshi K, Browdy T. Use of the Equity Implementation Model to review clinical system implementation effort, a case report. JAMIA 2000;7:91-102.

Mair F, Whitten P. Systematic reviews of studies of patient satisfaction with telemedicine. BMJ 2000;320:1517-20.

Ohmann C, Boy O, Yang O. A systematic approach to the assessment of user satisfaction with health care systems: constructs, models and instruments. In: Cappas C, Maglavera N, Scherrer J-R, editors. Medical Informatics Europe '97. Amsterdam: IOS Press. Stud Health Technol Inform 1997;43:781-5.

Supplementary Reading

Ammenwerth E, Kutscha A, Eichstädter R, Haux R. Systematic evaluation of computer-based nursing documentation. In: Patel V, Roger R, Haux R, editors. Proceedings of the 10th World Congress on Medical Informatics; 2001 Sep; London, UK. Amsterdam: IOS Press; 2001. p. 1102-6.

A before-and-after study with thorough examination of the quality of the nursing documentation records and user satisfaction, partly based on three questionnaires from the literature.

Hicks LL, Hudson ST, Koening S, Madsen R, Kling B, Tracy J, Mitchell J, Webb W. An evaluation of satisfaction with telemedicine among health-care professionals. J Telemed Telecare 2000;6:209-15.

A user satisfaction case study based on a previously validated questionnaire.

Jaspers MWM, Steen T, van den Bos C, Genen M. The Think Aloud method: a guide to user interface design. Int J Med Inform 2004;73:781-95.

Uses a short version of the QUIS questionnaire together with one developed by the authors to assess the level of user satisfaction.

Junger A, Michel A, Benson M, Quinzio LA, Hafer J, Hartman B, Brandenstein P, Marquardt K, Hempelmann G. Evaluation of the suitability of a patient data management system for ICUs on a general ward. Int J Med Inform 2001;64:57-66.

A case study, but unfortunately they have omitted to mention anything about the internal validity of their questionnaire, although the questionnaire is published in the article.

Lauer TW, Joshi K, Browdy T. Use of the Equity Implementation Model to review clinical system implementation effort. JAMIA 2000;7:91-102.

The article presents a method, the Equity Implementation Model, *to investigate and understand users' reactions to the implementation of an IT-based system, focusing on the impact of the changes such a system brings about for the users. The method has a research aim, but under certain circumstances it can be useful for more down-to-earth studies, for example, when there are special problems with user satisfaction.*

Murff HJ, Kannry J. Physician satisfaction with two order entry systems. J Am Med Inform Assoc 2001;8:499-509.

An extremely well-organized case study, which gives the impression that they are also in control of statistics.

http://qpool.umit.at.

This website, which is still under construction, aims to collect references from the literature to questionnaires that have been validated to a certain degree (last visited 31.05.2005).

Videorecording

Areas of Application

Monitoring and documentation as a means of analyzing how work procedures and the users' activities, respectively, are actually carried out or for investigation of complex patterns of interaction.

Used for:

- Data collection when it is practically impossible to get data any other way. This may be the case for studies of, for instance, ergonomic and cognitive aspects of the functionality of a system in practical use
- Studies of what/how work processes and user activities actually take place
- Studies of complex interaction patterns
- Supplement to achieve triangulations of other assessment methods (Kushniruk et al. 1997); see Part III
- Monitoring purposes and documentation of a sequence of events

Description

Anyone with knowledge of television knows what a videorecording is recordings of a visual representation of a sequence of events on a data medium.

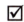

Assumptions for Application

To use videorecording in scientific or other formal contexts requires special background and experience in handling and interpreting videorecordings, including experience of field work in general (see under separate heading).

Perspectives

With the current technological developments videorecordings are in themselves not a technical problem in connection with assessment studies. The problems lie in defining the objective and the subsequent design, solving ethical problems, identifying pitfalls, and ways of analyzing and interpreting the data. The latter because a code to transcribe events on the recording has only been developed for specific purposes. Another challenge, if relevant for the study, is the fact that a videorecording contains not only physical acts and verbal communication, but also a large amount of nonverbal communication (body language).

Frame of Reference for Interpretation

Videorecordings as documentation or observation media do not in themselves need a frame of reference, but should they form part of a larger context, this context could have its own frame of reference.

Perils and Pitfalls

As an ordinary user, one should read dedicated literature before starting to plan a study based on videorecordings, as there are many circumstances to be considered. A few of the important ones are:

1. The Hawthorne Effect introduces a very big risk of bias during video studies; see Part III.
2. Furthermore, there is a risk that strong psychological factors and ethical problems make it inappropriate to use videorecordings of conditions/situations that are considered to be of a private nature.
3. Transcription of the recordings embraces many possibilities of interpretation and variation from plain punctuation and omission of part of the context in the transcribed verbal text to notes regarding behavioral or phonetic elements, and so forth.
4. The reproducibility of a transcript is usually quite poor.

Advice and Comments

-

References

Kushniruk AW, Patel VL, Cimino JJ. Usability testing in medical informatics: cognitive approaches to evaluation of information systems and user interfaces. Proc AMIA Annu Fall Symp 1997:218-22.

Supplementary Reading

Alrø H, Dirkinck-Holmfeld L, editors. Videoobservation. Aalborg: Aalborg Universitetsforlag; 1997. p. 9-27. (in Danish)
This book contains a series of articles on experiences and practical guidelines of what to do.

Ericsson KA, Simon HA. Protocol analysis, verbal reports as data.

Cambridge (MA): The MIT Press; 1984.

This book provides a thorough review of the literature on approaches to and problems of elicitation of information about cognitive processes from verbal data.

Kushniruk AW, Patel VL. Cognitive computer-based video analysis: its application in assessing the usability of medical systems. In: Greenes RA, Peterson HE, Protti DJ, editors. Medinfo'95. Proceedings of the Eighth World Congress on Medical Informatics; 1995 Jul; Vancouver, Canada. Edmonton: Healthcare Computing & Communications Canada Inc; 1995. p. 1566-9.

Kushniruk A, Patel V, Cimino JJ, Barrows RA. Cognitive evaluation of the user interface and vocabulary of an outpatient information system. Proc AMIA Annu Fall Symp 1996:22-6.

Patel VL, Kushniruk AW. Understanding, navigating and communicating knowledge: issues and challenges. Methods Inf Med 1998;37:460-70.

Keep an eye on the first two authors with regard to studies of the cognitive aspects and usability (they do not distinguish sharply between them). Although some of their articles are proceedings from conferences, they do use very little space to say a lot about methods relating to video-based studies and measurement of usability.

WHO: Framework for Assessment of Strategies

Areas of Application

The method may be applied for assessment of different (development) strategies, either individually or as a comparative analysis. Thereby, the method is particularly relevant early in the Explorative Phase for exploring the feasibility of basic ideas and solutions. Following this, it is obvious that the method may be applied for the same purpose when assessing ideas for further developments within the Evolution Phase.

Description

(Since the reference to this method is inaccessible, it will be described to the extent that the author is familiar with it and which sufficed for its successful use.)

The principle on which the method is founded is that every development or initiative for change may have several candidate solution models. Each of these solution models has its attributes, value norms, and philosophy, potentially ranging from conservative resistance toward change to revolutionary thinking. Each of the solution models will have their strengths and weaknesses, risks and challenges, as well as future viability. Consequently, they are also characterized by differences in feasibility and resource consumptions, and so on.

The approach is to prepare a table with different overall strategies as columns and issues or problem areas (functions or activities, features of the solution) as rows within the table. These problem areas typically constitute partial functions or areas of responsibility and activities within the organization. For a hierarchically structured table the top-level may be used to make the basic idea explicit, including the value norms and the philosophy of that particular model solution. Each cell within the lower levels of the structure will then summarize the features, assumptions, and consequences of the given strategy for the particular problem area. Examples are judgments of the consequence of a specific activity within the organization or the implications for areas of responsibility and competence within the organization.

During the evaluation of the different strategies, one may use a series of corresponding empty tables – for instance, addressing reliability/feasibility, resource consumptions, time scales, risks, assumptions, and so on. The first thing to search for during a combined analysis is potential showstoppers (there should be none, as it makes little sense to continue the elaboration of a given strategy when a showstopper has been identified). The rest has to be analyzed in its entirety, based on compliance of the value norms, strengths and weaknesses, policy and priorities, based on criteria defined for the solution by the organization.

The original description, aimed at large development projects within WHO and UNDP, operates with the following four strategies:

- *Preservation strategy*, which aims at minimizing the required change
- *Prioritization strategy*, building on a philosophy of continuous (incremental) and organization-driven change of structural aspects within the organization
- *Contract strategy*, which in principle reuses a lot from the previous strategy, but with an external steering mechanism
- *Laisserfaire strategy* – an anarchistic model assuming that things will happen by themselves. This strategy is based on the anticipation that actors within the organization will initiate activities and concerted actions by themselves and that these will lead to viable solutions in an appropriate way, simply because of common understanding and a common goal

One may define one's own overall principles for the strategies considered.

Assumptions for Application

The method does not include tools and techniques for the specific analyses and assessments. When these are too complicated for simple experience-based judgment, it is necessary to supplement them with relevant and appropriate tools and techniques. In any case, analysis of the strategies should be carried out by persons with a certain level of experience within the relevant application domain.

Perspectives

Within large organizations or organizations with conflicting stakeholder viewpoints it may be difficult to manage subjective aspects, personal interests, and hidden agendas, as well as the influence of a number of psychological and social factors, including that of informal power structures. In this situation, tools enabling a structured analysis, topic by topic and in a relatively objective fashion, will smooth the progress of establishing a rational decision-making basis. This is the advantage of the table like structure of the method.

The method is based on a reductionistic approach – that is, assuming that one may divide a wholeness into component elements and study these on an individual basis and subsequently make deductions about the wholeness on the basis of the combined characteristics of the individual parts.

Frame of Reference for Interpretation
(Not applicable)

Perils and Pitfalls
The aspect of time may be a pitfall of this method, as some strategies assume longer terms for their implementation than others. Thereby, the impact of and the return on the investment of the organization may differ significantly. Likewise with the feasibility of realizing a given candidate strategy. A principle of rating & weighting is normally not to be recommended whenever there are interdependencies between the different topics. Instead, qualitative rather than quantitative approaches to comparison are preferred.

As the method is based on a reductionistic approach, there is a danger that the aggregated conclusion for the wholeness based on individual conclusions for the component parts does not take sufficient account of mutual relations, interactions, and interdependencies.

It is important that all subareas within the solution space of a given strategy are defined in accordance with the same philosophy, value-norms, and principles.

Advice and Comments
The outcome of using the method may be combined with the *Logical Framework Approach* methodology (see separate description) for further preparation and formulation of subtasks within a solution model for a development project. Likewise, the *Logical Framework Approach* methodology may well be used to

elaborate on the description of each activity within the table, and precisely *Logical Framework Approach*'s approach for the identification of indicators and external factors may contribute to the risk management within a project.

References

Serdar Savas B. [Letter]. Copenhagen: WHO; 1994. Ref.No. KGZ/PH 201.

8. Other Useful Information

There is certain information that cannot be categorized under 'methods', but which should nevertheless be included because an understanding of these issues is valuable in an assessment context. In general, the area outlined in the table below is valid for all phases within the lifecycle.

Documentation in a Situation of Accreditation

Areas of Application

Planning of assessment activities in connection with the purchase of a 'standard' IT system, when the user organization is, or considers becoming, certified or accredited.

Note: *There is a difference in the way ISO9001 and ISO/IEC certification and accreditation work. In ISO9001 the organization itself defines the quality system and its object, whereas quality systems in, for instance, ISO/IEC 17025 standards are more fixed. Therefore, big differences may occur between quite specific demands for a given organization, so the following guidelines need to be adjusted to the actual department or hospital and its situation.*

Description

Many hospitals or hospital departments strive toward becoming accredited or certified (or they may already be so) in accordance with various quality control standards. It could, for instance, be ISO9001:2000, or ISO/IEC 15189, or 17025 (supported by national guidelines for their implementation and interpretation), or the Joint Commission on Accreditation of Healthcare Organizations. If you work toward accreditation or certification at the same time as you are about to introduce a new IT system, it is important to prepare as

227

well as possible for the planning and testing of the IT system from the start.

In this context there are a number of conditions to be aware of. The points below are drawn from the Danish version of the national guidelines supporting ISO/IEC 15189 and 17025 (see DANAK), so the reader is requested to make investigations on their specific local or national regulations and conditions. Consequently, this description can only serve as inspiration on some significant topics in one's own research for implications and assumptions.

A. There are differences in the assessment of off-the-shelf IT products (standard systems irrespective of the usual client adaptation) and that of custom-made IT systems. In the case of the latter, it is important to verify that all details work correctly and in accordance with the agreement. For the off-the-shelf system it may be sufficient to verify that all adaptations work and to verify that the system in its entirety works reliably, completely, and correctly (as per the agreement), and with an operational performance for which management can take responsibility. In other words, in standard systems there is normally no need to verify *all* details of the functionality in connection with delivery and installation of the IT systems, but one must be able to account for what has been tested, what has not been tested, and why and with what result.

B. It is not physically possible to test *everything* in connection with a technical verification of the correctness of the IT system's functionality. None of the ordinary standards, such as ISO 9001:2000, DANAK's RL10 (to support ISO/IEC 17025, for instance), or the American Joint Commission International Accreditation Standards for Hospitals, insist on a complete, detailed assessment by the client but require that the client can ascertain that everything has been tested either by the supplier or by the client.

C. In the Danish RL10 guideline there is a requirement for documentation of the test to be available, but it is not specified where and by whom this should be kept. Therefore, demands for access to the vendors' documentation of the system may arise.

D. There are no requirements for paper documentation of the test or reported errors, so this can be electronic.

E. The organizational structure and the responsibility of all parties involved must be crystal clear in relation to the operation and testing of the IT system and descriptions of procedures for reporting deviations. Delegation of tasks such as training and access control must be visible.

F. Subcontractors, including the hospital's own IT department (if they are the ones handling the technical operation of the IT system), are also subject to the requirements of DANAK's RL 10 guidelines if a user department is accredited according to the ISO/IEC 15189 or 17025 standards (see DANAK, Section 4.6.2):

> "If parts of the laboratory's computer work, for instance, back-up, are carried out by suppliers (who may be the laboratory's own computer department), the affected staff should be comprised by the relevant parts of the laboratory's quality system".

G. Assessment of an IT-based solution must include all the life cycle phases of the system, from requirements specification to phasing out. This means, for instance, that during the Explorative Phase it is necessary not only to ensure the quality of the requirements specification, but also to ensure that there is a frame of reference for later assessment, including consideration of its out-phasing or later replacement.

Assumptions for Application

People who need to handle issues of accreditation or certification in connection with an assessment project are advised to cooperate with people who are familiar with these issues; it is not difficult to deal with the accreditation issues, but one needs to know what to do.

It should also be a condition in a contractual relationship with a vendor that the vendor adheres to a given standard and/or to the terms of the client's accreditation/certification. This should be a well-defined, operational part of the contract.

Perspectives

It would quite clearly be physically impossible to test nontrivial IT systems for all details in the system in all its combinations purely because of the combinational explosion (see also under *Technical Verification*). It is therefore necessary to plan tests for the duration of its lifetime. This is not only applicable when there are new releases or version, but also when introducing functions that have not previously been used for that purpose in the organization.

Frame of Reference for Interpretation

Here the frame of reference is the actual standard.

Perils and Pitfalls

According to DANAK a possible subcontractor connected to the operation of the IT system must be the responsible to the department. This means that the department must at all times ensure that the IT system is securely tested and documented and that the operations under the subcontractor are carried out in accordance with accreditation requirements.

Advice and Comments

Conditions of great importance that need to be dealt with prior to formal testing in connection with the installation include aspects such as:

- The deviance reporting system, including:
  - Internal deviance reporting procedure(s), including:
    - Reporting systems, encompassing assessment of consequences and communication of this to those responsible for operations
    - Deviance reporting form
    - Description of who does what, who may and who must do what, how and when
  - Procedure for reporting one's own operation to the vendor and to the subcontractor, with follow-up
- Guidelines for:
  - What areas to test and criteria for acceptance
  - Protocol for the organization and contents of the test
  - Documentation of the test and its results

Furthermore, prior to taking the system into operation it is required that the following is described:

- The responsibilities of each and every organizational role player involved in the operation of the future IT system or the work procedures interacting with the IT system, including the system of registration and maintenance of competences
- The politics and procedures of the organization, including that of the document handling and configuration management

. . . and so on, describing all aspects that may influence the organization's ability to provide a flawless service.

See also under *Standards*.

References

The description above is the result of investigations by a working group concerned with accreditation and certification of the Copenhagen Hospital Co-operation's project in connection with the purchase of a Laboratory Information System, LIS-i, during the period November 2002-October 2003.

DANAK. Retningslinie RL10, Anvendelse af edb i akkrediterede laboratorier, Copenhagen: DANAK; 2002. Report No.: RL10. (in Danish)
> *(Last visited on www.danak.dk on 31.05.2005. Search for RL10).*

ISO/IEC. General requirements for the competences of testing and calibration laboratories. Geneva: ISO; 2005. Report No.: ISO/IEC 17025:2005.

ISO/IEC. Medical laboratories – Particular requirements for quality and competence. Geneva: ISO; 2003. Report No.: ISO/IEC 15189:2003.

Supplementary Reading

ISO/IEC. Information technology – open systems interconnection – conformance testing methodology and framework – Part 5: requirements on test laboratories and clients for the conformance assessment process. Geneva: ISO; 1994. Report No.: ISO/IEC 9646-5.
> *It is important to be familiar with this one in connection with testing an installed IT system prior to its operation when the organization is accredited or certified.*

Measures and Metrics

Areas of Application

Measures and metrics are used throughout the evaluation process, irrespective of whether it is constructive or summative. Planning of an assessment/evaluation study includes the conversion of an evaluation purpose to specific measures and subsequent establishment of metrics for their measurement.

> "You can't control what you can't measure. In most disciplines, the strong linkage between measurement and control is taken for granted."

(Shepperd and Ince 1993)

Note: 'Measures and metrics' is not a method, but it has been included in the Handbook of Evaluation Methods *because planning of an assessment/evaluation study includes precisely that of converting specific measures and then finding metrics for the measurement of each of them.*

Note: It does not make sense to talk about the use of resources in this context because this depends on which metrics and measures are chosen and combined for use in a specific method for a given study.

Description

There is a whole range of different measures and metrics, and many of them have been investigated in a number of standards. The problem with them is that as a whole they have been designed with technical people rather than the end user in mind. Nevertheless, they can be used as inspiration because if you understand a concept, it will often also have an analogous meaning for its day-to-day user.

Examples of measures (see references for details and specific metrics) are shown in the list below, where measures are partly converted to something relevant for the end user but without losing their original meaning. One must be aware that each of them can be made up of many submeasures before one gets an adequately full picture of a system's qualities.

- *Objectives Fulfillment*: The degree of fulfillment of the users' objectives when introducing a given IT system (see Brender and

McNair 2001) This measure consist of a great many of the following points, depending on the defined objectives of the system (see also the *Functionality Assessment* method).

- *Response Time*: This measure for system performance is normally used in the concept of 'the time elapsed from the moment the user presses the send button until an answer *starts* to appear on the screen'. Typically it is the response time that is used to measure the performance of an IT system, but there is another type of response time called 'throughput', which must not be forgotten.

- *Throughput*: 'The length of time from when a user (or another IT-based system) initiates an activity for the IT system to carry out until it is actually completed'. One example is the time lapse from a clinical user making an order for a blood test until this information is available to technicians in the laboratory concerned. Another example is the time lapse from the moment a technician approves an acute result in the laboratory until the answer reaches the patient's clinic. Although the data handling is electronic, it does not necessarily mean that it only takes seconds, like for the response time.

- *User Satisfaction*: This is directly related to the individual user groups' subjective opinion of the system. Please refer to the methods *Questionnaires* and *Interviews*, respectively, as they are the most commonly used methods to measure user satisfaction.

- *Usability* (see separate section): This has a number of subheadings, such as:
  - *Understandability*: The ease with which an IT system can be understood by the user (intuitively or explicitly with the aid instructions) to enable the user to utilize the system for a specific activity in a given context
  - *Learnability*: The level of training needed before a user can operate the IT system faultlessly
  - *Operability*: The ease with which the IT system to be operated by a user
  - *Usability compliance*: The degree of compliance with given standards for the design of user interfaces

- *Copability*: This measure is related to the individual user's ability to cope with his or her situation given the availability of a knowledge-based management tool – for instance, aimed at the management of diabetes (Boisen et al. 2003). It is closely related to *Usability* and *Utility* and varies as a function of learning the system's functionality.

- *Suitability*: The capacity to execute and support in a satisfactory way, a set of functions needed by a user to complete a specific action.

- *Functionality Compliance*: This corresponds fairly closely to a similar medical concept – that is, the capacity to function in accordance with a prescribed standard, which in this case could be a technical standard, the law, a single requirement, or even a requirements specification.

- *Accuracy*: The ability to convey the right (or the agreed) result of a transaction, for instance, an e-mail system sends an e-mail to the right (specified) recipient, or that as a user you get the same output on a given input every time. This measure may be used in its general form, and in particular it may be used to assess the accuracy of expert systems or decision-support systems. See, for instance, the overview in (Smith et al. 2003) and the section *Clinical/Diagnostic Performance.*

- *Precision*: The ability to deliver the same result from repeated measurements. The same is the case for this measure as for the previous one, so refer to the overview in (Smith et al. 2003).

- *Interconnectivity*: Technical (syntactic) aspects of communication between several IT-based systems.

- *Interoperability*: Semantic aspects of the interaction (cooperation) between several IT-based systems. For instance, when a patient's hospital address is changed in the patient administration system, its impact has to be immediately implemented throughout all the IT systems that are connected, such as the laboratory system or the X-ray system, so that the report to a service order will be sent to the relevant address(es).

- *Security*: The ability to protect data and information from unauthorized access.

- *Reliability*: The probability that an IT system's software works without interruption (breakdown) for a specified period of time and under specified conditions. Some submeasures include:
  - *Maturity*: that the IT system is free of programming errors so that there is no downtime because of them
  - *Fault Tolerance*: that the IT system as a whole can carry on working even if errors occur in one aspect of the functionality
  - *Fail-safe*: the ability to handle erroneous data in a sensible way. One example of an assessment in this context is the 'monkey test' – that is, when you get somebody with no experience of the IT system to use it
  - *Recoverability*: the ability to reestablish the normal level of performance and accuracy of data after a system breakdown with/without the intervention of an operator or vendor

- *Viability*: The ability to adapt to new conditions. The healthcare sector is constantly exposed to new initiatives and regulations, the development of new methods, and new IT systems that the old systems have to be made to communicate with. Therefore, it is important that implementation of changes can be carried out with minimal vendor assistance (i.e., *flexibility*), that it does not cost a fortune when software changes eventually have to be made (*maintainability*), and that one does not depend on the opinion and prioritization of several hundred other clients.
- *Testability*: The ability to enable the conduct of tests that simulate real operation without impacting on it.

Assumptions for Application

Measures and metrics are not in themselves difficult to work with, but each metric and measure has its individual assumption for application. The decision lies in which types of statistical methods to choose, for example, for the calculation and analysis because of the need by some methods for normally distributed data or independence between measures, and so forth.

User imagination is a requirement in order to correlate the measures to the purpose of the assessment task and the ability and experience to (re-)define each metric for the current practical application.

Some of the measures require technical insight and an understanding of the assumptions and pitfalls of the measures.

Perspectives

On the face of it, one would think that the perspective in relation to metrics and measures is that all the relevant measures can be expressed by a formula – that is, the metric, irrespective of whether the qualities measured are subjective or objective. Nevertheless, remember that methods and techniques can be so simple as to make it difficult to call them methods and techniques. Just think of the printed instructions on a carton of juice for how to open it.

Even the esthetics of an object can be expressed in operational measures – for instance, whether the beholder likes it (on a scale from 'repugnant' to 'irresistible') – as a subjective and intuitive measure (as opposed to formal). In terms of esthetics the metric is implicit, and it will require experts in a number of domains to even start to understand the perception of esthetics. However, one thing is certain: We will all be able to express our esthetic opinion of an object. It can be measured although the metric is informal!

Thus, there is nothing to stop us from defining metrics for the whole range of subjective and objective measures and their corresponding metrics. The point of subjective measures and metrics is that metrologically it is more difficult to get reliable results, and therefore people find it hard to accept them.

Frame of Reference for Interpretation

The frame of reference depends on the actual measures and metrics, and if they do have a frame of reference, it is described together with the metric.

Perils and Pitfalls

Every single metric and measure has pitfalls and perils, and it is necessary to assess these on an individual basis.

Advice and Comments

-

References

Boisen E, Byghold A, Cavan D, Hejlesen OK. Copability, coping, and learning as focal concepts in the evaluation of computerised diabetes disease management. Int J Med Inform 2003;70:353-63.

Brender J, McNair P. User requirements specifications: a hierarchical structure covering strategical, tactical and operational requirements. Int J Med Inform 2001;64(2-3):83-98.

Shepperd M, Ince D. Derivation and validation of software metrics. International Series of Monographs on Computer Science. Oxford: Clarendon Press; 1990. vol 9.

Smith AE, Nugent CD, McClean SI. Evaluation of inherent performance of intelligent medical decision support systems: utilizing neural networks as an example. Int J Med Inform 2003;27:1-27.

Supplementary Reading

DeChant HK, Tohme WG, Mun SK, Hayes WS, Schulman KA. Health systems evaluation of telemedicine: a staged approach. Telemed J 1996;2(4):303-12

The article is useful as inspiration regarding measures during the different phases of the system, from measuring efficacy during the early operational phase to measuring overall validity in its wider use.

Fraser JM, Smith PJ. A catalogue of errors. Int J Man-Machine Stud 1992;37:265-307.

This article reviews and discusses a number of biases and errors described in the literature and compares human performance with known norms of probabilities in statistically conditioned results, causal relations and logical conclusions.

Heathfield H, Clamp S, Felton D. PROBE project review and objective evaluation for electronic patient and health record projects. UK Institute of Health Informatics; 2001. Report No.: 2001-IA-611.

The purpose of this report is to guide those involved in an EHR. Appendix C contains a list of potential measures and where to get them as well as some relevant methods for their measurement.

Jeanrenaud A, Romanazzi P. Software product evaluation metrics: a methodological approach. In: Ross M, Brebbia CA, Staples G, Stapleton J, editors. Proceedings of the Software Quality Management II Conference "Building Quality into Software". Southampton: Comp. Mech. Publications; 1994. p. 59-69.

Sullivan F, Mitchell E. Has general practitioner computing made a difference to patient care? a systematic review of published reports. BMJ 1995;311:848-52.

A meta-analysis of 21 studies of the implication of practice systems in general practice –that is, a lead in to the many different ways of studying (measures and metrics of) largely equal systems.

Also see under *Standards*, for instance:

BIPM, IEC, IFCC, ISO, IUPAC, IUPAP, OILM. International vocabulary of basic and general terms in metrology. Geneva: ISO; 1993.

IEEE. IEEE standard for a software quality metrics methodology. New York: IEEE; 1992. Report No.: 1061-1992.

ISO/IEC. Information technology – software product evaluation – quality characteristics and guidelines for their use. 1st ed. Geneva: ISO; 1991. Report No.: ISO 9126-1991 (E).

Standards

Areas of Application

A number of de fakto and de jure standards exist, which each define a series of issues, like the contents of a User Requirements Specification, verification of an IT system, quality aspects of an IT system, as well as roles and relations between a user organization and a vendor in connection with assessment. They are an important foundation for work in an assessment context – for instance:

- IEEE 1061 deals with *Measures and Metrics*; for more details, see the separate section on this topic in this handbook.
- IEEE 1059 concerns elements that need to be included in the planning of an assessment activity. This should be used as inspiration right from the start of an IT project.
- IEEE 830 goes through a number of quality aspects for a requirements specification, which is highly relevant when the requirements specification functions as frame of reference for later assessment activities.
- ISO 9126 lists quality properties for an IT system; see also under *Measures and Metrics*.
- ISO 9646-5 contains a description of the roles and the interaction between the user organization and the vendor in connection with testing. Extremely relevant for those who are already accredited or certified.
- ISO 14598-1 is a key standard – that is, it defines the terminology and the relationships between the remaining standards in the series and ISO 9126. Furthermore, it contains the most important requirements for specifying and evaluation of IT systems.
- ISO/TC 212 points to a number of circumstances one should keep in mind in connection with assessments, including a checklist for assessing a requirements specification under preparation, planning of test activities, and assessing an offer or bid from a supplier.

Additionally there are also:

- FDA's guidelines for assessing medical equipment (*General principles of software validation . . .* 2002).

Description

There are a number of formal international standardization

organizations in addition to the national ones, which are often affiliated to trade organizations. ISO is the independent international one, CEN is the European standardization organization, and DS the corresponding Danish organization, while IEEE is the standardization organization under the Institute of Electrical and Electronics Engineers, Inc.

NOTE: *Assessment of resource requirements refers to the fact that it is usually a big job to understand the details and follow a standard instead of performing the same task in the 'usual way' or intuitively.*

Assumptions for Application

Generally speaking, standards are heavy reading because the writing is extremely compressed. They are written for specialists in the respective target areas. Some assumptions, therefore, may be hidden between the lines, and all explanatory text is omitted. In other words, experience is needed to find all the details and particularly to discover the implicit assumptions and consequences.

Perspectives

In general terms these standards are technology-oriented rather than user-oriented. But they are certainly worth going through as they provide much inspiration and can be used as checklists for a number of analysis, design, and specification tasks.

Frame of Reference for Interpretation

The standards are in themselves a frame of reference for a range of assessment activities.

Perils and Pitfalls

Precisely because these standards are technology-oriented, they should not be followed uncritically – or, rather, to make do with them alone – but use them as inspiration or as checklists and frames of reference, when, for instance, preparing a requirements specification.

New versions of the old standards and completely new standards are continuously being published. Therefore, one must keep up to date with what standards of relevance there are for one's own purpose – for example, via the standardization organizations' websites.

Advice and Comments

-

References

General principles of software validation; final guidance for industry and FDA staff. Food and Drug Administration, U.S. Department of Health and Human Services. 2002. *(Last seen on www.fda.gov/cdrh/comp/guidance/938.html, 31.05.2005)*

IEEE. IEEE guide for software verification and validation plans. New York: IEEE; 1994. Report No.: 1059-1993.

IEEE. IEEE recommended practice for software requirements specifications. New York: IEEE; 1993. Report No.: 830-1984.

IEEE. IEEE standard for a software quality metrics methodology. New York: IEEE; 1992. Report No.: 1061-1992.

ISO/IEC. Information technology – software product evaluation – part 1: general overview. Geneva: ISO; 1999. Report No.: ISO/IEC 14598-1.

ISO/IEC. Information technology – software product evaluation – quality characteristics and guidelines for their use. 1st ed. 1991-12-15. Geneva: ISO; 1991;ISO 9126-1991 (E).

ISO/IEC. Information technology – open systems interconnection – conformance testing methodology and framework – Part 5: requirements on test laboratories and clients for the conformance assessment process. Geneva: ISO; 1994. Report No.: ISO/IEC 9646-5.

ISO/TC. Laboratory information systems. Geneva: ISO. 1998. Report No.: ISO/TC 212/WG1 N41 Annex A.
(The sign 'TC 212/WG1 N41' means that this document is still the working document of a working group preparing the standard in question.)

Check current standards on the relevant websites:

(Please note that these links are just to the home pages of the organizations. From there you have to search their sites for any possible material of relevance.)

http://www.iso.ch/iso/en/ISOOnline.frontpage

(last visited 31.05.2005)

http://www.ds.dk
(last visited 31.05.2005)

http://www.ansi.org/
(last visited 31.05.2005)

http://standards.ieee.org/
(last visited 31.05.2005)

http://www.cenorm.be/
(last visited 31.05.2005)

Part III: Methodological and Methodical Perils and Pitfalls at Assessment

The number of experimental perils and pitfalls is scary. Nevertheless, within the literature on assessment of IT-based systems and solutions, sample cases were identified for most of them. The topic is simply too complicated, so one has to keep a number of details in mind all the time.

One further lesson gained from application of the framework is that experience with technology assessment within the medical domain does not necessarily suffice for exhaustive assessment of IT-based solutions. Therefore, prior, extended experience with assessment of IT-based solutions is needed for the planning and accomplishment of major assessment studies in healthcare informatics and telecommunication studies. Another experience is that application of the framework does not rule out the need for senior analytical experience on assessment studies.

In summary, the contribution of the framework is that of putting contents and structure to a meta-analysis, so the framework serves as a checklist of issues to be taken into account when planning or auditing an assessment study.

9. Background Information

The objective of the present part is to explore, whether known pitfalls and perils from other domains have analogues in the domain of assessment of IT-based solutions and to illustrate these flaws with examples from the medical informatics literature. A subsequent aim is to let the outcome of the analysis serve as a means for performing meta-analysis of assessment studies focused at the validity of such studies. The emphasis is on methodological and methodical issues within assessment studies and the interpretation of their outcome, and specifically on identification of pitfalls and perils in assessing IT-based solutions. Furthermore, the emphasis is entirely on the users' assessment of an IT-based system or an IT-based solution rather than on the developers' (technical) verification of the system.

The specific background of the present framework was the author's task as quality manager within the CANTOR (HC4003) Healthcare Telematics Project to perform a meta-analysis of a number of formal assessment studies, with the scope of learning from errors and problems. Given the preconditions of the active engagement within the project, collaboration with colleagues all over Europe, and the need to be objective and fair in the critique, while being exhaustive in the elicitation of lessons, it was necessary to develop an objective tool for the execution of this analysis task. This was accomplished and has been reported in (Brender 2001) in terms of the basic framework for meta-analysis of assessment studies together with its application on eight internal project assessment studies. The framework proved valuable for its intended purpose. Given the confidential nature of the proprietary software developed by the CANTOR project and the corresponding internal project assessment studies, there was unfortunately little that could be shared with a general audience. It was, therefore, decided to make further abstractions of the framework, in order to make it generally applicable for HTA studies, and then to apply it to the literature on assessment studies as a pilot verification.

Paradigmatic perils and pitfalls were searched for in the scientific literature. Within HTA studies in general, the effect that is searched for is often marginal but tangible, while for studies in other disciplines this may be substantial but elusive. Consequently, when analyzing for a given type of error known from another research field, it is necessary to make projections of the type of error described to see if an analogue may exist, and then search for sample cases within the literature.

The outcome was originally published as an internal project report in 2002 and later as a slightly refined version in (Brender 2003) which was also distributed at the HIS-EVAL workshop that led to the Innsbruck Declaration (see Ammenwerth et al. 2004). This present version is again slightly refined and updated.

9.1 Perspectives

To clarify the line of reasoning and the value norms behind the present framework, it is valuable to reiterate the perspectives of the author. For further details, see Section 2.4 in Part I.

> *"A perspective does not determine the answers to design questions but guides design by generating the questions to be considered"*
>
> (Winograd & Flores, cited by Kukla et al. 1992)

That is, a perspective is a holistic view on attributes and cause-effect relations within a system. The concept of 'perspective' (for a system development method) has been defined as *"assumptions on the nature of the working processes and how people interact in an organizational setting"* (Mathiassen and Munk-Madsen 1986). In a generalized version, the perspective is the implicit assumptions on (cause-effect relations within) the object of study. So a perspective is that aggregation of (conscious or unconscious, epistemological) assumptions of how things relate in combination with imprinted attitudes, which guides our decision making – for example, in a problem-solving situation (Brender 1999). Here, the object of study is assessment studies.

A few perspectives specifically regarding the development of the present framework shall be emphasized as follows:

First, contrary to domains like physics and chemistry, the domain of assessment of IT-based solutions is still emerging, and so is that of system development – at least for state-of-the-market when concerned with solutions that have a significant organizational element. Consequently, it is to be expected that a large number of trials and errors will occur, and one cannot blame the authors for the large number of experimental errors that stick out within the literature. There are only few cases where an IT system works perfectly and in full compliance with the needs of its organizational environment. Consequently, both the organization and the IT system have to mutually adapt pre- and postoperation. Moreover, technology evolves, but even worse is that the healthcare domain also evolves rapidly, and the IT-based solutions have to adapt accordingly. These concerns do not rule out the feasibility of assessment. It just means that one may have to freeze the intended adaptations during the assessment period to achieve a snapshot of the issue in focus. However, this strictly means that following a (short) period, the assessment conclusion may no longer be valid.

Second, a message from a study is not necessarily valid just because someone has made the effort to publish the results and has taken the responsibility as author(s), or it may be valid only in certain respects or to a certain level of significance. Neither does a statement from the authors that the method or the results "are validated" suffice if documentation is not provided. It may certainly be valid within the authors' context for their purpose, at their level of professional competence, or whatever but at the same time it may definitely not be valid otherwise. The reader is encouraged to make his or her own judgment.

Third, it is considered a rule of thumb that a work worth publishing has to be described *"in sufficient detail to permit its exact replication, the provision of information on its reproducibility (precision), and interpretation (inter- and intraobserver variation) and both how and whether 'normal' was defined"* (Jaeschke and Sackett 1989). In other words, it must be explained so others can repeat a study experimentally for verification purposes or for their own evaluation purpose. Otherwise, an assessment report will add little to the progress (maturation) of assessment as a domain and only contribute in terms of the authors' curriculum vitae and publication list. This is an element in rigorous scientific approaches. Even if the very strict demands in (Jaeschke and Sackett 1989) may not be feasible to fulfill in all cases, the scientific criteria do constitute a recommended target for scientific publications. However, this does not rule out the practical value of pragmatic and down-to-earth assessments.

Fourth, few assessment methods are well documented, mature, and proven valid and reproducible. Methods like the *Randomized Controlled Trials* (RCT) from the healthcare domain are promoted without fully acknowledging the difference in nature from medical and pharmaceutical technology to IT-based solutions that have a strong element of behavioral and other soft issues.

Fifth, this Part of the book primarily addresses measures of the effect (value or worth) of IT-based systems/solutions and excludes, for instance, economic aspects as an explicitly addressed topic. Moreover, it focuses entirely on assessment from a user perspective and excludes the developers' own technical assessment (benchmarking, debugging, . . .). It also excludes a distinction between different purposes for performing the assessment of a given IT-based solution, such as exploring its characteristics, evaluating its characteristics, or validating them.

Finally, rigorous scientific approaches must also be strived at within the domain of assessment in order to be able to convey messages with confidence. This is, of course, debatable. In practice, purely qualitative and/or subjective studies and other studies suffering from a number of the listed pitfalls and perils may still be of practical value within their own context: Those performing the assessment have an intention with the study (why else invest the resources?) and an intended use of the study outcome. What shall be debated in this respect is the appearance of studies within the literature, which don't contribute with a message to the audience. The literature should include only that which is solidly demonstrated as valid information and hence useful to others.

10. Approach to Identification of Pitfalls and Perils

A bias – *"the arrival at a conclusion that differs systematically from the truth"* (Jaeschke and Sackett 1989; Altman et al. 2001) – is the result of one or more experimental flaws within the design, accomplishment, or interpretation of the assessment study.

> *"What is required . . . is the recognition of potential confounders, followed by the incorporation of specific research design (or "architectural") strategies to reduce their impact and thus avoid bias."*

(Jaeschke and Sackett 1989).

> *"Bias is usually defined as a prejudice or partiality, whether conscious or not. This is in contrast to systematic error where no prejudice exists".*

(DeMets 1997)

In this paper, emphasis is on addressing all kinds of (unintentional) biases *and* systematic errors – together called 'pitfalls and perils'.

In order to achieve a candidate list of experimental flaws at assessment of IT-based solutions in healthcare, a synthesis and an abstraction was made on literature's description of paradigmatic experimental perils and pitfalls within medical science, natural science, and social science. Sources of inspiration are numerous; nevertheless, the main ones remain the following review papers: (Jaeschke and Sackett 1989; Wyatt and Spiegelhalter 1991; Fraser and Smith 1992; Sher and Trull 1996; Friedman and Wyatt 1997; and Coolican 1999). These reviews address different experimental approaches like field studies, cohort studies and case studies. Wyatt and Spiegelhalter (1991) explicitly and only address the experimental pitfalls and perils at the assessment of knowledge-based decision-support systems, comprising a specific subset of IT-based systems. The detailed interpretation of the meaning of each pitfall and peril within the original context as well as further examples are to be found in the original references.

The rationale of the basic approach has been to make a structured framework to enable and structure a fair and comparable analysis, based on scientific principles and documented knowledge. The structure was developed as an analogue to the SWOT technique by inclusion of a large number of experimental perils and pitfalls reported in scientific literature.

The sole purpose of the framework is that of structuring the information seeking and analysis to secure an objective analysis. The framework is inspired by and structured as analogous to a SWOT analysis, while a transformation of the four main concepts of a SWOT analysis has been turned into similar concepts of particular relevance for assessment studies. The framework was applied for verification purposes on a number of assessment studies within the CANTOR (HC4003) Healthcare Telematics Project under the EU Commission's Fourth Framework Programme, based on artificial experimental setups. Following the application in CANTOR, the framework was refined to accommodate the experiences achieved.

Finally, a review of case studies reported in the literature has been completed to add published examples to the identified types of flaws, thereby making it plausible whether analogies exist between the known types of experimental flaws and those observed in the literature on real-life assessment of IT-based solutions in healthcare. Within this process the contents of the framework was gradually refined and incrementally extended to accommodate new types of flaws identified.

An extensive search of methods and methodologies as well as case studies on assessment of IT-based system/solutions was accomplished previously; see (Brender 1997a, 1998, and 1999). The strategy then was to search for all combinations of concepts of 'assessment' (with synonyms: technology assessment, evaluation, verification, and validation), 'computer system' (with synonyms: IT, IT system, computer, computer-based system), 'methods' and 'methodologies', and 'case studies'. This search strategy was supplemented by search on a number of key players of the domain. The literature databases searched were PubMed and INSPECT, plus relevant databases of the local research libraries. Also included in the original literature study were two extensive databases of relevant literature that were acquired specifically for the assessment of knowledge-based systems and decision-support systems; see (O'Moore et al. 1990b; and Talmon and van der Loo 1995).

The above literature study was repeated to find newer cases and methods, with extensive use of PubMed's facility 'related references' for key papers, explicit search on authors of notable papers, and elicitation of key references from the notable papers. In case of difficulty in retrieving a paper, little effort was put into pursuing short publications (i.e., 2-4 pages), like proceeding papers. The reason being a general experience of lack of sufficient detail of the method and description of the results for the present purpose.

By application of this repeated and multiapproach strategy, the likelihood of the completeness of the framework being rather exhaustive with respect to types of experimental errors is rather high and depends mainly on the author's ability to identify all relevant (types of) flaws.

However, please note that reporting within this publication only includes examples of the best cases and bad examples to learn from or otherwise particularly relevant or paradigmatic examples out of the bulk of publications acquired. Thus, this publication does not reference the entirety of literature on assessment studies.

11. Framework for Meta-Assessment of Assessment Studies

The steps in the meta-analysis of an assessment study are as follows, based on the contents in Table 11.1: First, each element within the checklist of issues indicated under Strengths and Weaknesses is carefully searched for and analyzed in the mentioned order. To conclude that a given strength is absent or a weakness is present is a serious matter, and if found true, this may lead to the conclusion that the outcome of the assessment study in question is less reliable, if not more or less invalid. Therefore, an aspect identified as problematic unquestionably has to be argued and documented. This may be achieved by means of a list of associated notes, called "List of Clarification Points". Less certain problematic aspects may be indicated as question marks or by means of correspondingly weak phrases or statements.

Second, a cautious causal analysis might be accomplished to reveal as many as possible of the underlying perspectives and premises for the assessment study under investigation. Still, the scope of the present framework is not to support a full-scale causal analysis to identify the underlying cause-effect relations, even if it might bring forward further information to compensate for the problems already found. The reason is that one can only to some extent judge beyond the written text and into the information that lies between the lines. If decided upon, a causal analysis may be accomplished by means of approaches, ranging from simple ad hoc techniques or reviewing approaches to strictly formal methods digging into the raw material of the study or otherwise exploring the problem area. The purpose of such a step would be to rigorously document intimidations toward the study's own conclusion and the potential opportunities for resolving the problems identified. Moreover, the efforts to be invested in such a step shall naturally depend on the reviewer's role in relation to the assessment study (reader, auditor, decision maker or other user).

Finally, the entirety of information elicited for the assessment study is synthesized into a conclusion on the validity of the outcome and the authors' own conclusion through the topics listed under Opportunities and Threats within Table 11.1.

Table 11.1: Checklist of issues to take into consideration for an analysis of assessment studies.

Ratings for Strengths, Opportunities, and Threats are of a textual kind – mainly "Yes" and "No". Ratings for the individual Strengths and Weaknesses are: '+++' = "obstructive bias of this type apparently present"; '++' = "significant confounding factor of this type apparently present"; '+' = "minor confounding factor of this type found"; '-' = "no confounding factor seems to be present of this type, or it has been properly dealt with by the study team"; '?' = "not identifiable from the text".

SWOT Concept	Issues of concern	Study Rating

Strengths (explicitness of fault-preventive measures and initiatives within the study)	S1) Circumscription of study objectives
	   i) Delimitation of the investigation space
	   ii) Ambiguous or changing study objectives
	   iii) Stakeholder analysis
	   iv) Targeting the methodology/method to the study aim
	
	S2) Selecting the study methodology/method
	   i) Subjectivity versus objectivity
	   ii) Assumptions for methods' application
	   iii) Application range
	   iv) Circular inference
	
	S3) Defining methods and materials
	   i) Construct validity of methods, techniques, and tools
	   ii) Prophylactic grounding
	   iii) Prognostic measures
	
	S4) (User) recruitment
	   i) Diagnostic suspicion
	   ii) The (un-)used user
	
	S5) (Case) recruitment
	   i) More than one population included as the subject of investigation
	   ii) Compliance between application domain and target domain
	   iii) Use of artificial scenarios or setup
	
	S6) Frame of reference
	   i) Placebo effect
	   ii) Hawthorne effect
	   iii) Co-intervention
	   iv) Before-and-after study
	   v) Carryover effect
	   vi) Checklist effect
	   vii) Human cognition/recognition of cases
	   viii) Usability and user acceptability
	   ix) (Adverse) confounding effects	

	S7) Outcome measures or end-points	
	i) Constructive assessment	
	ii) The substitution game	
	iii) Complex causal relations	
	iv) Comparing apples and pears	
	v) Technical verification of outcome measures	
	S8) Aspects of culture	
Weaknesses (perils and pitfalls that should be considered at the study design or interpretation)	W1) The developer's actual engagement	
	i) Beyond the developer's point of view	
	ii) Unstable technology	
	W2) Intra- and Interperson (or -case) variability	
	W3) Illicit use	
	i) Assessment bias	
	ii) Evaluation paradox	
	W4) Feed-back effect	
	W5) Extra work	
	W6) Judgmental biases	
	i) Hindsight or insight bias	
	ii) Judgment of the probability of events	
	iii) Judgment of performance	
	iv) Miscellaneous judgmental biases	
	W7) Postrationalization	
	W8) Verification of implicit assumptions	
	i) Matching of study and control groups	
	ii) Implicit domain assumptions	
	W9) Novelty of the technology – technophile or technophobe	
	W10) Spontaneous regress	
	W11) False conclusions	
	i) False-negative studies	
	ii) False-positive studies	
	iii) Competing risks	
	W12) Incomplete studies or study reports	
	i) A publication dilemma	
	ii) The intention to provide information	
	iii) Presentation of the future	
	iv) Exhaustion of the data material	
	W13) Hypothesis fixation	
	i) Publication bias	
	ii) Randomized controlled trials	
	iii) Action-case research	
	W14) The intention to treat principle	

	i) Constructive assessment	
	ii) Action-case research	
	W15) Impact	
Opportunities (options for elicitation of (partial) validity of conclusion despite problems identified)	O1) Retrospective exploration of the existing data material	
	O2) Remedying problems identified – beyond the existing data material	
	i) Triangulation	
Threats (risk assessment regarding obstruction of conclusion)	T1) Compensation for problems	
	T2) Pitfalls and perils	
	T3) Validity of the study conclusion	

Shading a cell in the table column 'Study rating' may be applied to indicate that the issue of concern is "not applicable for the study in question". Similarly, a number in this column shall refer to an item on a numbered list of notes following the table (List of Clarification Points), with the purpose of documenting and discussing a given problem.

Note that the review process reported below nowhere includes the second step, as the purpose was not to dissect case studies within the assessment literature, but to find illustrative examples.

When viewed in a Quality Management perspective, Strengths address flaws that typically are implemented at the strategic level planning. Weaknesses indicate flaws implemented at tactical or operational levels of planning and interpretation stages. Opportunities address the feasibility of and opportunity to alleviate problems identified during a follow-up at the tactical level. Threats address the conclusions on global validity at the strategic level of the follow-up. However, these distinctions are implemented in the table without making the details explicit to the reader, as it is merely a practical basis for structuring the technique and for securing completeness and consistency.

Strengths are characteristics built into the overall study design, corresponding to the basics of planning, plus explicitness of fault-preventive measures/initiatives within the study design. Similarly, Weaknesses are related to the actual implementation of the study and include an inventory of perils/pitfalls to look for within the data collection, analysis, and interpretation. When looked at in practical terms, Strengths are aspects that one would normally expect to be described primarily in a Methods & Materials section, while Weaknesses to a larger extent would appear from a Results section. In particular there is a strong correlation between the different aspects of Strength and Weaknesses within the above

SWOT-variant approach: a nonfulfilled Strength aspect may imply a severe Weakness, and most Weaknesses may be prevented by awareness during the design of the assessment study, and thus serve as Strengths.

Opportunities are concerned with options for problem solving – that is, extension of data analysis or further data collection to recognize and/or remedy identified problems. Then, Threats will constitute the overall risk judgment of the study under analysis, with the purpose of validating whether, given the problems and options identified, the study's conclusion fulfills the study objectives or whether there are biases severe enough to obstruct the conclusion. In practical terms, Opportunities are dedicated to attempts to explore a combination of the sections of Methods and Materials and the Results to see what might exist that is not presented. Finally, Threats will analyze the entirety, reflecting the Discussion section in this part of the *Handbook of Evaluation Methods*.

The following discusses the four aspects in more detail.

11.1 Types of (Design) Strengths

The list of issues under 'Strengths' emphasizes characteristics built into the overall study design with the scope of exploring whether a number of known pitfalls and perils are present. Therefore, one would normally find these in the descriptions within a Methods and Materials section. Included in this topic are issues relating to circumscription of the task, focusing of the objective(s), analyzing preconditions, establishing the methodology and selecting the global set of methods and techniques to be applied.

11.1.1 *Circumscription of Study Objectives*

First of all, one has to ask the question "What is the scope of the study?" Is the case study report written to convince someone of the qualities of a given system (a marketing objective), or to present the value of a given development or assessment approach (a scientific objective), or just to fulfill a contractual/political obligation? Who is the target reader? Do you write to convince yourself, to justify resources spent, or to bring a message for others to learn from?

Unclear objectives or hidden agendas for an assessment study may compromise or squeeze the assessment activities into one particular structure rather than design a dedicated approach for each of the questions asked. Dedicated assessment approaches – all things being equal – are normally the more efficient and/or effective approaches.

11.1.1.1 Delimitation of the Investigation Space

Often, the objectives of a study imply a huge investigation space, like "measuring the effect of . . .". In such a case, it is important to make explicit what the actual focus shall be, in a way that is well balanced with the stated objectives.

It is indeed appropriate to have a broad scope as a starting point, but it should be boiled down to something practical, or the message may be lost in a mist of data and information. The bias in this respect is concerned with the inability to provide a clear and focused answer to the information needs expressed in the global question.

One way to boil down a broad scope to something feasible is to take a hierarchical approach to the formulation of the study objective. This is clearly done and reported in the study of Østbye et al. (1997), though not formulated that way: Their motivation explicitly states an interest in determining the future dissemination strategy of the IT system (for penetration of the market) and to *"gain experience with a variety of evaluation methods to be used in similar, future studies"*. This leads to its overall aim *"to identify and quantify important effects of . . ."*, which again was immediately boiled down to the study's overall aim *"the focus of the study was on the benefits of these functions to the users, . . ."*. Thereby, they circumscribe the task implicitly (excluding the adverse effects) and explicitly (excluding the economic costs). All of this is comparable to the definition of the objective at a strategic level. The implementation of the methodological approach in terms of methods, metrics, and measures constitutes an operationalisation of the study at a tactical level, while the practical implementation of the study in terms of work procedures and prescriptions is perceived as the operational level planning. All three levels are described in an abstract and concrete way, and implementations and further delimitations are nicely argued in their 'Materials and Methods' section. From this perspective, the study is convincing, although only a very few measures are used to explore the strategic and tactical level objectives. So far, so good, but at the end of the paper a third objective suddenly appears: *"One of the high-level objectives of the study was to "contribute to the establishment of an evaluation culture at the Central Hospital.""* One might call it a hidden agenda, although in this case, it is of a constructive type. Nevertheless, even if there may not be a conflict in the present case, ambiguous study objectives or multiple objectives are normally not to be recommended (Jaeschke and Sackett 1989).

The study of Crist-Grundman et al. (1995) addresses four questions in their (formative) evaluation:

1. How can nursing practice be supported?
2. What are the implications of nursing participation?

3. Which areas of nursing practice are impacted?"
4. Is there evidence that the system provides a powerful new tool to improve quality and continuity of care?

Each of these four study objectives is huge, and none of them is even discussed in the paper, which actually provides a fair amount of detail on what has been done. This brings us to a question about the meaning of the term 'evaluation', which is so often used at random within the literature. In short, evaluation is the act of measuring quality characteristics[9], which is precisely what Crist-Grundman et al. (1995) do: The study provides examples of their findings and argues these findings but provides no measures, in compliance with their intension of a formative development. Still, even if the study has to be interpreted as an explorative study applying formative assessment, it has insufficient detail on measures to provide convincing evidence toward a reader as regards the conclusions on such huge study questions.

11.1.1.2 *Ambiguous or Changing Study Objectives*

Jaeschke and Sackett (1989) state that failure to identify whether a study is asking an explanatory, a pragmatic, or a treatment question may be fatal to both the internal validity and generalisability. Similarly, it may be perilous to not be aware of whether the study is a feasibility study, a pilot study, or an exhaustive study. Even worse (for summative assessments as opposed to constructive assessment), there may be attempts to shift from the one to the other – at any stage from designing to writing the conclusion on the outcome. In constructive assessment, changes of objectives (for instance, represented in terms of a user requirements specification or similar agreement) are the rule, being executed in a needs-driven fashion that reflects the changing needs, constraints, and conditions. Any study design has to take subtle account of the constraints and preconditions, and this normally has to be openly presented in a report on the study in order to enable a fair judgment by its audience.

A change of focus was not explicitly observed anywhere within the literature. That is, no one confessed, neither explicitly nor implicitly. Nevertheless, quite a large number of publications on assessment of IT-based systems appear as mere 'add-on' (summative) assessment studies for which the outcome won't make any difference or will imply only small changes to the system or project.

A prime example of a study with a meta-perspective on what they are doing and how the assessment works within the entirety is (Gordon and Geiger 1999). They hypothesize that a *"Balanced Scorecard methodology would provide an effective framework . . . to manage implementation of an EPR"* and monitors its role and

---

[9] See the formal definition of *evaluation* in Part I.

success within the implementation project in terms of a number of performance measures linked to each of the objectives while triangulating measures to explore the validity of the hypothesis originally stated.

11.1.1.3 Stakeholder Analysis

The omission of a stakeholder analysis may severely bias an assessment. One example given in (Brender 1997a) may illustrate this: At the design and development of an electronic healthcare record for anaesthesia meant for medical preconsultation prior to operation, the user requirements were elicited from the anaesthesiologists. However, while the nurses were implicitly expected to add specific patient information, they were never asked for contributions or comments to the requirements specification. So when the prototype system was ready for assessment, the nurses refused to operate the system ("it is not our system!"). A simple stakeholder analysis might have resulted in the involvement of the nurses as well and thus avoided the conflict situation.

By coincidence, the author of the present report was recently, within two months, among those attending two presentations of the same EHR system. As none of these presentations are documented in detail in the literature, this example shall only serve as an illustration: The individual responsible for the assessment of the system presented its aims, methods, and results; addressed the clinical benefits and effects of the systems; and concluded that the EHR as a result of this now is in the process of being distributed to all other clinical departments as well. The other – a representative of the clinical laboratory of the same hospital – presented the case story on integration with the laboratory information system as viewed from their perspective, a story that makes your hair stand on end, revealing a lack of influence on matters related to the presentation of laboratory service reports toward the clinical end users: Only one sampling event can be presented per day. This may be acceptable in psychiatry and geriatrics but presumably not in paediatrics and intensive care, and others. A legal statement on the case is beyond the scope of this paper. Yet, it was obvious that the positive statement put forward by the administrative party needs greater nuances. Also, this inconsistency could have been avoided by performing a stakeholder analysis prior to the assessment study.

11.1.1.4 Targeting the Methodology/Method to the Study Aim

The actual assessment objective is of paramount importance. An example is the huge difference between "quantifying the potential benefit" versus "demonstrating the general usability . . . by quantifying the effect of the use", in which the ambition of the former is higher than that of the latter. Normally in HTA, one addresses the additional benefit implied by the new technology as compared with the traditional technology and approach, rather than proving only that a system is applicable, which corresponds to the latter. There is a strong bias in case the one is aimed to prove the other.

Another example is the distinction between 'efficacy', 'efficiency' and 'effectiveness'[10], so nicely discussed by Wall (1991) and Goodman (1992). It is a decision whether one wants (1) a circumscribed, in-depth, well-defined, and well-controlled study addressing the effectiveness or (2) a balanced study of averaging, population-based conditions, which address efficacy yet with a number of inherent variables. The latter is usually the case for randomized controlled trials (Goodman 1992). One point of caution in this respect, often not recognized, is related to the generalisability (external validity) of the study conclusion inherent to the sources of variance and the study population included (Wall 1991; and Goodman 1992). Nolan et al. (1991) explore and discuss a number of sources of variance inherent specifically to knowledge-based systems and decision-support systems.

11.1.2   Selecting the Methodology/Method

It is necessary that the study method tie in closely with the study objectives (Friedman and Wyatt 1997). Picking the wrong approach will, for whatever reason, answer a different question.

11.1.2.1   Subjectivity versus Objectivity

Some methods are designed to achieve subjective measures; others are designed to achieve objective measures on the object of investigation. All things being equal, objective studies tend to create greater credibility among the audience. Yet, techniques that focus on subjective aspects seem to prevail in the literature on assessment of IT-based systems in terms of questionnaires and interview investigations. However, even if they seem so easy, they are prone to perils and pitfalls as well as perspectives and hidden assumptions. Below, a couple of examples are explicitly addressed, with aspects of subjective approaches in general.

A large number of pitfalls, perils, and biases are inherent in the questionnaire approach, like culture and an innumerable number of psychological factors (Andersen and Enderud 1990; Fivelsdal 1990; and Coolican 1999), judgmental factors (see Section 11.2.6), postrationalization (Section 11.2.7), and so on.

Examples of psychological factors may be unwillingness to report on certain questions (e.g., due to sensitivity or prestige involved), intermixing or conflict

---

[10] See these concepts in the footnote page 172

between the official version and a personal opinion, fatigue at large questionnaires, mood at the time or context of responding, or lack of introspection or self-awareness. There are many ways to avoid these pitfalls, and therefore it is of relevance to be able to inspect the questionnaire used in a study.

Questionnaires are tools, and tools need verification with respect to construct and content validity before application (see also Section 11.1.3.1). Beyond this comes the problem of translation within multilingual studies and of monolingual, multinational studies, like English questionnaires applied in Denmark, where most of the population does speak English as a second language but not as bilinguals. It is not valid per se to apply a questionnaire in a foreign language, and it is not easy to translate a questionnaire while preserving the meaning in case one wants to make a multinational survey.

Triangulation of methods in (Kushniruk et al. 1997) clearly indicates the problem of interviewees' biased judgment when applying a questionnaire approach and thus illustrates some of the psychological biases in questionnaires.

Moreover, standardized questionnaires for the assessment of user acceptance have been developed; see the review and recommendations in (Ohmann et al. 1997). Unfortunately, this study does not address the methodological pitfalls of such questionnaires. Furthermore, three years later, the authors developed yet another questionnaire for assessment of user satisfaction for a dedicated purpose (Boy et al. 2000). Thus, the usability of the first mentioned standard questionnaires might not have been satisfactory for all purposes, which adds to the question of standard questionnaires as a satisfactory approach for assessing user satisfaction or acceptability.

To a large extent interview techniques suffer from the same perils and pitfalls as questionnaires but some approaches allow interaction and iteration, verification and elaboration of responses until a question is understood and answered. Fairly objective techniques do exist for analysis of the acquired and transcribed text, such as the Grounded Theory approach. However, interpreter reliability is a major concern for structured interviews, as the reliability depends both on the ability of the interviewee to report accurately and consistently and on the quality and ability of the interviewer to facilitate this process (Sher and Trull 1996). The outcome even depends on the professional background of the interviewer and his or her organizational relation to the interviewee (Rosenthal 1976; and Sher and Trull 1996). It is therefore of relevance to know the prior experience of the interviewer.

Expert opinions are also subjective measures. It is therefore recommended to acquire a second opinion from a panel of independent experts (Keen et al. 1995) in order to take into account bias from hidden agendas or other motives. An unbiased comparison is necessary if one wishes confidently to be able to say something about the technology assessed (Bryan et al. 1995). Different kinds of consensus approaches for expert opinions may partly or fully compensate for the subjective nature of singular expert opinions, like that outlined in (Goodman 1995).

11.1.2.2 *Assumptions for Methods Application*

It is good practice within the domain of statistics to verify whether the known assumptions for application of methods, techniques, or metrics are fulfilled or made probable. The same is not always the case in other domains, like technology assessment of IT-based systems, even if each method, technique, and metric does have implicit and explicit assumptions about the nature of their application (Brender 1997a and 1999). Further, the implicit assumptions have to be verified after elicitation, either by judgment or by formal proof, depending on their nature.

Assumptions for application of statistical techniques could be a chapter in itself, as the assumptions for applications are so often broken. An example of explicit assumptions is the assumption of normal distribution by many parametric statistical tools for data analysis. Such assumptions are normally explicitly described in statistical textbooks – often spelled out in detail. Still, the assumption on the nature of the numbers processed is commonly violated: A t-test assumes a normally distributed population with observations from a continuous scale. The responses to questionnaires normally are discrete (an ordinal scale) and definitely not expected to be normally distributed. Unfortunately, even recent literature of evaluation studies includes a vast number of examples of this basic violation of assumptions. The subtraction of ordinal scale measures for pre- and postobservations, like in (Gamm et al. 1998a), are still from an ordinal scale, and thus the t-test is (still) not applicable. Similarly, the calculation of the standard deviation for measures from an ordinal scale in (Boy et al. 2000) is a violation of the assumptions for calculation, where quartiles or percentiles could have been used instead. Although it is not entirely clear how Murphy et al. (1994) calculates a derived score from the ratings in a pre- and posttest questionnaire, they do generate a score that seems no longer to be ordinal, and, if so, their use of the t-test may be applicable.

Another example is independency of measures. Rating & weighting approaches formally assume independent variables. A rating & weighting approach was applied in both (Einbinder et al. 1996) and (Celli et al. 1998) for the selection among vendors in a purchase scenario. However, functionalities in an IT-based solution are in general not expected to be independent, and a given functionality may be replaced completely by another innovative approach. An example is the cleaning of irrelevant orders in a requesting system (like requesting para-clinical services): Two extreme alternatives are (1) an administrative tidying up of superfluous orders after a certain timelag and (2) active receipt control at the arrival of the patient or sample, followed by an automated removal of not executed orders. Depending on the formulation of the rated measure as the presence of number 1 (or 2) a third alternative in terms of an embedded (implicit) solution for the receipt control will rate the global solution low. Thus, the method applied not only assumes independent variables, but also that the set of functions pointed at constitute the optimal solution. In this case one should apply the outcome as a guideline but not as the golden truth when selecting between solutions.

Independency of measures is a relevant issue also when preparing and processing questionnaires, an issue that is normally not visible from a presentation of the method. Thus, a questionnaire approach is not valid per se.

Tacit, implicit assumptions constitute a danger to every assessment activity. Examples of hidden assumptions of methods are, for instance, assumptions on (cause-effect relations within) the object of study, like the assumption for most diagramming techniques that the work processes modeled may be schematized in a hierarchical fashion with defined interrelations and interactions (see, e.g., Brender 1999) or that it is a valid approximation for the application purpose. Assumptions for the application of a method may formally be violated, yet the implications may be minimal or inconsequential. Thus, in practice, the important factor is that the author demonstrates his or her awareness of this issue by proper notice and handling. It is not necessary to provide the full measures but to provide a statement, like *"The assumption of . . . was evaluated by . . . prior to use"* (McNair 1988). Then, the reader knows that verification of assumptions has been done, and the rest is only a matter of trust.

Finally, the assumption for a valid conclusion of a case study is the construct validity of the assessment tools applied (see this concept in Section 11.1.3.1). There are so few studies that report on their efforts to verify the construct validity that it is worth mentioning (Murphy et al. 1994) as an example to follow; see, however, also Section 11.1.3.1.

When the application of a 'standard' method is reported convincingly in the literature, it may still be relevant to make a random verification of one or more elements of the tools. For instance, when translating a 'standard' questionnaire from the literature for one's own purposes, the verification of the construct validity is important if not mandatory (see also the discussion in Section 11.1.8 on cultural aspects).

11.1.2.3   *Application Range*

Application range is the range of conditions within which the system will be applicable. In this respect, a number of biased cases are known from the area of decision-support systems or algorithms/models; see, for instance, the examples in (Bjerregaard et al. 1976; and Lindberg 1982) and the discussion in (Friedman and Wyatt 1997).

'In-vitro' studies and 'in-vivo' studies are both important, but one cannot replace the other, and there is a strong bias in interpreting one as equal to or replacing the other. The concept of 'in-vitro' studies stands for studies performed in an experimental setup, whereas 'in-vivo' studies refer to studies conducted in a fully operational environment. One should be aware that in-vitro studies are often chosen, precisely because a realistic setup or real-operation cannot be established for the assessment purpose. Such a lack of reality cannot normally be fully compensated for. An example is presented and discussed in Section 11.2.6.1, in terms of the study of Wiik and Lam (2000), in relation to another problem of that study. Thus, such studies are focused efforts and shall be interpreted as such.

11.1.2.4 *Circular Inference*

Circular inference arises when one develops a method, a framework, or a technique dedicated to a specific (population of) case(s) and applies it on the very same case(s) for verification purposes. In medicine this corresponds to a situation where an algorithm is developed on the basis of a population of cases and the algorithm is tested for validity by means of the same cases. Another example is when an algorithm is evaluated by means of successive cases and these cases are then used for the refinement of the algorithm.

When the population of cases includes only one member, as is often the case in development and assessment of an IT-based system, the risk of circularity is slightly different. If one has a case and prepares a dedicated framework/method for assessment of certain aspects within that case, then one has a circular inference if one, on the basis of that sole case, concludes that the framework/method is valid rather than only applicable. An example of the framework/method may, for instance, be a questionnaire that is developed specifically to elicit information about a given case. There may be nothing wrong with the measures provided or with the general conclusion of the case study. One may apply the questionnaire and elicit data as well as measures in a number of respects, and one may convert this to information. However, one cannot conclude from such a case study alone that the framework (or similarly a method or technique) is valid. At the utmost one can conclude that it seems to work in practice. It requires independent indicators of internal validity (like a frame of reference, triangulation of methods or cases, or alike, or other approaches to verify the construct validity) to conclude anything beyond that. Consequently, in such cases one should hesitate and conclude only that the methodology – or the method or the framework – "was suitable as applied", may have "worked well for the case at hand", and "has indicated that . . .". Only the successful application of the methodology in full will for other cases be able to increase the probability of its validity to a level of proof.

One example is seen from (Brender and McNair 2002): The assessment approach and ideas within the assessment methodology applied have gradually matured in a chain of projects, while the assessment tools are novel and their development dedicated for that particular application. So the methods and tools are developed and verified on the same case. Consequently, as noticed by the authors, there is a risk of a 'circular inference' bias no matter how well the tools worked for the case at hand. Special for the case is that it was implemented as case-based action research (see this concept in Mathiassen 1998), implying that the researcher is actively engaged within the practice situation in close collaboration with the prac-tice team and interacting with it. This type of research is experimental in an incre-mental, iterative, and error-based refinement approach, implying that the role of the researcher is of an interfering type with an intrinsic relation between the research and the practice – the worst possible indicator of a circular inference if it is not consciously and carefully dealt with. Whether or not there is a circular inference in such a case study depends on the actual conclusion and awareness of the authors but at the same time depends on the context within which the methods and tools are developed and applied as a function of time. This type of bias constitutes a built-in peril of constructive assessment as well as of case-based action research, where the methodological foundation changes in a dynamic fashion depending on the case itself (McKay and Marshall 2002; see also the discussion in Section 11.2.14.2). And that is why a frame of reference for comparison or a multimethod approach (triangulation of methods) is so valuable.

Another example, a borderline one, must be discussed, (Timpka and Sjöberg 1998). They apply a well-structured approach for the evaluation based on a rigorous and renowned subjectivist approach to the data analysis – the Grounded Theory – yet with the slight deviation already at a fairly early stage of the analysis that *"concepts from theories were applied to the findings already at . . .".* The paper concludes, *"The results suggest that . . . takes place at three distinguishable social arenas".* It is precisely these 'arenas' that were inspired by theories from the literature and incorporated intentionally into the data analysis coding scheme. It is therefore suggested that the conclusion of that study should be somewhat weakened, even beyond the verb *"suggest".* An alternative approach, like a falsification approach, might have been an approach similar to the role of a null-hypothesis in a statistical analysis; the null-hypothesis here being that the theories adopted are valid concepts within the analytical approach. Then, their conclusion might read something like "the results achieved from application of the analytical method did not contradict the null-hypothesis, and thus the theories adopted from the literature seem applicable within the present analytical approach. In other words, the suggestion that . . . takes place at three distinguishable social arenas cannot be rejected".

The problem seen from this discussion is of a general nature and inherent in numerous studies. Whether or not a given study applying the above approach is subject to the bias of circular inference is a matter of the awareness of the extent to which the methods and approach applied and the data achieved provide a solid basis for the conclusion, as well as whether this is reflected in the discussion and the conclusion.

Note that operationalisation of a method or methodology normally is not per se affected by this bias.

A development methodology/method based on an organizational learning approach by nature constitutes a similar type of circular inference: The lessons are incorporated into the basis for the further process. This approach and philosophy is the very idea and intention behind formative assessment, and it has the purpose of optimizing the ongoing development process and/or the quality of its outcome.

11.1.3 Defining Methods and Materials

When reporting from an assessment study, one should remember that one is not reporting for oneself, but bringing a message to someone else. Moreover, when one reports the outcome of an assessment study, one is often tempted to put more emphasis on the results or conclusion than on other parts of the reporting. However, bringing insufficient information bears the risk of making the reader suspicious toward the justification of the conclusion as a whole and thus letting down the entirety. To be convincing, the method and materials need to be described in sufficient detail to exclude uncertainty about the approach, methods, and metrics/techniques applied. That is, as a rule of thumb the description of methods and material should adhere to the guidelines usually applied for scientific studies (see, for instance, the website http://www.icmje.org/index.html, which covers the Vancouver Rules for scientific manuscripts).

There are methods at two levels: One contains methods inherent within the object of investigation, and the other contains methods applied to accomplish the (assessment) investigation. The former is not necessarily needed in full detail in the description of an assessment study, but the latter is definitely needed. For an IT-based system the former corresponds to a description of the development methodology and methods, while the latter comprises the assessment methodology. Pretty often, publications include both, which implies the risk of sitting between two chairs – neither is described in sufficient detail – or perhaps the implementation is – while the assessment performed is meant to make the success visible but has the opposite effect due to insufficient information. The right balance between the two descriptions is delicate. As regards the assessment study, the reader does need sufficient details also of specific system or implementation details to be able to judge the causal mechanisms leading to the observations and conclusions reached. The balance between descriptions of the development and the assessment is delicate, however nicely achieved, while taking little space in, for instance (Southon et al. 1999). In contrast, an extended system description followed by something like a ten-liner description of the evaluation and its conclusion has very little value for a judgment of the validity of the assessment conclusion. The reader in such cases is left with virtually no details to justify the conclusion of the assessment study.

The risk of insufficient description of methods is that a reader may presume that the conclusion is untrustworthy due to lack of information. One can take a look at (Kushniruk and Patel 1995) to see that even for a conference proceeding, which is normally a short publication, it *is* possible to outline the approach taken at a sufficient level of detail to be convincing for the reader. So the length of a publication is not the only issue.

11.1.3.1 *Construct Validity of Methods, Techniques, and Tools*

Questionnaire studies, of which thousands exist, are a paradigm example of methods that tend to be generated ad hoc and in a dedicated fashion, without providing the reader of such a study with neither information on its contents nor on any measures of confidence in its internal and external validity (correctness, accuracy, or precision and generalisability). So we will use these as examples to illustrate the issue of construct validity or internal validity.

An example – almost a model exemplar – with an exhaustive description of their assessment approach and verification of the technique applied is (Murphy et al. 1994), – the mere awareness of the issues of relevance makes it convincing. They say, *"First, preliminary analyses were performed to evaluate the reliability and construct validity of the newly developed attitude scale"* and *"Content validity of the items was established with a panel of five experts . . . using rating scales and narrative comments. Items were reviewed for their relevance to the common characteristics of . . . and for readability"*. The text is interpreted in the sense that the draft questionnaire was applied and commented by a panel of experts (but experts in what professional domain?) and that the questionnaire was subsequently assessed by statistical means. Such an investigation of the draft questionnaire is not common in the literature, but it ought to be. However, even if this paper constitutes a model to follow, be aware that this also has its problems: The combination of content validity, relevance, and readability versus the combination of construct validity and reliability are not the same. Content validity is related to issues like the representativeness (coverage and completeness) of the topic investigated, while construct validity is related to issues like the correctness, coherence, and consistency – that is, the capability of the structure to capture the qualities intended. Similarly, reliability is related to *"the ability to perform a required function under stated conditions for a stated period of time"* (Dybkær et al. 1992) – that is, related to availability and repeatability (closeness of repeated measurements), which is not the same as relevance and readability. This dispute shall, however, not in itself, break up an impression of an otherwise detailed study, as it just shows that the issue of exhaustiveness in assessment studies may be painful and that questionnaires are not easy and reliable tools per se.

The study of Chin and Haughton (1995) demonstrates in a similar way a strongly convincing insight into statistical techniques for analysis of data elicited through a questionnaire survey, and it has a lot of data. It seems to be a solid study. This is a good starting point for another illustration of the concept of construct validity. Two comments: First, they seem to have little awareness of the concept of construct validity of a questionnaire, or, rather, there is no explicit sign of verification of the construct validity of the questionnaire within the text. Second, surveys on users' subjective perception of the benefits of IT in hospitals are indeed appropriate as the scope of a study. However, asking those responsible for purchases and management of such systems may be dangerous with respect to the construct validity of the assessment questions asked, depending on the perspective of the study. We have not acquired the questionnaire of the study, and it would require a major investigation to verify the next issue, so let it just stay as an illustration that is not necessarily true of the case at hand: The point of illustration is related to the question "What can a manager answer reliably on behalf of the entire organization?", and the danger resides with the conclusions. The referenced study explicitly and intentionally focuses their study questions toward the management level *("[I]nvestigates the benefits ..., as perceived by . . . responsible for . . . and the management of the systems")*, and the authors of the study seem to be very well aware of the danger in concluding, as they don't conclude beyond what one might reliably expect from managers in most cases. Perfect! It would have been problematic if they had asked for the managers' opinion on, for instance, benefits to the staff, end-user satisfaction, patient satisfaction, and impact on specific workflow aspects or work practices. Thus, the issue at stake (when the questionnaire has not been verified with respect to construct validity and reliability) is "What are the chances that the target group can answer the questions reliably?"

11.1.3.2 *Prophylactic Grounding*

Any assessment method and methodology has its strengths and weaknesses, pitfalls and perils, and characteristics as regards the dependability of the number or type of observations, for instance. Even a small discussion of these issues, such as in (Østbye et al. 1997), will, to the reader, demonstrate an awareness that adds considerably to the value of the outcome, as it demonstrates that the methods are not just applied as is, like statistical measures often are in medical scientific literature and ad hoc questionnaires in assessment of IT-based systems (see Section 11.1.2.2). Depending on the quality of the presentation in general, an awareness of that kind will give the competent reader a hint that the right skills are part of the foundation of the study. Therefore, a description of the study design that includes explicit considerations of a preventive nature is considered a strength. Actually, the entirety of issues relevant under this topic is correlated to the union of all the issues within the present paper.

11.1.3.3 Prognostic Measures

This aspect is concerned with whether the description of the study design includes explicit considerations of a prognostic nature, like power considerations (Friedman and Wyatt 1997). For instance, investigators tend to ignore that the probability of an extreme outcome decreases as the sample size increases; see, for instance, (Fraser and Smith 1992), meaning that confidence in the conclusion is highly dependent on the sample size. This is where, for instance, the power functions used in statistics may prevent overinterpretations (applicable at, for example, the planning of randomized controlled trials also for IT systems, but not for in-depth studies of a single case).

Investigations using too small a sample size may exhibit vulnerability to the extreme, or to other confounding factor(s), and may reveal itself in terms of, for instance, the appearance of two subpopulations.

Insensitivity to the sample size has to do with whether for the sample size one may expect to reveal the characteristics of the population of subjects included. One cannot always merge two populations (for instance, from two different departments of users) to achieve a larger sample size. Or at least before doing so, one has to verify that the characteristics of the component populations are identical, for instance, that they exhibit similar distributions of the individual measures. For usage of IT-based systems, organizational differences, as well as motivational factors and other soft human aspects are key factors for the hospitality and acceptance of the system, and therefore two different departments may reveal very different population characteristics. This is carefully handled in (van Gennip and Bakker 1995), while the data within (Gamm et al. 1998a) are merged into one study group, and the reader feels insecure about potential differences in characteristics between the sites involved or of the risk of subpopulations within the outcome measures, which might impair the conclusion. This is further discussed in Section 11.1.4.

It is rarely feasible at assessment of IT-based solutions to apply a large number of cases in order to fulfill the need for a high level of confidence in its outcome. However, in case there is an awareness of this relationship within the interpretation and discussion of a study, like in (Østbye et al. 1997), and if the conclusion is presented cautiously, the study may gain in trustworthiness. Moreover, to make the preconditions of an assessment study clear might give the readers another basis for acknowledging even a slight information gain achieved.

Again, it is the signs of awareness of pitfalls that make the reader convinced of the value of the efforts invested and the conclusion stated.

11.1.4 (User) Recruitment

This is related to the *Attribution error* in (Fraser and Smith 1992), where it is described in a more general way as *"the tendency for attributors to underestimate the impact of situational factors and to overestimate the role of dispositional factors in controlling behaviour"*. The sample (here of users) must be representative if not typical with respect to the characteristics of the population about which one wants to generalize the results. There is a risk of an unintentional bias when the selection of participants within a study is not randomly performed, - a problem also pointed at by, for instance, Jaeschke and Sackett (1989); Wyatt and Spiegelhalter (1991); Friedman and Wyatt (1997); and Coolican (1999). For instance, participants who are likely to be able to carry out the study are often unintentionally selected before those who are less likely to perform. Therefore, the subjects of the investigation need to be well defined in terms of inclusion and exclusion criteria (Wyatt and Spiegelhalter 1991; and Friedman and Wyatt 1997).

In medicine there is a tradition for defining explicit inclusion / exclusion criteria of cases (patients) to be involved in a study (see the 'case recruitment' below), while a similar specification of inclusion and exclusion criteria with respect to the physicians to be involved often are less explicit but are definitely a clear demand in assessment of an IT system (Wyatt and Spiegelhalter 1991).

All of these problems are implicitly clear from the study of Gamm et al. (1998a), addressing end-user satisfaction. The reader doesn't know the inclusion and exclusion criteria of users, and doesn't know the response rate or characteristics of users actually involved in the evaluation study. We know that pre- and postobservations are matched but not whether or not the physicians involved constitute decision makers (such as chief physicians or physicians at a consultancy level), for instance. It does make a difference for the attitudes and expectations in the pre-investigation study; whether they are domain experts or novices/trainees or whether the physicians during long-term use were exposed to a preinstallation period at all. The issue at stake is that physicians constitute a group of professionals with rapidly changing positions and a long-term specialist training (Brender 1997b). Moreover, we don't know whether the observations are different between novices and experts, as suggested by, for instance, Dreyfus and Dreyfus (1986); Beuscart-Zéphir et al. (1997 and 2001); and Patel and Kushniruk (1998).

Considerations of inclusion and exclusion criteria must be explicitly described in a study report. When a population is composed of more than one subpopulation (for instance, different institutions from different countries and with the risk of applying different culturally dependent professional schools, like in cross-national studies), one has to verify whether these subpopulations stem from the same original population before a conclusion can be made from merged data material. The presence of a consensus process within a study or of certain types of training implicitly tells us that the involved participants do come from different institutions, and thus that the subpopulations are (or at least were) nonhomogeneous. The risk is that a harmonization or learning effect based on the functionality applied would be misinterpreted as an effect of another kind.

11.1.4.1 *Diagnostic Suspicion*

"Knowledge of the trial subject's prior exposure to the test manoeuvre may influence both the intensity and the results of the search for relevant outcomes" (Jaeschke and Sackett 1989). In medical diagnosis, it does make a difference to a physician to know that the patient in front of him has a history of a certain condition when searching for specific information, as this may immediately narrow down the diagnostic space or focus the investigation – thus the title of this bias. It is called a bias because it has an influence on the efficiency of the diagnostic process, which sometimes may not be a desirable player in an assessment study addressing a specific question.

A direct analogue in assessment of IT systems may be the history of the system in terms of vendor, development methodology, or even market rumors. Such information may definitely bias a user's judgment in a purchase situation.

11.1.4.2 *The (Un-)Used User*

A subtler analogue to the 'diagnostic suspicion' would be a situation where the users carrying out the assessment study have been deeply involved in the development work, as they are gradually trained in the functionality and peculiarities of the IT-based solution (see Section 11.1.4.1), partly through extensive debates and partly through access to prototypes – for example, at demo events or after the technical installation and setup. They know the system, know the flaws and the history of efforts to compensate, so they know their way around the problems – or perhaps because they have been told that it cannot be otherwise. Users who have a deep prior knowledge of the system may unintentionally cover up some problems that new users will experience and immediately react to. Consequently, they may appear blind toward certain problems because they have decided on a solution themselves or have become acquainted with the functionality. This is especially troublesome for rapid prototyping and when the theme of investigation is as soft as usability and user acceptance of an IT-based solution. The implication as regards the interpretation of, say, the functionality or usability in this respect is that the performance of the 'used' and the 'un-used' users will reveal two different populations of data. New users might be more critical or handicapped at first, but they will also learn and eventually get used to it. Therefore, the question is what information is addressed by the assessment study, and if relevant, these aspects should be given explicit attention or dedicated efforts should be made to take them into account.

Consequently, it is of importance during the detailed planning and implementation of an assessment study to take into account the extent to which the users that are to be involved have prior knowledge of the system and to match this with the intention of the assessment study. This goes beyond that of taking into account the effect of mere computer literacy – that is, different starting points of different user groups, as is the case in (van Gennip and Bakker 1995).

11.1.5   (Case) Recruitment

This is closely related to the concept of representativeness and *allocation bias*, addressed by Wyatt and Spiegelhalter (1991) – for instance, in terms of the composition of (sub-) groups of patients with specific disease patterns. However, each and every exclusion criteria delimits the *generalisability*, which then becomes a drawback that works in the opposite direction (Jaeschke and Sackett 1989). Still, the subjects of investigation should be well defined in terms of inclusion and exclusion criteria. One can normally not generalize beyond the setting of the assessment study.

When the text of a study report states that 80% of the patient stream normally is 'normal', then a baseline reference database that includes *"28 single disease patterns and 2 borderline negative reaction"* (like in Wiik and Lam 2000) is incomparable to a real-life patient stream. It may be okay for a demonstration of benefits of some sort to apply such a population, as for the case study referenced, but not for an intended real assessment.

Even a slight bias – for instance, due to lack of explicitness in the composition of the subjects of investigation within the study – may imply that the outcome is not applicable either at normal practice on the premises of the study location or at similar settings elsewhere.

The means to prevent the risk of a bias within the recruitment of cases is to apply a combination of the above-mentioned inclusion and exclusion criteria, such as "the complete stream of patients that are characterized by the defined criteria" and of randomization. Thus, the issue of dedicatedness of the subjects has to be explicitly stated. A special topic of concern may be the longitudinal cohort studies, which, as Jaeschke and Sackett (1989) point out, often suffer from lack of control of which case is included in the test group or in the control group.

11.1.5.1 More than One Population Included as the Subject of Investigation

The presence of different populations is explicit and nicely dealt with in the study of van Gennip and Bakker (1995): They know they have two different study populations and keep them separate in the result presentation. However, also note the pitfall described in Section 11.1.6.9. The danger is to merge such groups before investigating whether they are from the same population. An analogous example is the merger of populations of physicians and nurses unless their group characteristics are in control.

11.1.5.2 Compliance between Application and Target Domains

The concept of 'case' may for assessment of IT systems refer to a target domain involved or a target organizational type rather than to a patient type, as is the case in the medical domain's normal interpretation. There is a difference in applying an IT-based solution in a geriatric department (which then serves as the case) compared to an intensive care unit, irrespective of whether the target organization is specifically named or is named as a general-purpose functionality. These two target domains differ significantly with respect to complexity. Therefore, it is important to describe the target domain and the application domain in sufficient detail to enable the reader to judge for himself or herself whether the similarities of the application comply with the target domain in order to suffice for the study purpose and its conclusion.

A variant of this issue is seen in (Murphy et al. 1994), in relation to the compliance between the area of expertise and the usage of this expertise for a specific purpose. For verification of their survey instrument, the study used *"a panel of five experts from the Patient Care Information System Task Force of a multi-hospital corporation"*. However, we don't know the area of expertise of these experts. Are they experts in conducting assessment studies or, for instance, in clinical medicine, or what? Moreover, it is not clear from the text precisely what they did (*"Content validity was established with . . ."*) – in other words, whether they were trial respondents or auditors. Therefore, it is not easy from the text to judge whether the area of expertise was the right one for the purpose, but as the study in general seems solid, we have less reason to question the suitability of their approach, and so we just use the case as an illustrative example.

11.1.5.3 Use of Artificial Scenarios or Setup

When performing constructive assessment during a prototyping development, it is normally necessary to use artificially constructed cases dedicated to the stage of the prototype functionality. Similarly, it may be necessary to apply an artificial setup for assessment – for instance, at an early assessment of a completed IT system or of a product IT system. In such cases, one should realize that there may be an enormous difference between a real-life IT-based solution and application of artificial scenarios or an artificial setup (see also Nowlan 1994), and that artificial setups may be meaningless for certain types of behavioral studies (Coolican 1999).

These are some of the particular dangers:

1. The user may exhibit an altered behavior within an experimental setup. Beuscart-Zéphir et al. (1997) demonstrate (as also discussed in Brender 1997a and 1999) that there is a discrepancy between expert user's description of his or her work practice and the observed work practice, and found that this divergence was much larger for a highly experienced person than for a novice. Their explanation is that – for cognitive work, at least – the novice operates more or less according to the prescribed procedures (the one that they are told as novice users/trainees), whereas apprenticeship implies the mastering of a momentary mental image (unconscious) as a means for accomplishment of a task through shortcuts and alternative procedures. The study of Beuscart-Zéphir et al. (1997) points at a plausible explanation in terms of expert users expressing the prescribed procedure (the way they tell trainees) rather than their own real procedure. The users are incapable of expressing their mental image of their own work processes. This phenomenon complies with the well-known knowledge engineering problem of getting expert users to explicate their knowledge accurately and completely and also the change in behavior as a function of apprenticeship (Dreyfus and Dreyfus 1986; Patel and Kushniruk 1998; and Beuscart-Zéphir et al. 2001). Thus, if a user in a teaching session can adapt his or her procedures to the prescribed procedure, he or she may also do so in an experimental setup, where there is a focus on approach.

2. The experimental setup and artificial scenarios are out of the real-life context. In a real-life context, the work of healthcare staff tends to comprise many parallel activities and great variation (see, for instance, Brender 1997a and b and 1999), while the experimental assessment setup may to a larger extent allow each activity to proceed in an undisturbed, sequential manner, thereby biasing the assessment of, for example, effectiveness and usability.

Many cases reported in the literature constitute quasi-experiments, in the sense that the design attempted to mimic a real application within a kind of laboratory setup. This may be caused by project conditions that rendered it impossible to manipulate the environment to the extent required to conduct assessment within a real-life operational environment. Moreover, the conditions of an assessment study may prohibit a number of features normally required for proper conclusion on validity and generalisability of a study, such as random assignment of subjects. In such a case, it does not always make sense to prepare a baseline measure or a model of the existing system as the frame of reference. Instead, an exploratory situation analysis providing a multifaceted picture of the usability with a causal analysis of problems identified might be a feasible approach for concluding on the usability of the IT-based solution in question with the anticipated future use as the frame of reference.

11.1.6 The Frame of Reference

The statement *"Therapeutic reports without controls tend to have enthusiasm, and reports with enthusiasm tend to have no control"* is credited to Jaeschke and Sackett (1989). Subjective statements made by the target users are definitely valuable – as are the results based on (human) interpretation – because the target users are the ones to make the final judgment of whether or not they like or want the system. Nevertheless, a subjective statement cannot replace hard documentation when it comes to reporting on an assessment study within the literature because the reader cannot judge the full context in which the assessment has taken place and therefore cannot necessarily transfer the subjective conclusion to his own situation. In such a case, the reader is dependent on his knowledge of the authors and his personal trust in their judgment.

Studies that ignore or do not accurately take into account the need for having a proper frame of reference for measuring change may be strongly biased; see also the extended discussion on baseline data in (Assmann et al. 2000). This again is closely correlated to the question that the assessment study is designed to answer. If one intends to demonstrate the benefit of something new, be it the effect of a new pharmaceutical treatment or the introduction of an IT-based function, a frame of reference for measuring that change is essential for documentation of the actual change or benefit. Otherwise, how can one distinguish the effect introduced from the effect of merely doing something to treat a patient, so the patient gets better no matter what has actually been done (Wyatt and Spiegelhalter 1991) – the placebo effect? Thus, an analysis of this issue for an assessment study should address whether the study design includes proper consideration of a frame of reference.

Measuring the frame of reference may be particularly difficult when the focus of the assessment is a particular process within an organization – like a training or education process, a Continued Quality Improvement (CQI) process, or a consensus-making process. First of all, it is difficult in itself, simply because of the interference with other processes within the organization. Second, a frame of reference for training/education, for instance, is complex because it may not only be a matter of a shift from a manual system to an electronic system, but at the same time it may include a complete change of teacher, teaching materials, and/or even of educational principles. So an analysis of cause-effect relations in a study of effectiveness, efficiency, or efficacy of a teaching/education system is somewhat complex. Similarly, when focusing on a CQI-managed system/organization, one might use the number and type of events handled as an indicator for quality or effectiveness of the new system (the less CQI events handled, the better the system); however, if the new system – after a period of adaptation and maturation – demonstrates a significant increase of CQI events handled, this may actually be due to a decrease in effectiveness or to an increase in efficiency of the CQI approach. The one is harmful to the organization, whereas the other is advantageous. See also Section 11.1.7.3.

The paper of Einbinder et al. (1996) presents a tool for evaluating clinical information systems at the time of purchase. In other respects the publication is characterized by its clarity but suffers from a complete lack of assessment of the proposed approach other than a subjective judgment saying, *"We found our evaluation tool . . . to be an effective mechanism for structuring clinician participation . . . and for comparing different clinical information systems."* Without any kind of (formal) assessment of the evaluation tool other than one application, and without any kind of frame of reference for formal comparison, unfortunately, all that one can conclude is that their approach was applicable to their case. The reason is that we don't know whether the system finally selected was a success, and we don't know what kind of problems subsequently occurred. We know only that *"Clinician response to this process has been favourable"* but not how this was observed, rated, or otherwise measured. The conclusion of the study, *"is an effective and efficient way of distinguishing among candidate . . . systems"*, is not supported by documentation within the presentation. The authors seem not to be aware of this inability of the readers to draw the same conclusion from what is presented. One might excuse the paper by the limited space for proceeding papers, yet the publication ends with an empty half page. The number of open questions is simply too big, so it's up to the reader to judge the credibility of the referenced technique for evaluation of tenders. Nevertheless, this does not preclude that it is valuable as inspiration for others in a similar situation, and this may have been the scope of the publication.

11.1.6.1 *The Placebo Effect*

The placebo effect (that is, the effect from merely doing something to treat a patient and the patient gets better no matter what has actually been done – often called a 'control group') is a well-known experimental bias in medical and pharmaceutical assessment studies (Friedman and Wyatt 1997; and Gluud 2005) but less known in the domain of IT-assessment studies.

A study design that applies the individual user's own baseline performance as the frame of reference for judging an improved performance potential is perilous, unless one knows the pitfalls. It compares to a before-and-after-study, where, for instance, the intermediate change may be installation of a (new) IT-based system, focused attention, or training. The absence of a true control group rules out the possibility of controlling each and every interfering factor, such as the mere effect of a change in a working environment leading to new/changed tasks, as, for instance, that pointed out by Bryan et al. (1995) and Keen et al. (1995), related social changes or restructuring the patterns of responsibility and competences, prolonged attention, and so forth.

It is not an easy task to design an experiment that will take into account all experimental pitfalls in this respect. However, assessing an improvement in performance against one's own baseline is secondary when the reader is unaware of how much can be achieved with similar efforts invested in other means or approaches for the 'old' organization. Some methods are goal-free and hence do not have a frame of reference. However, for other methods a statement like "the frame of reference is nonexistent" is sometimes nonsense and shows that the scope of the study has not been made sufficiently clear or insight into the basics of assessment studies is more or less absent. For instance, an expert tutor may normally perform training ad hoc, and this personalized expert tutoring *does* constitute a baseline frame of reference for assessing the effect of introducing an IT-based learning tool – of course, depending on the scope of the study. In such cases an approach in which the participants serve as both control and study group may sometimes be applied. That is, the effect of the learning tool is assessed in two different areas, manually in the one and IT-supported in the other and with a crossover approach, like that suggested in (O'Moore et al. 1990a). A very nice crossover design is found for the histo-pathology study in (Wiik and Lam 2000), studying changes in intra- and interobserver variations in three different sub-domains of histo-pathology: One pathologist from one of the three organizations involved was recognized as the expert within one of the subdomains. Besides this, a number of nonexpert specialists were involved from each organization. In this way, each expert served as the frame of reference in some respects, and as one of the nonexpert specialists in other respects of the same study, thereby eliminating the placebo effect and establishing a solid frame of reference approach.

11.1.6.2 Hawthorne Effect

The psychological effect of being observed is widely known from assessment studies. Humans tend to change or improve their performance if they know they are under observation (Wyatt and Spiegelhalter 1991; and Friedman and Wyatt 1997). There are a number of variants of this bias, from being observed by a superior to being part of a team of colleagues or explicitly being the subject of investigation. Sometimes the Hawthorne effect is the actual effect strived at – for instance, in programs of continuous comparisons of the level of excellence between organizations as an element in a quality assurance program, a common practice for quality control within laboratory medicine (de Verdier et al. 1984).

A Hawthorne effect may be inescapable, as also discussed above, but then it should at least be *balanced*, so that the groups compared are observed at the same strength (Wyatt and Spiegelhalter 1991) in order to establish a proper frame of reference for judging the potential effect of the subject of investigation.

An example of a measure that may be valuable and that may be impervious to the Hawthorne effect is seen from the study of Allan and Englebright (2000): Measures of the pattern of overtime. The reason is that such an investigation may be kept blind to the participants/employees, and/or it may be elicited after the global assessment event via the archives of the organization.

11.1.6.3 Co-Intervention

When dividing a study group into a control and a test group, it is important not to perform additional procedures on one of the groups in order to be able to discriminate the treatment effect from other effects and thereby investigate the add-on value of the intervention of interest (Jaeschke and Sackett 1989). Similarly, in case there is only one study group, the object of investigation, it is important not to perform other (major) change activities in parallel in order not to confound the investigation as a whole.

The study of Hetlevik et al. (2000) is one example of a thorough case study, randomizing the practices involved, but note that with their procedure the control group remains completely untreated, while the intervention group gets an IT system, as well as training and follow-up in several different ways along the way. In other words, it is *not* just the impact of the decision-support system that is measured.

Even if it is a well-executed study, there are similar problems in (Shojania et al. 1998), but one year later, members of the same research group present another study – of another IT system – without co-intervention problems, (Kuperman et al. 1999).

The study design of Østbye et al. (1997) applies a control group as the frame of reference. The intervention ward was exposed to a complete analysis, design, and implementation effort, while the control ward was not. This may imply that the effect measured includes not only the effect of the system introduced, but also the effect from the attention on the organization (a Hawthorne effect – see Section 11.1.6.2 –partly compensated for by the control ward approach). Moreover, an effect may arise from inspiration for changes induced by an analysis of the organization's work procedures, and so forth. Data from a longitudinal survey of the overall workload on the organization in question shows that the workload on the organization does not change as compared to the control ward. However, it is not clear from the text whether compensation for the extra workload generated by the implementation has been made; if not, the resource consumption for the implementation project may turn out to be a confounding factor in itself, because it *is* a competing activity. So the statement that the clinical workload is the same does not necessarily make the two organizations comparable with respect to the global workload.

It is indeed difficult to separate the different types of effects, and such a separation need not be the only desirable scope of an assessment study. A gain in efficiency or effectiveness may derive from the implementation project's process itself rather than as an effect of the new IT system. In the case study of Østbye et al. (1997), a solution to prevent this discussion might have been to carry out the same analysis, design, and implementation process in both wards, while delaying the actual operation in daily practice for one of the wards (by random selection as actually done within the study) until the 'after' study had been completed.

In conclusion, it is of importance that only the independent variable is changed or manipulated.

11.1.6.4   Before-and-After Study

Before-and-after studies, which may be efficient in particular for small, circumscribed systems, may not be a solution for major, highly integrated IT-based solutions, like PACS systems, because at the point when the system is operational a number of other factors may have changed, impeding the comparison of the 'before-state' with the 'after-state' (Bryan et al. 1995). A switch-back approach with repeated shifts from the old to the new system and back to the old system may be a solution to the problems in a before-and-after study, as discussed for PACS systems by Bryan et al. (1995). That way, the effect of doing something is gradually induced, and bright ideas from the one system are allowed to propagate into the other system until a new steady-state baseline situation has been achieved. Ultimately, one may assess the difference in efficiency or effectiveness or whatever between the two systems. This was tried at an early stage to assess the effect of a knowledge-based system, and is briefly mentioned in (Wyatt and Spiegelhalter 1991). A major problem for switchback approaches is that it may not be feasible to switch completely between the two systems (Bryan et al. 1995) – for instance, switching between a manual, paper-based system and an electronic solution.

Friedman and Wyatt (1997) are reporting a special kind of bias, which they call 'second look' bias, for laboratory experiments with decision-support systems based on written cases. The problem arises when the user is asked first to read the case and give his or her conclusion as a kind of baseline measure and then give a second conclusion while using the decision-support system. The reason is that the 'before use' and 'after use' conclusions are incomparable because of the extended decision-making period for the 'after use' scenario.

11.1.6.5   Carryover Effect

This bias is a contamination effect, (Wyatt and Spiegelhalter 1991; and Friedman and Wyatt 1997), concerned with the transmission between the study group and the control group of, for instance, knowledge gained by using the new IT system. That is, what one learned in the study group might be beneficial and hence exploited also for the control group. This is most likely to occur for systems that have an educational effect (Wyatt and Spiegelhalter 1991).

Sometimes this effect is deliberately exploited, as suggested in Sections 11.1.6.1 and 11.1.6.9, to take into account problems with achieving a frame of reference. However, in other cases this effect constitutes a bias. As an example, one may imagine a situation, where more than one IT-based system are introduced and assessed in parallel. Then, what one learns from using the one may have a biasing effect on the outcome of the other system's assessment outcome, and vice versa.

11.1.6.6   Checklist Effect

This bias is concerned with the effect of introducing new means in combination with the introduction of a new IT system, like a checklist or a questionnaire (Wyatt and Spiegelhalter 1991; and Friedman and Wyatt 1997). A way to escape this bias and isolate the effect of the IT system is to introduce the same means within the control group (Wyatt and Spiegelhalter 1991).

11.1.6.7   Human Cognition/Recognition of Cases

In case a classification of objects/cases include replicate occurrences of the objects/cases – for instance, in order to study intraperson variability, like ECG examinations and histo-pathological preparations (in medicine) – the human ability to recognize pictures and objects may be highly significant. This problem is probably not marked for novices but may be highly significant for experts, as the mechanism for their diagnostic ability is the visual pattern recognition.

The ability to recognize such patterns will naturally depend on the characteristics of the images, like coloring, shape, size, and distribution of image objects. This will reduce the impact of recognition for a domain with a large number of regular objects spread uniformly over the whole image. This type of pitfall emphasizes the 'insight bias' discussed previously: One small trick is to blind the details of the protocol so that those not involved as classifiers arrange the practical details. Another trick would be to let the image sets have different sizes (even if they are identical but rotated, etc.) by omission of a couple of images or addition of a couple of redundant copies. Alternatively, when having a candidate sample at hand, it might be feasible to make multiple images of the same sample (image sets) by locating alternative areas of interest, some of which may be even less pronounced in their patterns.

Most of these concerns were explicitly handled in the study of Wiik and Lam (2000). The examples and the above approach for handling them are taken from this study. The study deals with two pathological domains in order to measure the learning effect of an IT-based learning tool on the intra- and interperson variation of the diagnostic performance: autoimmune serology and histo-pathology. As implicitly said in the previous paragraph, this bias may be less pronounced in autoimmune serology, where each image includes thousands of blood cells evenly distributed over the image. The same is not the case for their study of histo-pathological samples, and a note was made in this respect for the cancer histo-pathology domain by one of the participants who observed this phenomenon. The risk of this bias was known by the study designers as judged from the efforts actually put into this topic (turning, mirroring, and randomizing the images, but based on the exact same images). Considering that this bias may potentially weaken or even completely ruin the outcome conclusion, it is considered a weakness of this study that the potential of this bias is neither discussed nor verified in the data analysis. One may use (Marcelo et al. 2000) as a model example of how one can handle the problem of recognition – at least for some applications: they make six representative snapshots from each case and use these individually.

11.1.6.8   *Usability and User Acceptability*

This topic is controversial because of the frame of reference. The down-to-earth frame of reference *is* the users' judgment of the usability of the system in an authentic use situation, where *quality* is defined as follows:

> *"[T]otality of features and characteristics of a product or service that bear on its ability to satisfy stated or implied needs."*

(ISO 8402)

The new ISO definition of quality has lost parts of the subjective element in its interpretation in order to become more operational in an assessment context: *"[D]egree to which a set of inherent characteristics fulfils requirements"*, where requirements are *"need or expectation that is stated, generally implied or obligatory"* (ISO 9000:2000).

So the proof of the pudding is in the eating, correlating to the question "When the usage is becoming serious, will the users then accept this and that detail of the functionality?" On the other hand, users are flexible, tend to adapt, and, when asked, humans tend to rate the usability of a system in a very positive light despite actual serious problems (see Section 11.2.6). Consequently, their rating is not always trustworthy for others but requires awareness and explicit attention from the study designers.

On the other hand, given the definition of the concept of 'quality' there is no objective frame of reference for the assessment of usability and user acceptance. It is a methodological issue to discover exactly what we are measuring or against what, and what the final criteria to be used are for judging and concluding on the usability and user acceptability.

The question marks raised on the value of questionnaires are valid also for assessing the usability or user acceptability of IT-based systems and leave the domain of assessment in a vacuum. What else to do or how? Just stop publishing them – unless the publications have a valuable novel contribution for others to learn from. At least, they are not valid per se for judging the validity of a developmental hypothesis or approach.

11.1.6.9 (Adverse) Confounding Effects

Whenever differences or relationships are observed in results, it is always possible that a variable, other than the independent variable, has produced the effect (Coolican 1999).

Even with a proper matched control group, one may observe adverse effects that introduce confounding factors in the assessment study, such as a change in working methods (van Gennip and Bakker 1995). Their study included three hospitals, each with two matched wards as pairs of cases, and all were assessed in an identical way before and shortly after introduction of the new system. The one hospital involved computer-literate end users, the other two hospitals computer-illiterate users, in order to be able to measure the effect of prior computer experience. However, the computer-literate case was explicitly noted to change working methods during the assessment, yet the study does not report to what extent the other two did the same. Such a change of pattern cannot be expected to produce a black-and-white effect or an on-and-off effect, so some or several measures may be affected and thus become unreliable. In the study referenced, the problem may not be serious because the assessment took place only weeks after the installation. Thus, the two cases without computer literacy would probably not have succeeded in adapting to it and identified and exploited new options within that timeframe. Nevertheless, the study may be used to illustrate the pitfalls of confounding factors, while also pointing to the time factor as an issue of concern.

The assessment of an IT-based solution is complex. For instance, if the effectiveness of healthcare increases, then the number of bed days for a single patient is reduced. However, as long as there are patients waiting, this just means that a new patient will occupy the bed, implying that the throughput will increase, which again implies a higher workload in other respects such as the initial diagnostic effort and so on. Reduced waiting lists will enable booking of more nonacute cases, which in itself is a new pattern of cases. At the same time, strategies for handling and prioritizing waiting lists may change as a function of political, administrative, staff, or research-related issues. Each change will propagate itself into the organization and induce a number of uncontrolled effects, with second and third generation of induced effects, as suggested by the model for organizational change of Leavitt (1970). All of these effects signify potential confounding factors in the holistic system constituted by an organization.

Bryan et al. (1995) say, *"In principle, a contemporaneous comparison of hospitals operating using PACS within hospitals using film-based radiology systems is feasible"*. However, as also discussed by these authors, a suggestion of randomly allocating hospitals or patients to either of the two groups has to be handled cautiously. The reason for promoting caution is that the organizations introducing the PACS will change for many reasons and in many directions as discussed above. This may have uncontrolled effects that evolve as a function of time, while the control group may be fairly constant. A better approach might be to include all hospitals in the development effort (which actually was their ultimate goal for the system), while coordinating the stage of implementation and letting them switch into a partial application of the system only. If the IT-supported parts differ from hospital to hospital (comparable to the approach suggested by O'Moore et al. (1990a) and Wyatt and Spiegelhalter (1991)), they may serve as each other's control group, while being fairly comparable with respect to nonobserved aspects. This is, however, easier said than done with IT systems with wide organizational coverage, as system implementation constitutes a huge organizational effort.

11.1.7 Outcome Measures or End-Points

It is of paramount importance that the actual set of outcome measures is well composed and complies with the information needs drawn from the study objective. So when designing an assessment study, its measures should address the ultimate intension with the object and the phase of the study, as also discussed in Sections 11.1.2 and 11.1.3.3. An example worth mentioning is the distinction between measuring the aid of a decision-support system and the effect on clinical outcomes from introducing the decision-support system into the clinical decision-making process (Wyatt and Spiegelhalter 1991).

Moreover, see the extended discussion of different measures of efficacy, effectiveness, and efficiency in (Wall 1991).

11.1.7.1 *Constructive Assessment*

For constructive assessments, outcome measures may be applied as indicators in terms of tuning points or preventive measures, as seen from the study of Herbst et al. (1999). Its purpose was to increase the likelihood of success in a constructive assessment approach. This study provides us with an example of a solid two-step approach for the identification of outcome measures for constructive assessment, based on an interview approach that in its first step focused on aspirations, expectations, and predictions of potential problems, resulting in ten global issues to pursue in the assessment activities (Herbst et al. 1999). Also, consensus approaches may be applied with benefit for such purposes. However, there is a pitfall in this respect: How to assure the reader of the completeness and validity of the selected (outcome) measures, as there may not be a set point that may serve as an ultimate frame of reference for the desirable outcome.

The very nature of constructive assessment necessitates that it is dynamic and changes according to options. We may not be in a position to know how the IT system would have been had we used another development and assessment approach or other measures. The approach taken by the authors provides some guarantees for the completeness of issues, but only a subsequent analysis of failures ultimately experienced will demonstrate its completeness and validity.

In conclusion, a distinction must be made between choosing outcome measures as tuning points for the system development efforts (constructive assessment) or as indicators for the final system's performance (summative assessment). They may be selected according to the same rules but play different roles in the global process.

11.1.7.2 *The Substitution Game*

This aspect is concerned with whether the study design accentuates risk factors rather than causal relations. According to Jaeschke and Sackett (1989), in general terms, the substitution of changes in a risk factor, not established as causal, for its associated outcome will constitute a pitfall. Medical examples come from studies of coronary heart disease, where many of them claim to be efficacious on the coronary rate because of an effect on one of the risk factors. Consider for instance, the models for understanding co-morbidity (co-occurrence of disorders) by Sher and Trull (1996) as an analogue example from medicine: (1) one disorder may cause another; (2) both disorders may be co-effects or consequences of a common cause or process; (3) mutual (reciprocal) causality; (4) co-occurrence as a chance result attributable to the high base rates within a particular setting; and (5) co-occurrence because of overlapping or similar criteria.

As regards the area of IT systems assessment, an example might be an IT-based learning system, where serious problems with interperson and interinstitutional variations may originate from a number of sources (causes), ranging from lack of standardization or harmonization activities to insufficient education and training. In such a case, professional conservatism among the specialists or their motivation might be risk factors, or different professional schools may bias the inter- and intraperson variation and cover other problems.

The concept of risk factors is not entirely clear for systems development and assessment. That which in one context constitutes a component factor within a cause-effect mechanism may in another context constitute a risk factor. Therefore, it is necessary to discuss the concept of risk factors a bit further to identify the implications for formative assessment.

Risk is defined as *"the possibility of loss"* (Hall 1998), and a risk factor is therefore a variable that controls the possibility of loss. In a systems development context, loss is synonymous with failure and is normally only partial. As an example, within the requirements analysis and design phase, user involvement, and hence motivation, is decisive for the success of the final outcome and therefore is viewed as an element in a cause-effect relationship, whereas hidden agendas, political agendas, or competing activities may constitute risk factors. However, at the assessment of effectiveness or efficiency, motivational factors constitute risk factors. In the methodology of (*Handbook for Objectives-Oriented Planning* 1992), risk factors are handled in terms of external factors (external to the elements in the causal mechanisms, yet impeding one or more of these component elements), and this may be the best way to understand the concept of risk factors in relation to the pitfall stated by Jaeschke and Sackett (1989).

The reason that accentuation of risk factors rather than causal relationships comprises a pitfall is that the interference mechanism may be very complex and with an obscure correlation between the risk factors and an outcome measure, and thus confuse the interpretation of the outcome. Consequently, while carrying out assessment activities, it is necessary for the project management to be in control of the risk factors, or at least be able to monitor them so that they don't turn into confounding factors interfering with other cause-effect relations. Monitoring or controlling the risk factors throughout an assessment activity enables other factors of relevance and their causal relationship to be explored. Thus, if not having an explicit model of the causal relations between different factors within the target object, it is at least necessary to have a model of risk factors while designing the assessment study.

Given the interpretation of Jaeschke and Sackett (1989) in relation to 'the substitution game', a large number of assessment studies in reality may suffer from this bias – namely, a large number of questionnaire studies on user satisfaction as they address the motivational factors explicitly rather than the causal mechanisms leading to satisfaction. Studies like (Gamm et al. 1998a; and

Lauer et al. 2000) address the users' attitudes, expectations or reactions to implementation of an IT system and thus potentially suffer from this problem. However, the difference between the two approaches is that while Gamm et al. use a questionnaire approach to achieve their primary findings and then interviews to search for explanations to elaborate their findings, Lauer et al. use a method (the Equity Implementation Model) explicitly addressing events that are used to analyze and get an understanding of the resistance or acceptance by users. Whether the latter approach succeeds in revealing the causal relations or otherwise handles these within the process of analysis is not fully clear from the paper, but without doubt it is an approach worth considering as an alternative to questionnaire studies.

Being in the middle of this discussion one should not forget the definition of quality in Section 11.1.6.8. Users' perception of usability and user acceptability is strongly linked to their implied needs, which include not only nonstated functional needs, but also subjective feelings and opinions. Thus, the human subjectivity may indeed be relevant as target measures in themselves, as strongly stated by Gremy et al. (1999). So we have a paradox. The perils and the consequential needs of awareness in this situation are related to attempts of interpreting the linkage between the outcome and assumed causal effect mechanisms behind the outcome.

In conclusion, the issue of an assessment study focusing on risk factors rather than indicators of causal relations is not simple. The danger is inherent to statements that interpret the linkage between the outcome and an assumed causal effect mechanism leading to the outcome.

11.1.7.3   Complex Causal Relations

An example of relevance, beyond that discussed in Section 11.1.6.9, is assessment of an IT-based system that is meant to improve a system of Continuous Quality Improvement (CQI), as studied in (Wiik and Lam 2000). A CQI system performs quality management by continuously looking out for problems, while pursuing identified problems in order to solve or alleviate these. It is confusing that a facilitation of the CQI may imply more problems to be handled and therefore appears to increase the number of actual problems. Consequently, one has to await a stable new situation before an effect on a CQI system is measured. However, a question is "When is an improvement due to an improvement of the CQI system or just a consequence of a lot of other things being done at the same time?", like analyzing, implementing, and installing an IT-based system. An indirect effect may originate from a mere change within the organization. The discussion demonstrates that assessment of the effect of an IT-based system on CQI is very complicated, and a better approach in such a complicated case might be to carry out an in-depth case study rather than a case-control study.

11.1.7.4 Comparing Apples and Pears

When comparing groups, there is always a risk of comparing incomparable groups of objects of investigation. Thus, this issue has to be emphasized as a point of concern while considering the study design.

A sample case is the introduction of electronic healthcare records (EHR) on a ward, for which the baseline mode of operation was entirely paper-based. Laboratory Information Systems have been common for decades, contrary to the EHRs. Thus, computer-generated (electronic) reports of laboratory services are correspondingly common, while electronic communication of these reports is not necessarily so. Comparing the efficiency of electronic communication of laboratory service reports with a baseline functionality constituting a human transportation of computer-generated reports does not always provide new information, while an assessment of the impact on clinical performance in the broad sense certainly makes sense.

This example is obviously a paradigm example cut out in carbon. Real-life examples may be much, much more subtle, like in (Gamm et al. 1998a). They performed a study with a pre- and a postinvestigation of user attitudes, where they focused on users' expectations in the preinvestigation and actual attitude in the postinvestigation in a number of ways. However, even if they applied a multimethod approach, there is a different focus for each of the two phases, and it is not clear to the reader how the pre- and postobservations are matched and determined. Yet, the fact that it is a multimethod study partly or fully compensates for this shortcoming and increases the reader's confidence in the conclusion. So the case referenced need not be invalid for this reason – the reader just doesn't know.

Another situation to look for is a study applying the same system for several cases (e.g., several hospitals or departments). When installing such systems it is common to customize them to the actual application and the local organizational environment. Thereby, one has to bear in mind that for some cases there is a risk of comparing apples and pears, rendered even worse when there is six months or more between installations, like in (Gamm et al. 1998a), as precisely half a year is a commonly used interval between versions and major updates of systems. This, of course, depends on the study question addressed. Nevertheless, an awareness and handling of this issue in a visible manner within the reporting will increase the reader's confidence in the study conclusion.

11.1.7.5 Technical Verification of Outcome Measures

In medicine it is customary to certify the quality characteristics of the outcome measures; see, for instance, the list of common measures in (Jaeschke and Sackett 1989): Sensitivity, specificity, receiver operating characteristic curves, and likelihood measures, however, not to mention the huge number of other metrological quality measures (see, for instance, Dybkær et al. 1992; and BIPM et al. 1993). In contrast, the domain users of an IT-based system or tool tend to trust that the system performs all actions and calculations in a correct, complete, and consistent manner, or that to live with potential problems is acceptable. This is definitely not a valid assumption per se. In case the IT system calculates a specific measure, correctness of the outcome measures may with some justification be assumed for off-the-shelf systems but not for prototype IT-based systems. Moreover, one may assume a simple summation or calculation to be correct but definitely not a measure like the Kappa-value for a prototype system explicitly addressing intra- and interpersonal variation in professional performance, as done in (Wiik and Lam 2000). In this case, it would have been a matter of adding (1) the formula and the literature reference for the Kappa-value and (2) a statement that the correctness had been verified by the users prior to the study – for example, by hand or by application of statistical tools.

The quality of the outcome measures presented is imperative for the interpretation of the outcome of an assessment study. Therefore, outcome measures need to be well defined and verified with respect to their quality characteristics, including general behavior like sensitivity (the degree to which the measure is influenced by various variables and assumptions). All of this has to be visible in the study description, especially when the study is assumed and pretends to be quantitative by nature. All that is necessary in a publication in order to convince the reader is a statement as simple as "technical verification of the system prior to the assessment of . . . revealed no bugs that will hamper a conclusion made on the basis of the present findings". No study fulfilling even this basic information need was found so far, nor was any fulfilling the more extended requirements.

11.1.8 Aspects of Culture

Our understanding of the concept of 'culture' may be expressed shortly this way: *"By cultural behavior, we mean the stability across generations of behavioral patterns acquired through social communication within a group, and valued by the group"* (Maturana 1987, cited and discussed in Demeester 1995). Culture is the style of working in the field or the mental, tacit (learned) behavioral pattern behind the style of working (Hampden-Turner and Trompenaars 1993 and 1997; and Trompenaars and Hampden-Turner 1997). Thus, culture is guiding the preferences; culture is what comes before starting a discussion of strategy, and so forth, in a chain of causal events toward problem solving. When specifically talking of the interpretation of culture in an organizational context it means "the acquired preferences in problem solving", where problem solving should be understood in the broadest sense and not only as problem solving in a profession oriented perspective.

Inability to take cultural aspects into account may imply a huge bias in the planning, execution and interpretation of an assessment study. This bias is called 'ethnocentrism' by Coolican (1999) and is concerned with *"interpreting the behavior of another culture as one would interpret that behavior in one's own culture".*

The discussion above specifically points to management and decision-making issues as being particularly vulnerable to cultural differences. The consequence is seen in (Fröhlich et al. 1993), which so clearly demonstrates that even within Europe (European Union) there are huge differences in our way of doing things, merely by showing the outcome of an investigation on types of involvement in systems development and implementation for different categories of employees. This implies that what is a valid conclusion in one culture may certainly not apply to another cultural setting. Specifically for the healthcare sector, Kaplan (2000) discusses the need to take culture seriously into account in terms of an organization's history and current circumstances.

The discussion in Section 11.1.7.2 on user involvement and motivational factors is a paradigm discussion biased by a Western cultural perspective on how things work: The master thesis work by Malling (1992) clearly demonstrates that one of the reasons why a modern development approach applied to a major systems development project in Thailand failed was that the end users refused to get involved due to the decision-making pattern within that culture, strictly in contradiction to trends and demands in Western cultures.

Consequently, particularly careful planning must be applied when generalizing studies – for instance, questionnaires across country borders and also between organizations or professions: *"Culture can be as different from one organization to the next just as surely as it can be different from nation to nation"* (Kaplan 2000).

11.2 Types of (Experimental) Weaknesses

The scope of this section is to outline a number of potential pitfalls and perils that are correlated to data collection, analysis, and/or interpretation.

11.2.1   The Developers' Actual Engagement

This section pinpoints some biases that may arise as a result of the developers' engagement in an assessment study, depending on their actual role and interests. All of this does not mean that one should exclude the developers as collaborators and hence authors of the study report. On the contrary, one has to be fair toward one's collaborators, and those contributing also have the right to the credit for that. However, it means that when reporting a study, one should be strict and open about the relations and agreements between the two (or more) parties as well as about the type of engagement or role of the parties.

Note that the concept of 'developers' here also includes potential consultants on organizational changes and similar external people.

11.2.1.1   Beyond the Developer's Point of View

"The developers of an information resource usually are emphatic only up to a point and are often not predisposed to be detached and objective about their system's performance"

(Friedman and Wyatt 1997)

Moreover, the relationship (for instance, in terms of a desire for a future contractual or strategic relationship) or interdependency between the developer and a user organization may be of a nature that prohibits an objective study or study reporting. Or even worse, confidentiality agreements in a contractual relationship may prohibit certain details from surfacing in a report, in which case the credibility and/or the scientific value of the study may be severely reduced. When not explicitly stated by the authors, a first place to look is in the list of authors and affiliated organizations.

When the developers are deeply involved in an assessment, the readers may rightfully question the impartiality of the entire process and the outcome measures, and thus also the conclusion. Therefore, a description of stakeholders participating in an assessment study is important for the interpretation of an assessment study. It is of utmost importance that the reader knows the role and influence of the developers (and beyond) on the approach, data processing, and interpretation. A prime example in this respect is provided by Kaplan and Lundsgaarde (1996), as they, in a few words, make this clear to the reader: *"Both researchers were from outside the institution; they were asked to perform the evaluation by the system developer"*. Perfect, but even more perfect would have been if they had also stated their terms for publishing their findings.

Even the mere presence of the developers may change the behavior of the participants in a way comparable to a Hawthorne effect or a feed-back effect (see Sections 11.1.6.2 and 11.2.4).

11.2.1.2 *Unstable Technology*

Some types of technology, like surgical expertise, may unintentionally evolve during the assessment period (Jaeschke and Sackett 1989). Similarly, evolution of supportive technology, adaptation, and further exploitation of the options enabled by the applied technology may take place (Fineberg 1985). For IT-based systems, this is not restricted only to changes in the organizational environment, including second order changes or adaptations induced by the new technology (like that presented in (van Gennip and Bakker 1995); see Section 11.1.6.9). Included here are in particular changes within the IT system itself.

Again, there is a difference between summative assessments and constructive assessments. There may be a serious error in a summative assessment study if the IT-based system is changing during assessments, while changes in the IT system (or its design or specifications) is the very nature of constructive assessment approaches as seen from, for instance, the study reported in (Gordon and Geiger 1999). They rightfully kept the method applied stable while the project used it as a constructive support of the design and implementation process. Had they also changed the method during the study, a moving target bias (for the assessment) would have resulted.

It is nice to see the honesty in this respect in the discussion within (Wiik and Lam 2000): *"During the . . . experiment, regular contact was made through telephone and e-mails between the lead laboratory at . . . and . . . (comment: the developer). Thereby fine-tuning of the functionality of . . . was undertaken to meet the detailed requirements of the end users. Although it was initially planned to use experience from . . . , delay in the delivery of the software prevented this transfer of experience"* (end of citation). It means that the technology indeed was unstable and changed during the assessment study that was meant to be summative. Consequently, the outcome of the study reflects a constructive and a summative assessment at the same time. The extent to which this wrecks the outcome of the study is unknown. It may even be that the outcome is slightly underestimated as compared to what might have been the outcome had the tool been ready when the assessment started. In a concrete summative assessment case the impact from an unstable technology may be nondrastic if only details are iterated, and this can be handled in the interpretation of the assessment outcome. However, this way of sitting between two chairs is definitely not to be recommended under normal circumstances, and one has to be extremely careful when interpreting the outcome.

Another legitimate type of active engagement by the developers in an assessment study is that sometimes it is necessary to remove obstacles to the assessment. This is especially valid for constructive assessments where the development activities are still ongoing. Yet, removing obstacles should not be intermixed with an improvement of functionalities in reporting an assessment study, unless intentional. There should be no gray zone between these two extremes (for summative assessment studies).

For summative assessments, it is preferable for the interpretation of the assessment study to freeze the functionality of the IT system while assessing it and call technical assistance only when needed. The developer may then in parallel carry out technical developments on known problems and provide the evaluation team with a new version at the end of the assessment study. A postverification activity can then investigate whether the new version lessens the identified shortcomings, and a PostScript statement may be added to the conclusion of the assessment report.

A challenge for the meta-analysis of assessment studies is that it may not be easy to find such information on the developers' engagement. It may, for instance, be implicit in the text under methods, results, or discussion, like in (Wiik and Lam 2000) rather than explicitly described up-front like in (Kaplan and Lundsgaarde 1996).

In conclusion, when reporting from an assessment study, it has to be clear to the reader whether, why, and how the developers of an IT-based solution are engaged, as this has implications both of a methodological kind and on the interpretation of the study outcome. Therefore, it is recommended that all assessment studies explicitly state the involvement and role of the different stakeholders within the assessment study.

11.2.2   Intra- and Interperson (or -Case) Variability

People are different, professional practices are different, organizations are different, and cultures are different. Depending on the assessment methods applied (subjective ones naturally being the most vulnerable), innumerable factors may contribute to an observer bias, originating within the interaction between the observer and the object of investigation (Coolican 1999); consequently, it is relevant who performs which parts of a study.

Moreover, this variability is relevant not only among the observers within a study, but also to the participants: Even if two organizations are of identical type, like two clinical wards, and even if matched by characteristics, the professionals working in the two organizations have different backgrounds and contextual environments for the interpretation of what is presented to them. This is obvious in connection with cross-border studies and has deep roots of origin in professional practices (Nolan et al. 1991; and Brender et al. 1995); while within a region or within neighboring departments differences may reflect variations in the technology applied or the choices made and the evolution of local practice.

Consequently, the intra- and interperson variation may become a serious problem when a case includes only a limited number of users or cases. Thus, the merger in (Wiik and Lam 2000) of two users from one organization with one user from a similar organization in another country into a study population of three subjects is considered as seriously biased, unless the two subsets are thoroughly investigated for matching characteristics. However, this effort is not visible within their report, notwithstanding that it is not easy to match the characteristics of two subjects with those of one subject to a level that will lend credibility from a logistical or statistical point of view.

In contrast, the study presented in (van Gennip and Bakker 1995) demonstrates in this respect a great deal of awareness of pitfalls in the interpretation, like extrapolations and variability among the cases, matching of controls and study groups, and so on.

A bias from intra- and interperson variation may be especially influential when the user group comprises physicians (see also Section 11.1.4). The reason being that in a ward there are normally just a few physicians, ranging from chief physicians to consultants, to senior registrars and registrars, of which some may be in a short-term specialty training position or he or she may be in a specialty training scheme in another specialty, just acquiring the necessary generalist training, – all of which makes a difference. In (Gamm et al. 1998a), the six sites involved comprise outpatient clinics from rural and urban areas in the United States, and includes 22 physicians (*"and physician assistants"*) from these six sites (in the longitudinal study: 12 physicians from three sites). A pretty extensive study has been accomplished and reported within (Gamm et al. 1998a). However, it is not possible for the reader to get a feeling of the homogeneity and comparability of the sites in terms of physician characteristics, nor of the pattern of replies as a function of apprenticeship. It may make no difference as regards the conclusion, or there may be internal patterns within the data impairing the interpretation – the reader is powerless to judge this.

In conclusion, when one theoretical model is applied for more than one organization that serve as cases in a case study, a strong awareness of confounding factors in terms of inter- and intraperson variability is necessary.

11.2.3   Illicit Use

Illicit use or lack of use of the system will introduce a bias (Wyatt and Spiegelhalter 1991). In medicine and medical decision-making, lack of compliance to the research protocol is an example, while for IT-based solutions this includes not only the lack of compliance to the assessment protocol, but also a lack of compliance with user manuals. Hence, this bias is relevant for all types of IT-based systems.

Illegitimate use may appear as misuse, abuse, or even sabotage, all of which may give a severely damaged image of a system's performance or its functioning. Such bias may not be intentionally illegitimate, but it could also arise as a consequence of inadequate training or follow-up on the changes in an organization.

It is natural for users to invent new applications of the system or to exploit the new system's options in what some may perceive as illicit ways, but this may actually be a sign of the opposite (see, for instance, van Gennip and Bakker 1995). There is, however, a grayzone where the deviations included merely are a natural variation within the work procedures, as Gruding specifically points out:

> *"A wide range of error handling, exception handling and improvisation are characteristic of human activity . . . People know when the 'spirit of the law' takes precedence over 'the letter of the law' ".*

(Gruding 1991)

Such changes or variations will perhaps be even more pronounced for IT-based systems (Keen et al. 1995), as such systems/solutions are never finished. As a result, the object of investigation for an assessment study may truly be a moving target. To get a long-term perspective, one may just think of the changes implied or the revolution of practice following the introduction of the photocopying machine, which is comparable. In an organizational setting this merely reflects the dynamic nature of an organization, as seen in Section 11.1.6.9.

Consequently, this effect is not necessarily to be considered as entirely negative, but it may definitely bias the interpretation of the data from an assessment outcome should the authors not be aware of this phenomenon. Moreover, it is worth noting that this bias is highly susceptible to time and therefore more likely in longitudinal studies; the more the users get used to a new system, the more innovative they are likely to be, implying that any symptom of alternative usage patterns must be searched for within the data material.

11.2.3.1   Assessment Bias

The feeling for the belief in an information source (IT-based system), whether negative or positive, may bias the outcome (Friedman and Wyatt 1997). While carrying out an assessment study, the participants may start collecting extra data to prove themselves right and the system wrong or vice versa (Wyatt and Spiegelhalter 1991). This bias is particularly relevant for the assessment of expert systems and decision-support systems, where for instance a system's diagnostic performance is compared to the performance of a user group, like expert physicians. Moreover, this bias is particularly likely if the participants have strong preconceptions about the value of the system (Wyatt and Spiegelhalter 1991) or fear of making errors. The increased data volume may augment the diagnostic effectiveness of the control system by enforcement of the decision-making basis, but it will decrease the corresponding cost-effectiveness of the control group. One should monitor for this bias. This may be achieved through a longitudinal measurement of certain indicators, like size of the decision-making basis (for instance, number of tests per diagnose should be invariant).

An analogue for other types of IT-based solutions may consist of individual initiatives to perform parallel bookkeeping by means of the previous paper-based system or just in terms of paper notes in the users' pockets.

No example of measures of this type has been identified within the literature.

11.2.3.2   Evaluation Paradox

A special type of 'illicit use' may arise in a field trial of decision-support systems and may therefore be of special relevance for studies of such systems: Some users may be reluctant to rely upon a new technology until it has been proven valid and beneficial (Wyatt and Spiegelhalter 1991; and Friedman and Wyatt 1997). The consequence may be that the system is not fully applied as intended, resulting in different kinds of illicit use – for instance, the 'assessment bias' (see Section 11.2.3.1) or a lack of conformity to the protocol (see also Section 11.2.14).

11.2.4   Feed-back Effect

The philosophy of providing concurrent feed-back is the philosophy behind the enabling mechanism of a learning process. Moreover, intentional usage of the feed-back effect is explicitly the philosophy of critiquing decision-support systems, as in (van der Lei 1991), where for instance the constant feed-back on pharmaceutical interferences or necessary investigations in certain cases is intended for the gradual training of the user, with the scope of reducing the frequency of undesirable events. So the feed-back effect is not considered wrong per se.

Still, the feed-back effect sometimes does constitute a bias, as discussed by Friedman and Wyatt (1997). An example is when the feed-back interferes with measures of the diagnostic accuracy of medical decision-support systems compared with a group of physicians (Wyatt and Spiegelhalter 1991). This bias may also be induced because of the implicit training by the system of relevant measures to perform in general.

Another example of this bias for assessment of IT-based solutions in general is a scenario, where there is an interaction between the developers and the users during the assessment. The developer's presence may be needed for technical reasons during assessment of prototype systems; however, the developers should be kept under control. An interaction between the developers and the users may unintentionally compensate for problems in a learning mode and may in a short-term perspective hide serious problems. Studies on usability are particularly vulnerable to the involvement or presence of the developer: When a problem is identified within the ergonomics or within the cognitive support or functionality of the IT system the developer may by his extended knowledge of the system immediately introduce a shortcut or an explanation to the problem. The effect of providing concurrent feed-back thus compares to an accelerated training of the users in using the system in the right way. In healthcare, the throughput of physicians on a ward may be pretty large, so it does matter to what extent training in the new solution is needed and consequently the impact of feed-back on the conclusion may be significant. The problem is that the system is not assessed on its own – that is, the usability or user acceptability might be overestimated. The impact of this bias depends on what one wants to assess by the study, – the short-term usage (corresponding to immediately after a purchase and installation of a commercial system) or the long-term usage (the users know all the shortcomings and inconveniences and compensate by the mode of usage). Naturally, the long-term effect will tell whether it is worth pursuing a commercial development, and, therefore, this type of bias may be considered less significant in a long-term study of an effect. A remaining problem for a long-term study is that the reader of the conclusion cannot judge the up-front struggle with the system in case the assessment focus is on usability and acceptability.

If the users are not trained well enough before the assessment, the system's own reactions will serve as a feed-back mechanism and provide training to the users.

One way to identify a feed-back effect might be to look for a time dependency within the data material.

11.2.5   Extra Work

Assessment studies often lead to extra workloads for the participants. This may naturally imply increased efficiency in the participants' work at the expense of his or her effectiveness (Wyatt and Spiegelhalter 1991) with a consequential underestimation of the assessment outcome, signifying a bias. Therefore, it is just perfect that a study like (Østbye et al. 1997) explicitly includes data of the workload before and during the introduction of the new system and the assessment activity and compares its findings with the control group's workload. However, see also the discussion in Section 11.1.6.1, where the problem of competing activities is raised: only one of the groups is engaged in the development and implementation work, while the control group is not. It is not visible from the study whether compensatory resources are introduced into the organization in order to avoid the effect of extra work.

11.2.6   Judgmental Biases

Human judgment is not always reliable. There are a number of situations, where the judgment of probabilities makes a trick with the human belief, based on interfering psychological factors. In particular, Fraser and Smith (1992) go into details with a number of variants concerning people's ability to judge probabilities of events, a subject that is extremely important in studies applying subjective or fuzzy measures. They themselves state that not all of these biases are fully documented within the literature, or that the context of their appearance may not be fully known.

Similarly, Rosenthal (1976) reviews a number of studies dealing with behavioral biases, like biosocial (e.g., the effect of age, sex, and race of the experimenter), psychosocial (e.g., emotional effects), situational effects (e.g., experimenter's experience), and the effect of the experimenter's own expectations. Except from the situational factors, which are included in Section 11.1.2.1, the other biases are judged less significant when assessing IT-based solutions.

11.2.6.1   Hindsight or Insight Bias

There is a risk of a bias, when dealing with nonblinded events. Informing people about the outcome of an event increases their post-hoc estimate of the probability of that outcome (Fraser and Smith 1992). Furthermore, when the process/action under investigation is fully open to the parties involved, they may overestimate the effect when this is not objectively measured (Jaeschke and Sackett 1989).

A sample scenario is a training or examination situation, at which the trainees are given the task of classifying objects. The trainees don't posses the expertise to be able to classify fairly objectively, so in case they know the composition of the study population prior to the classification efforts, there will be a bias toward the known a priori probability of each class. Such a case is seen in (Wiik and Lam 2000), where groups of histo-pathologists by means of an image-handling IT-based tool are asked to classify a number of patient cases with melanocytic lesions, with the global purpose of measuring changes within the inter- and intragroup variability as a function of time. Only one of the pathologists had precisely this domain as his area of expertise. Two problems appear in the case study in this respect. First, the population of samples includes only pathological samples, and only samples of melanocytic lesions. Second, the number of samples is smaller than the total number of possible classifications in the taxonomy of melanocytic lesions. In such a setup, all classes in the study cannot be expected to mimic the a priori real-life frequency, nor will all diagnoses appear. Therefore, when the domain is known, the line of reasoning among colleagues will unintentionally put focus on those classifications that are more likely than others. Furthermore (and not known for this case), in case it is the nominated expert who collects and composes the set of cases dealt with, the frame of reference will also be biased, because he or she knows which diagnoses are included and which are not. In a real daily life practice, every sample would be unknown and thus the span of the sample outcome would be much larger. Consequently, the measures cannot reflect a real-life variation within and among groups of pathologists.

In short, the setup of assessment has to be designed according to the question asked of the study, and if that is concerned with the effect in real practice, then the study has to mimic the real practice situation – or one has to be aware of and judge the impact from this bias.

11.2.6.2   *Judgment of the Probability of Events*

People's judgment of probabilities of events differs from the empirically observed frequency (Fraser and Smith 1992).

Østbye et al. (1997) report from their study that 78% of ward users subjectively reported that they called the laboratory less often than before installation; however, the (objective) investigation of actual telephone activity shows that there is no clear change. At the same time, the study reports compliance between the subjective and objective measures of telephone activity for the laboratory users, thereby indicating that there may be confounding factors in one (or both) of the study groups. So this is obviously a relevant bias to take into account when assessing how often certain events take place.

11.2.6.3   *Judgment of Performance*

An experiment with triangulation of methods (see the concept in Section 11.3.2.1) revealed that humans in a questionnaire survey may actually rate the usability of a system in a very positive light despite actual serious problems revealed by triangulation with an objective investigation accomplished in parallel (Kushniruk et al. 1997): A questionnaire as well as a videorecording were elicited. At first, one might explain the difference as diverging opinions between the researchers and the users on what are serious problems. However, their observation is consistent with what others have observed as well, as noted by Kushniruk et al.

(1997). Also note the comment on the similar, biased judgment in (Østbye et al. 1997), where 78% of the users reported a given change, but this change was not reflected in a parallel objective measure.

Further, the findings of Beuscart-Zéphir et al. (1997) indicate that one has to be careful not to address situations that enable a respondent to answer in a prescriptive manner rather than to correlate to the realities in his or her actual work procedures; see Section 11.1.5.3.

11.2.6.4 *Miscellaneous Judgmental Biases*

A. *Connected events*: Errors are likely to appear in the judgment of the probability of tied events (including multistage inference and testing the conditions for a rule of the type "if . . . then"), in the judgment of connected or associated, but independent events, and in the judgment of association (i.e., probabilistic dependencies) at occurrence or nonoccurrence of events (Fraser and Smith 1992)

B. *Overprediction*: People tend to give similar predictions to situations with different degrees of uncertainty (Fraser and Smith 1992)

C. *Miscalibration*: People are over-confident in their own judgment of general-knowledge items of moderate or extreme difficulty (Fraser and Smith 1992)

D. *Illusion of control*: This is concerned with the perception of control over objectively chance-determined events – that is, distinguishing skill situations from chance situations (Fraser and Smith 1992)

E. *Confirmation bias*: When measured, instances expected to be positive instances tend to show a bias toward such a positive outcome (Fraser and Smith 1992, page 289). An example from an image or ECG classification study shows that knowing beforehand that all images or ECGs are pathological will a priori make the classifiers exclude the class 'normal' from the solution space searched, even if this class outcome is part of the span of classes

F. *Differential treatment of positive and negative information*: People process information more efficiently if it is presented in a positive form than if it is presented in a negative form (Fraser and Smith 1992). An example is the ability to process text that includes "not known" as compared with "unknown" – or, even worse – double negations

11.2.7 *Postrationalization*

Much knowledge (or awareness) is tacit, implicit and inaccessible to consciousness, and external pressure to provide answers may lead to postrationalization (Barry 1995). The tacit nature of not only past events but also of present activities implies that findings may be incomplete or biased. Conventional methods for evaluation, such as questionnaires and interviews, include a bias caused by users' limitations in recalling their experiences (Kushniruk et al. 1997), and the same is the case when trying to recall one's motivation or line of reasoning.

Postrationalization may in particular affect the elicitation of causes for observed phenomena, while exploring observed phenomena during the data analysis, because once an event or a state has passed, it is more difficult to reflect on the view at the time of the event/state (Barry 1995). For instance, Kushniruk and Patel (2004) illustrate the problem of inconsistencies found by means of triangulation with videorecording versus questionnaires presented some time after the events. This does not imply that unconscious problems and causes are not relevant or not feasible to address – they may certainly be. Moreover, we may postulate that *the* major problems and causes are the ones most likely *not* to be forgotten, but postrationalization is a strong bias and definitely necessary to have in mind at the design and implementation stages of assessment studies.

11.2.8   Verification of Implicit Assumptions

Not all assumptions are as explicit as those normally defined for application of well-known methods (see Section 11.1.2.2). Implications of decisions made are another type of assumptions, as shall be seen from the following.

11.2.8.1   Matching of Study and Control Groups

Case-control studies are prone to one special type of bias (Jaeschke and Sackett 1989): Cases with a particular characteristic under investigation (like exposure to something) are gathered, and then matched with a group of controls that have not been previously exposed. The risk of a bias here is related to a potential skewness when matching cases and controls. Consequently, it is relevant to identify whether and how much effort the authors have invested to actually verify a correct matching of cases in order to avoid confounding factors (see also Section 11.1.6.9 and the review in (Sher and Trull 1996) of means for analyzing case-control issues). As shown by Østbye et al. (1997), it may be that fairly simple means or measures are needed to convince the reader of matching case and control groups.

11.2.8.2   Implicit Domain Assumptions

Cross-border studies and studies that involve more than one organization have a number of implicit assumptions. A number of studies have clearly demonstrated the effect of epidemiology on the clinical effectiveness of decision-support systems (see, for instance, Bjerregaard et al. 1976; and Lindberg 1982).

Furthermore, the study of Nolan et al. (1991) reports from an investigation of a standard medical procedure applied as the basis for the development of decision-support systems or algorithms at three different European sites. Their study demonstrates that in addition to the epidemiological factor, terminological differences or different interpretations of specific terms within the standard procedure are key factors, hampering the transferability of such systems. These confounding factors are especially risky for cross-border studies and comparative investigations and are perceived as a bias within the data – also valid for the target readers to bear in mind when interpreting the conclusion of a study. It may arise from differences in terminology systems and is not only restricted to medical procedures. Questionnaires and theoretical models or otherwise stand-alone written material are victims of the same kind of diverging interpretations. Therefore, it is important to search the data volume for signs indicating that such hidden assumptions have been verified if the verification is not included in its entirety. And, therefore, it is necessary that applied procedures, tools, and techniques are clearly documented in a study report.

11.2.9 Novelty of the Technology – Technophile or Technophobe

Effects of prior inadequate technical literacy (Wyatt and Spiegelhalter 1991) may constitute a severe bias in an assessment study; see also the section on '(un-)used users' (Section 11.1.4.2). Several aspects are at stake in this respect.

First, prior inadequate technical literacy may have several causes. One is lack of exposure to that technology, and in that case, the motivation or psychological barriers are not a problem. A learning curve, however, may interfere with the interpretation of the performance of the system. Conversely, insufficient literacy may originate from technophobia (fear), causing the behavioral pattern to take a variety of forms, ranging from hostility or prejudice to apathy or lethargy. At both extremes, the performance (benefit, usability, or . . .) will be underestimated.

Second, with the knowledge that a problem exists in an organization and that traditional means will require overwhelming investments of one kind or another, it is natural to look for new technology as the rescuer (technophile), implying the risk of a bias, and consequently, that the performance is overestimated. A proper control group approach may prevent this type of bias.

One way of looking into the data for this bias may be to look for subpopulations either characterized by different patterns of motivation or lack of prior literacy. Alternatively, when similar groups from two or more organizations are involved, one may search for characteristics that differ. Unfortunately, a reader will normally not be in a situation enabling such an inspection, and in that case, it is valuable to search for information that (1) indicates whether and how cases or users have actually been matched, and how the validity of this match has been verified after the event or (2) a description of exclusion criteria for noncomplying subjects (see Section 11.2.14), followed by a description of the appearance of such subjects.

11.2.10 *Spontaneous Regress*

Symptoms, signs, and other manifestations of disease may spontaneously regress, making even useless interventions appear worthwhile (Jaeschke and Sackett 1989). The same is valid in organizations, where long-lasting problems may disappear, either spontaneously or when other seemingly independent events take place, like the leave of a superior. This type of bias may be further enforced in assessment studies of IT-based systems, as the number of cases included within a study may be only one or a few, implying that averaging by means of large numbers of subjects (cases) cannot be achieved. Consequently, this phenomenon is definitely relevant to consider when interpreting assessment studies.

This discussion emphasizes the one in Section 11.1.7.2 on the need of having a model of the causal relations within the object of investigation. With such a model one may identify cases of spontaneous regress as inexplicable on the basis of that model, like in medicine where even chronically ill patients sometimes unexpectedly become well. Such cases will normally be recognizable within the data material of a study as extremes of one kind or another and may be explored as such. If there is more than one of a kind, they will reveal themselves as a (minority) subgroup within the study material. So, vice versa, if there are subgroups within the data material, one should investigate for this phenomenon; see, for instance, the suggestions by Brookes et al. (2001).

11.2.11 *False Conclusions*

11.2.11.1 *False-Negative Studies*

When the outcome measures cannot detect actual changes or differences among groups, there is a risk of Type II Errors (false-negative studies, concluding that a treatment is not efficacious when, in fact, it is) (Jaeschke and Sackett 1989; Friedman and Wyatt 1997; and Coolican 1999). The actual sample size is definitely one source of this type of error, so, again, when the discriminative power of the outcome measures is known, a power function may indicate the sample size required to avoid this type of error (see Section 11.1.3.3).

11.2.11.2 False-Positive Studies

On the other hand, there is also a risk of false-positive studies (Type I Errors), which conclude that a treatment is efficacious when, in fact, it is not (Friedman and Wyatt 1997; and Coolican 1999). One of the pitfalls in this respect is that it is alluring to seek and present those measures out of the totality of outcome measures that are in favor of the scope or hypothesis, at the expense of objectivity. It is safer that the design of an assessment study be based on an approach that (1) attempts to reject the hypothesis or (2) applies measures that broadly characterize the qualities of the overall solution. It is a pitfall for a reader of a case study report that assessment studies often don't present each and every measure acquired and analyzed. Particularly, in this respect, it is important to choose a representative set of measures when filtering what to submit. It is necessary that the report on an assessment study provides a glimpse of the entirety and not only a potentially biased selection. This is not only a matter of objectivity, honesty, or lack of awareness, but may be enforced simply by limited space allocated to the presentation, which so often is the case during conference proceedings, for instance. Still, it is feasible to present a lot of data in a short text, as seen from (Kushniruk and Patel 1995). Alternatively – in case of insufficient space – a glimpsed statement may be as simple as "No other significant findings (or benefits, or . . .) were found from *** measures of ***". Such a statement will give a hint as to the depth of the study and the proportion of findings to support the data presented and its conclusion.

11.2.11.3 Competing Risks

When a major event precludes the subsequent occurrence of a lesser event, then the latter cannot be explicated on its own (Jaeschke and Sackett 1989). A medical example would be a longitudinal study, where the death of a proportion of the participants is covered by the risk of stroke. For an analogue of the assessment of an IT-based system an example could be the malfunctioning of one part of the system that prohibits determination of performance for the system as a whole. Therefore, sequencing events, and in particular unforeseen events observed in a study, should always be analyzed in respect of their implications.

11.2.12 Incomplete Studies or Study Reports

One can compare reporting practice in medical informatics with that of the medical arena: In medicine, a report on the history of a single interesting patient is normally not published unless the case and the outcome measures are outstanding and thoroughly documented, while this type of reporting often takes place in medical informatics literature.

11.2.12.1 A Publication Dilemma

In the medical informatics arena, a problem often encountered is studies with a biased focus on presenting the implementation of new technological opportunities, while scarcely reporting on the assessment of the system or solution developed.

There is a publication dilemma in many studies reported in the literature: A description of a development issue or method that one finds relevant for others to learn from may gain little appreciation by the target audience until its value is documented in terms of an assessment study. However, documentation of such an assessment takes a tremendous effort and contains sufficient information for a publication in itself. So what to report – the development or the assessment? Neither can do without the other.

As viewed from an assessor's point of view, one example out of numerous publications suffering from this dilemma is the otherwise sound study of Allan and Englebright (2000), where the presentation approach leaves too little space for documentation of the assessment results. The evaluation results in the referenced case are both quantitative and seemingly strong and convincing – had the assessment results stated not been completely lacking in a description of the methods for judging them.

11.2.12.2 Intention to Provide Information

Of course, it is useful to assess the benefits of an IT-based system, the way that Kaplan and Lundsgaard (1996) did it: *"Interviewees were asked specifically about benefits they thought the Imaging System provided"*. Their study was explicitly planned with this limited scope. However, what about the other half of the story – the neutral aspects and especially the drawbacks of the Imaging System? Friedman and Wyatt (1997) call this skewed presentation 'intention to provide information' bias.

In theory, one single shortcoming of an IT-based solution may be so severe that its entire use is threatened. Consequently, a reader may rightfully doubt a conclusion, which says *". . . indirectly assessing the first three of Hillman's five stage assessment hierarchy . . .: imaging efficacy, diagnostic efficacy, and therapeutic efficacy. These efficacies were believed by the physicians to give positive results in the last two stages: improvements in patient outcomes, and cost effectiveness"* (Kaplan and Lundsgaard 1996). Whether this is a likely prognosis or not is up to the reader to judge from the findings presented. Nevertheless, telling half the story does not leave the readers with a feeling of trust in the solution and that the system if installed in their department will have no major obstacles. In the present case, this feeling of a study bias is strengthened by the explicitly mentioned fact that the study was ordered by the developer of the system.

11.2.12.3 *Presentation of the Future*

The study of Galfalvy et al. (1995) so nicely and gradually elaborates the study purpose from an overall objective of studying the effectiveness to a focus on a combination of six specific assessment questions, each with descriptions of methods and procedures. However, the reader is left in a state of not knowing whether the approach and the methods applied are valid and useful. The major problem with their publication is that it constitutes a description of what is going to take place in the future: *"... will be followed ...", "will be prepared ...",* and *"So far, only results of the first survey of providers are available".* Such a publication may primarily serve as inspiration for others who want to address the same assessment question and prepare a similar dedicated approach, but there is no guarantee of the value of the approach.

Yet, this is to some extent an agreed practice for conference proceedings, as the final outcome may succeed in being presented at the conference itself and thus be of momentary value (but not lasting value) to the audience of the conference. However, this practice definitely diminishes the value of the written proceedings, and this is aggravated by the fact that the final outcome seldom is published in its entirety.

11.2.12.4 *Exhaustion of the Data Material*

It is necessary that the data material and the observations presented are exhaustive in order to explain all observed phenomena. For example, the data material collected may unexpectedly reveal two or more (distinct or cogent) subpopulations. In such cases, the data material needs to be further explored for plausible explanations. The appearance of subgroups may be real or just statistically coincidental (Feinstein 1998). Which of the two is the answer has to be explored (Brookes et al. 2001), even if subgroup analysis sometimes is a risky business (Smith and Egger 1998), partly because we are normally not dealing with marginally different user and case groups in assessment studies, as is often the case for RCT in medicine.

One explanation may be that the subjects of the investigation originate from two different subgroups that differ in apprenticeship or professional background, as discussed in a previous section. Another explanation could be that the investigators (e.g., interviewers) belong to two populations, or that other unforeseen factors/biases influence the one group but not the other. When concluding that two or more seemingly identical organizations in an investigation are actually different, one has to consider the potential of a bias from terminological, methodological, cultural, epidemiological, organizational differences, and so on, as previously discussed in Section 11.2.8.

11.2.13   Hypothesis Fixation

Hypothesis fixation occurs when an investigator persists in maintaining a hypothesis that has conclusively been demonstrated to be false (Fraser and Smith 1992). When a specific hypothesis is addressed (rather than an explorative investigation), this hypothesis should be explicitly stated and shown as an integrated part of the assessment protocol. It is definitely relevant to consider this type of bias in studies on assessments of IT-based solutions.

A prime example illustrating this bias in general may be the fixation of the Middle Ages on a model of the universe, where Earth is flat and at the center of the universe; today we know that this theory was wrong. Nevertheless, it was persistently pursued and with cruel means.

An example from assessments of IT systems may be the hypothesis that a given expert system/decision-support system is clinically useful. Another example of a hypothesis is that an IT system is as useful in a new organizational environment as it was in the one that originally designed and implemented it – that is, that the system/solution is transferable. The latter seems to be an implicit assumption behind the marketing of new IT systems. These are examples related to the object of investigation, but a third example may be the hypothesis that a given methodology/method is generally applicable, like a system development method or the RCT assessment method. These and a couple of other issues of relevance for the hypothesis fixation bias are discussed in a number of subsequent sections.

11.2.13.1   Publication Bias

Publication bias *"is a bias in the published literature, where the publication of research depends on the nature and direction of study results"* (Royle and Waugh 2003). Another kind of publication bias outlined by these authors is 'location bias', affecting controversial results and results that contradict existing knowledge and therefore is to be found in less prestigious journals or published in the gray literature (proceedings, technical reports, dissertations, book chapters, etc.) if at all successful in being published. The authors review four studies, which compare the effect of inclusion or exclusion of the gray literature in meta-analyses. The conclusion was that scientifically published trials showed an overall greater treatment effect than gray trials, thereby illustrating the publication bias. The corresponding phenomenon in publication of the assessment of IT systems in healthcare may be that the literature does not provide a rich picture of the validity of evaluation methods. This might be the reason behind the phenomenon of missing publications, like that observed and discussed in Section 11.2.12.3.

A major problem is probably that the validity of a method or a hypothesis is not black and white but may be drawn from a continuum on a scale of gray tones. Within the literature a hypothesis, such as the validity of a particular assessment method, may never be concluded to be less than successful, simply because the method may be successful in some respects and less successful in other respects. However, failures are rarely published, and, even worse, journals are often not willing to publish negative outcomes (Egger et al. 2001).

Moreover, a method/hypothesis may not be exhaustively investigated as a method, as is usually the case in other professions. So its application may never be repeated and published by others than the developers. How will it then be feasible for assessment designers to know the level of confidence that one can put into a given method when there is no tradition of publishing malfunctioning methods or approaches?

Finally, as the validity is not black and white, valuable information may still be achieved from application of a given hypothesis or method.

Still another version of publication bias is the bias in the references applied in a publication. Many authors ignore publications in languages that they do not read, publications from other professions, or publications that are not available in their local library. Some authors deliberately omit the gray literature as references. Others have a bias toward recent references to demonstrate that their insight into the literature is up-to-date. And still others tend to reference viewpoints supporting their own hypothesis or conclusion. The latter is clearly of the worst kind. In previous times it was good practice in a scientific publication to show one's knowledge of the literature. However, considering the increasing amount of literature it is no longer feasible to be fair to the literature as a whole. What is important remains to be that one is balancing the pros and cons in one's presentation of the literature and that one is fair toward the material applied as well as toward the material known of.

11.2.13.2 *Randomized Controlled Trials*

It has been stated more than once that randomized controlled trials (RCT) are the strongest approach for assessing the effect of an IT-based system – for instance, by Johnston et al. in 1994 (referenced by Friedman and Wyatt 1997). This statement may be valid when the objective is to study clinical efficacy of a decision-support system, but it is not necessarily so when the objective is to study the clinical usability of such systems, as also discussed by Friedman and Wyatt (1997). However, to maintain the hypothesis that RCT is the strongest approach and consequently *the* approach to pursue when justifying or documenting an investment in an IT system, but it will leave out a whole number of valuable solutions from being promoted. Thus, the present discussion of RCT is intended to serve as an illustration of the bias of hypothesis fixation rather than a discussion of particular problems specifically inherent in RCTs. For that purpose the problems in RCTs shall be discussed briefiy.

The purpose of randomization in medicine is usually to overcome a number of biases that are inherent in the selection or allocation process or the service process itself. One may randomize at the application level (e.g. a hospital using a given IT system), at department level within such a hospital, for selection among the users included or the patients dealt with by the IT –system, respectively, the alternative services (Wyatt and Spiegelhalter 1991).

A major problem in assessing IT systems is the shortage of case sites. This makes it virtually impossible to randomize the entire development or implementation and assessment process. In (Østbye et al. 1997), randomization was applied for the selection of one out of two candidates of the intervention site, with the looser nominated as control group. This draw has the advantage of circumventing potential maneuvers caused by hidden agendas or other biases from surfacing, thereby avoiding an allocation bias. Still, it is only with hesitation that the study can be characterized as a true randomized study because the draw cannot achieve what it would normally do for another purpose of randomization, namely that of averaging each of the characteristics of a study population and a control group. If the two sites are truly identical, then such a randomization is a good choice, but it is an illusion to think that it can compensate for inequalities in such a small population.

Another problem with RCTs for assessment of IT-based systems is the significant changes within the organizational environment that are brought about by implementation of the IT system itself. In reality this means that the two systems are no longer really comparable despite their prior characteristics and the randomization; see the discussions in (Bryan et al. 1995), specifically when applied to PACS systems.

An insight into what is taking place may introduce psychological biases, as seen from a number of biases dealt with in the present part. In medicine one can often blind medication/treatment of patients both toward the patient and toward the healthcare professionals, thereby double-blinding the study in order to combat those biases. This approach is often coupled to RCTs. However, one of the major assessment problems of IT-based systems is the inability to blind the studies at all, which is caused by the inevitable transparency of the allocation. In other words randomization cannot be applied to combat the large number of biases by means of blinding, due to a lack of possibility of blinding an assessment study (see all the references to (Wyatt and Spiegelhalter 1991) in the present Part).

Thus, holding onto the statement that RCT is *the* standard against which IT systems should be measured compares to a hypothesis fixation. RCTs may definitely have tremendous value for some types of systems, such as expert systems, decision-support systems, or educational systems. However, other approaches may *have* to be applied for other types of systems, depending on the nature of the system and also on the nature of the assessment questions asked.

11.2.13.3 Action-Case Research

The potential of a 'hypothesis fixation' bias has to be considered particularly carefully for action-case research because of the very nature of the action-case research approach that iterates in an incremental and error-based refinement fashion. The researcher may in a sequence of projects apply the methodology or method and each time refine it according to the previous lessons, while often not being able to apply it stringently – for instance, due to the patterns of responsibility for the IT-based solution in operation.

It is in this hypothesis that the hypothesis fixation for action-case research studies will reveal itself in terms of symptoms of diverging lessons and refinements at subsequent applications. If a convergence of the experiences cannot be obtained, the researcher should abandon his own theory or make a major revision. The problem is that for research of the action-case type within system development or assessment, each application and refinement step takes normally two to three years or more.

Unfortunately, this type of bias will be very difficult to identify within the literature because of the sequential application being distributed over a long time span and equally because of the length of time before other research teams begin to report their experiences with the methodology/method. One way might be to search for previous, successive studies performed by the same group on the same subject/object, which never succeeds in finalizing and concluding. So, if a publication states, "In this paper we discuss the challenges we faced and the means by which we plan to meet these challenges", two years after presenting "preliminary results of the surveys and plans for the . . . future . . .", then one might suspect something to be wrong.

11.2.13.4 Conclusion

The very nature of assessments of IT-based solutions makes it very difficult indeed to judge the existence of a hypothesis fixation bias in general. It will perhaps take ten years of experimental work with a given theory, before one can judge whether this bias might be present – the main problem probably being that not all theories are adopted by others and applied for verification purposes.

11.2.14 The Intention to Treat Principle

Once an assessment study is going on (or preferably before that), one has to decide what to do with the cases that do not comply with the protocol. Shall the patients who didn't do as prescribed be excluded from the data (Wyatt and Spiegelhalter 1991)? In pharmaceutical trials, it is considered appropriate to plan with a set of criteria for what to do with the patients who do not take the medicine as prescribed. The reason for doing so prior to the study is that otherwise a bias may occur in the process of judging whom to exclude and whom not to exclude – when one knows the outcome (fully or partly). In pharmaceutical studies this is relevant not only for the patients, but also for the physicians and for the entire sites (in case of multisite studies).

The analogy for assessment of IT-based solutions is obvious. The analogy to cases and patients naturally would be users or user organizations in the assessment study. The answer to the question stated above is that it depends on the aim of the study: Is the scope to identify the maximal benefit achievable with the new technology (efficacy) or the average benefit of it in a real situation (effectiveness)? Normally, the answer would be the latter, but there might be exceptions. In any case, at the design of an assessment study concerned with an IT-based solution one has to decide on what to do with the cases that do not comply with the protocol. A deviance may, for instance, be that a user abstains from specific steps of a prescribed procedure. The inclusion/exclusion criteria should be explicitly stated under methods, as previously stated in Section 11.1.4, to be easily found by the reader when relevant.

The bias of also including cases that do not comply with the protocol (e.g., in order to increase the data material) is particularly relevant at the assessment of the validity of knowledge-based systems and decision-support systems. However, some variation is natural and to be expected, but it has to be monitored during an assessment study in order to stay in control of the events so that the outcome reflects the intended objective (see also the discussion in the section on 'illicit use').

As part of the presentation, all kinds of deviations should be stated, and the authors should explore and explain the actual reasons for omissions or exclusions, as the causal reasons behind such deviations are plentiful and may provide a rich picture of the system. It is relevant to know, for instance, whether participants are deliberately excluded after some (objective) criteria or whether an actor abstained, on his own volition, in the middle of a study. Parts of this information might be highly relevant for the interpretation of the outcome (like the following explanation for dropping out: "I don't want to waste my time on that" versus "I couldn't find the time"). To be convinced, at least in the present context, the reader needs to know in detail how many participants were excluded and for what reason. And the reader needs to be convinced that these rules are defined to a reasonable extent prior to the completion of the study and not designed after the event – in order to achieve convincing results.

Consequently, due to the natural variation aspect one has to conclude carefully as regards the presence of this bias. The bias, which is definitely relevant to look for, is concerned with the explicitness of relevant criteria prior to the execution of the study.

Note that there are two special cases for the 'intention to treat' bias, both concerned with the intention to continue even if the original plans were deviated considerably: constructive assessment approaches and action case research. For both of these special cases, the intention to treat bias has to be considered with careful attention to the balance between preconditions for the case and confidence in the interpretation of the outcome.

11.2.14.1 Constructive Assessment

The intention to treat principle is a built-in necessity for a constructive assessment project. Constructive assessment is characterized by a willingness to deviate considerably from the original plan as a function of the process and the results achieved, while supporting tools and techniques have to be designed, adapted, replaced, or refined to accommodate interim changes; this together with a supportive philosophy compares to constructive assessment. It is not always feasible to design fully compliant research projects for the application of theories, methodology, and methods at each step within fully controlled trial applications, especially not for assessment of large IT-based solutions. Neither may it be feasible to make studies on a multitude or even on a certain number of cases in parallel to average the outcome. One may have to take the one or just a few cases available, apply the methods to the extent feasible, maneuver within the space of compliance and deviations before one can elicit lessons from experiences gained and use these to make adaptations of the methodology/method and then try again.

11.2.14.2 Action-Case Research

The type of application-oriented research called action-case research (see the concept in Mathiassen 1998) is experimental in an incremental, iterative, and error-based refinement approach. The researcher is engaged in the practical application, and thus there is an intimate relationship between the application and the research. It is a must to always do what is best and to make interim corrections because in real-life cases the researcher has to respect the patterns of competence and responsibility/liability within the application domain as well as incidents occurring and thus has to adapt rather than strictly obey the original plan. The progress in terms of research conclusions may consequently turn out to be small.

Again, the intention to go on despite deviation from the plans is a built-in obligation.

The paper of McKay and Marshall (2002) discusses the pitfall of action research, 'post hoc action research', at which the actions in a development project are initiated without a founding research question and a theory to guide its exploration. As long as they are not published, the lessons learned are merely the outcome of a trial and error approach. There is nothing wrong with such a consultancy-like approach. However, there is the potential of a pitfall residing when striving to publish the lessons as a scientific research paper, unless properly handled. Our own action-case research, summarized in Part I, Section 4.2, has a strong theoretical foundation to guide the real-world problem situation and hence constitutes a model of the type that McKay and Marshall recommend. They provide a checklist of questions to assess the validity of action-case research.

Another potential pitfall in this respect arises in the situation mentioned in (Swartz and Remenyi 2002) of researchers doing action-research within their employer's organization. There is the advantage of readily accessible information, but there is also the potential of a pitfall in the schism between the objectiveness, rigor, and neutrality required by a researcher and the loyalty toward the employer. This is related to the problem previously discussed in Section 11.2.1.1. The paper of Swartz and Remenyi (2002) discusses how this situation may be handled. Further, it is of utmost importance that the reader knows the role and influence of the researchers within the case and that the research process is auditable in the presentation of its outcome.

11.2.15 *Impact*

Whenever a new information resource is introduced into an environment, there can be many consequences, of which only some relate to the stated purpose of the resource (Friedman and Wyatt 1997). During an exhaustive assessment, it is important to look not only for the intended effect, but also for side effects, whether adverse or beneficial, as so nicely demonstrated in (van Gennip and Bakker 1995). Even an awareness of this phenomenon in the data analysis of a study report will render a study more valuable.

11.3 Types of Opportunities

The issue in question in this section is to explore what might potentially be done to remedy, compensate for, or correct the biases identified, whether these were really overlooked, deliberately not included in the presentation, or unavoidable due to the project preconditions. The notes (the List of Clarification Points) previously established during the analysis of Strengths and Weaknesses provide the basis for such an analysis. The effort starts with an analysis of the problems actually identified – be they small or large.

Note that a supplementary and retrospective exploration of the data material has to be managed with the same cautiousness in respect of pitfalls and perils as the original study because some data lose information if (parts of) the context is lost, such as their meta-data. A large number of the perils and pitfalls discussed in the previous two subchapters may arise merely as a question of insufficient information in the presentation of a study. Therefore, it is worth investigating whether more information may be revealed.

11.3.1 Retrospective Exploration of (Existing) Data Material

The List of Clarification Points is carefully analyzed against the information already provided in the study (as a norm, primarily in the Methods and Results Sections) to see whether the *existing* data material is likely to include data and information that will clarify the issues raised or enable a reduction of the impact of the problems identified if further analyses were initiated.

The first option to be explored is whether, given the methods applied in the study, it is likely that additional, nonreported data exist that may remedy some of the problems identified or clarify some of the issues raised. One may consider whether the study is of a nature that will enable further investigation activities to be pursued, like elicitation of more information from the bulk of data generated. This is often the case in the medical arena, where the subject under investigation normally has a medical record supposedly complete with regards to all relevant information. Similarly, an IT-based system may often generate huge amounts of data during operation, and some of this may turn out to be valuable in a supplementary investigation in case they are stored as a backup of the system's operation or as a partial copy on paper, and so on.

The study of Gamm et al. (1998a) is a fine example of a study with potential problems (see Sections 11.1.4 and 11.2.2) that may be further explored: The in- and exclusion criteria for users may be revealed, the response rate or characteristics of users actually involved in the evaluation study may be defined, the actual number of different user categories may be revealed, and the potential of influence by level of expertise on the outcome may be explored. Fairly easy.

Another example is the data obtained by interview techniques – for instance, if they exist on a tape or a transcript. Interview techniques suffer to a large extent from the same perils and pitfalls as questionnaires; see a previous section. Yet, when relevant for the study conclusion, fairly objective techniques do exist for the analysis of the text acquired from interviews, such as the Grounded Theory Approach. Although laborious, it may be applied after the event to remedy a potential lack of confidence in the study conclusion.

11.3.2 Remedying Problems Identified – beyond the Existing Data Material

Are the problems identified of a kind that may be explored or clarified retrospectively by eliciting further data? If the problem area turns out to be insufficiently covered – say, by the inability of the data to explain phenomena observed – it might be worth looking at options to get more data. Based on the List of Clarification Points, an analysis should be completed in order to establish to what extent and in what respects the study type enables further investigation activities to be pursued in terms of complementary investigations.

Sometimes it is feasible after the event to carry out additional inquiries or investigations while preserving the study conditions and noting the risk of post-rationalization and confounding factors (see Sections 11.2.7 and 11.1.6.9). An analogue from the medical domain is the efforts that might be put into carrying out additional biochemical investigations on samples preserved for precisely that purpose. Examples from the medical informatics domain may be interviews of the respondents and the people involved, or supplementary questionnaires, or even elicitation of more data. An inspiring example can be found in (Østbye et al. 1997), who used telephone consumption as an explicit measure, as in some cases it is feasible to retrieve information on the use of the phone from telephone companies or bills, or the like. Similarly, in a case study of an IT system, the verification of correctness of any outcome measure (see Section 11.1.7.5) that is judged significant for the study conclusion may be accomplished afterward, provided that the system has not changed in the interim. For instance, the study of Wiik and Lam (2000) uses kappa statistics; however, kappa statistics are not just obvious to everyone, and a reference to the formula applied is necessary for a reader with the relevant insight to be able to verify that the statistics are appropriately used and thus that the measures are valid (see also Section 11.1.2.2).

Thus, after the event, one may still have options for remedying some of the problems identified.

11.3.2.1 Triangulation

Triangulation constitutes a rigorous scientific approach to compensate for weaknesses in the study methodology by application of different approaches for measuring the same characteristic. This should, however, not be confused with a multimethod approach applied solely for getting a multitude of measures in order to achieve richer information on different characteristics of the object of investigation. We would prefer to distinguish between real triangulation and a multimethod approaches.

Triangulation can be used at different levels in a methodology: methods, measures, and data triangulation, as well as investigator and theory triangulation (Ammenwerth et al. 2003).

Triangulation of methods that include an investigation of potential divergences within the outcome will increase the confidence in a study tremendously. In some particularly vulnerable studies, triangulation might (partly) compensate for the lack of confidence caused, for instance, by a missing baseline frame of reference. The advantage of using triangulation is that it may compensate for weaknesses in the methods applied, where stronger methods are not available or feasible to apply.

The study of Gamm et al. (1998a) applies a multimethod approach, but it was not fully clear whether it was a real triangulation, as it says, *"In tandem with the surveys, interviews . . . provided additional detail and context for interpreting the survey results"*. However, a parallel publication of the same group on the same case (?) says, *"Additional validation of instruments and confidence in findings are pursued through a comparison of questionnaire results with interviews and observation . . ."* and *"Triangulation of qualitative and quantitative methods . . . provides some additional confidence"* (Gamm et al. 1998b). So it seems to be a triangulation also in the first referenced study. This just shows how important details of the wording are for the interpretation of a study.

Triangulation of measures is used for mutual verification purposes (see, for instance, Gordon and Geiger 1999), in which it is explicit that measures from application of one method are correlated with the outcome of the other methods providing specific measures of user satisfaction *("We correlated these findings . . ."* and *"representative focus group statements were paired with associated survey findings")*. Although the same level of explicitness as regards the actual use of multiple methods is not the case in (Østbye et al. 1997), the mere presence of the awareness presented by the authors will still increase the readers' confidence in the outcome.

Triangulation of measures may also be used for analytical purposes. For instance, Keen et al. (1995) use the concept at an assessment study of an investigative type (or constructive type) addressing cause-effect relations within the pattern of outcomes. The deviations exposed by the triangulation may be applied to elaborate the understanding of the subject of investigation.

Triangulation of data corresponds to repeated applications of methods and measures. This type of triangulation may be accomplished as repeated applications on the same case but at different periods in time or on a new case. In the former case, one has to be aware of the problem of organizational change as a function of time, while organizational differences are an obvious issue in case of the latter. Moreover, in the case of triangulation of data, it is also relevant to take into account intra- and interobserver variations, corresponding to variation in the interviewees' mood in an investigation of staff's attitudes in a user satisfaction study, for instance.

11.4 Types of Threats

All in all, an analysis of Threats is concerned with a synthesis on the possibility of assigning credibility to the study, while taking into account the entirety observed for the study. Therefore, a major part of the basis for the analysis in this respect is often the information provided and discussed within the Introduction and Discussion sections of the assessment study report itself.

The purpose of the present section is merely to guide the reader through this analysis and its interpretation.

11.4.1   *Compensation for Problems*

The issue here is a judgment of the likelihood that the Opportunities can compensate for the problems identified. This issue is related to the possibility of judging the validity of the conclusion of the assessment study, based on the prospect for remedying the problems on the List of Clarification Points, as reviewed in terms of the activities prescribed under Opportunities.

Is the study under analysis of a nature that will allow further investigation? If the study is of an explorative nature, of an experimental kind, or constructive, then the case may already be far, far ahead in the next iteration, and the questions raised may be irrelevant or superfluous in the new context. Or when you get your hands on the report of an assessment study, it may be years old and thus not worth or feasible to pursue.

Is it worth digging deeper? If you are a decision maker using the information provided, then definitely "yes". If you are a referee on a report on assessment, then definitely "yes". If you consider applying the IT system assessed, then definitely "yes". If you consider applying the method, then "perhaps". Alternatively, if you just happen to have the report in your hands, then "no" – just take advantage of the lessons learned from it, and use the information provided as a stepping-stone.

Any assessment study has to be judged also in a larger context. Often, when reading a study report retrospectively, one would ask "Why haven't all the problems identified within a given assessment study been taken into account prior to the assessment studies? They must have known". This is not necessarily (only) caused by a lack of skill. First and foremost, the most important reason may be the preconditions of the assessment. There is always a limit to the resources available, both as regards the number of heads at the different skill levels and their actual availability for a given period of time, and as regards the relevant cases to be included. It is therefore important to be aware of the implications of the preconditions and to judge these against the level of ambition reported for the study. Sometimes, a smaller, more focused study will gain more (valid) information than the grand studies that were designed but not fully accomplished.

In conclusion, given the Strengths, Weaknesses, and Opportunities in the light of the above discussion, what is the likelihood that the Opportunities may remedy the problems identified?

11.4.2   Pitfalls and Perils

While designing a study, it is up to the managers/participants to judge the potential implications of each and every pitfall and peril – that is, to consider whether or not it is a confounding factor. If there is a risk of a bias, it is necessary to consider what the implications on the outcome may be and subsequently take all necessary precautions to take this into account at the detailed planning, execution, and/or interpretation of the study. Similarly, it is necessary for the reader of a study's concluding remarks to judge whether or not given biases are handled or taken properly into account at the interpretation of the study conclusion.

Is there an awareness of the pitfalls and perils observed, and are the corresponding issues present? In itself, the mere awareness of potential confounding factors may reduce their effect, and, thus, the presence of such awareness may constitute a preventive measure. The mere presence of an awareness tends to indicate that sufficient skill may be available to combat, circumvent or interpret data while taking these dangers into account, thereby making the study conclusion more reliable. A prime example like (Østbye et al. 1997) explicitly discusses the strengths and limitations of their study. This ought to be the case for all reports on assessment studies.

Equally, the complete absence of an awareness of potential dangers may in itself constitute a major threat to the trustworthiness of a study, given – of course – the trustworthiness of the study as a whole. Simply for that reason the advanced reader does not get sufficient information to judge with confidence the generality and validity of the conclusion. This is one of the reasons why a ten-liner evaluation description within a number of papers in the literature lends little credibility.

Finally, the discussion of pitfalls and perils, and good and not so good aspects, in a study report inevitably will reveal the depth of the authors' knowledge of experimental design of assessment studies – a factor in the judgment of the study's credibility. And as Coolican puts it:

> *"We should be able to indicate in the discussion of our study just where our design has weaknesses, where we did not have control and, therefore, how limited we are in assuming that our independent variable really did affect our dependent variable. We should be able to point out possible differences between our groups, and differences in their experiences, which might be responsible for any differences in the dependent variable which we identify, making it difficult to attribute these differences solely to the change in the independent variable."*

(Coolican 1999)

It is in the discussion of the results that the researcher reveals his or her level of understanding of assessment in a larger context.

11.4.3 *Validity of the Study Conclusion*

Does the study comply with its objectives, given the information elicited at the meta-analysis? This is the ultimate question that will answer whether the conclusion is valid or whether it is likely to become valid based on further investigations or analysis. The answer to the question is a holistic judgment based on a synthesis of the entirety of findings according to the above investigations.

The fact that an intervention is highly efficacious in one situation does not necessarily *guarantee* its efficacy in another scenario (Jaeschke and Sackett 1989). Therefore, it is relevant also to judge the extent to which a generalization of the study conclusion is valid beyond the actual study accomplished and the problems identified in it. Such an extrapolation is relevant for a judgment of the application range of the study conclusion. For instance, it depends on (1) delimitations of the space of the investigation, (2) an analysis based on the List of Clarification Points to highlight nonconclusive problem areas within the study, (3) characteristics of neighboring domains or applications, or (4) something completely different. One cannot blame a planning activity that could not produce a better solution due to the conditions.

When compromises made are consequences of conditions for and within the study itself, these assessment studies should formally be interpreted as pilot studies – in other words, *"the initial step in the identification of new technologies that are worth testing with more rigorous scientific methods"*, as Jaeschke and Sackett (1989) put it. Pilot studies do also have a value in themselves. The importance lies in whether or not the authors of the study are aware of their own perspectives and their premises when interpreting the data into a conclusion.

Still further, some studies do themselves extrapolate the conclusions to a level that may be questioned. Given that they only address half the story (see Section 11.2.12.2) and the findings of Kushniruk et al. (1997) (see Section 11.2.6.3), it is questionable whether one can extrapolate to the efficacy from a judgment of benefits alone, and even further to the cost-effectiveness, as suggested in (Kaplan and Lundsgaarde 1996) (see Section 11.2.12.2). In other words, the external validity (generalisability) is a major concern as regards the conclusion.

A study may be of value at one of many levels, depending on the role of the readers. In case the role is that of referee or auditor, rigorous scientific values have to be judged against the intended application of the study report (publication, marketing of the subject of investigation, constructive input for initiatives of change, etc.). Otherwise, it is up to the reader to judge the value for himself or herself. This could be in terms of inspiration for own assessment work, for example, as a buyer.

All in all, it is important that a study is factual and objective, that there is an awareness of perils and pitfalls, and that the conclusion does not exceed the limits of the study and its sources of bias.

12. Discussion

The essence of the contribution of the present part is (1) the transformation of known pitfalls and perils from other experimental disciplines to the domain of evaluation and Technology assessment of IT-based solutions in healthcare, (2) the abstraction and structuring of the information into a framework that guides its application, and (3) the review of a number of assessment studies reported in the literature to identify some examples of good and bad design of Technology assessment studies of IT-based solutions. The framework is designed with the scope of supporting at meta-analysis of assessment studies in a checklist fashion, and consequently, the framework is of value to others for assessing the conclusion of reported Technology assessment studies of IT-based solutions. However, even if the framework is designed for a retrospective analysis of case studies, the knowledge gained may also be applied prospectively as a checklist of issues – with examples – to take into account at the design stage of assessment studies.

The author's personal experience is that medical professionals may be highly competent with respect to technology assessments of pharmaceutical or medical technological solutions but lacking in experience of assessments of other types of solutions. Tremendous efforts and many creative and highly competent ideas may be put into the design of assessment studies, while violating a number of experimental rules and recommendations. Thus, the experience is that evaluation of IT-based solutions is a profession in itself, which cannot compare with that of designing technology assessments for pharmaceutical products or clinical techniques and tools. The reason may be that it is not that obvious to make the links from known experimental pitfalls in HTAs to the corresponding ones for the assessment of IT-based solutions in healthcare.

Worth noting here is the differentiation between science and pragmatism. First, for practical or other reasons, it may not be feasible to design the perfect assessment study for a given case; therefore, it is preferable to design an assessment study in compliance with the preconditions. Second, even if one or more biases may be present, their actual influence may not be significant enough to wreck the global picture of the IT-based solution. Third, the efforts invested in an assessment study have to be balanced against the information gained and the intended effect of the conclusion; if no consequence is to be taken, then why assess at all? Finally, even if it is unfeasible to accomplish the perfect assessment study both in principle and in practice, the resources to be invested have to be balanced against the information gained. Then, oppositely, if the information gain is minor from a practical perspective or the scientific benefit is insignificant, why bother spending resources on publishing it?

A couple of lessons are obvious from the present report. First, assessment of IT-based solutions is not a simple task, and second, the pitfalls and perils are not necessarily present among the knowledge base of the medical domain users. These arguments further emphasize the need for an independent knowledge base to be available at technology assessment studies of IT-based solutions. Finally, the framework does not rule out the need for senior analytical knowledge specifically related to assessment studies. The subject is simply too complicated, and one has to keep a number of details in mind all the time. Therefore, the contribution of the framework is that of putting structure and contents to such an analysis.

12.1 A Meta-View on the Study of Pitfalls and Perils

The purpose of the study on pitfall and perils was to explore whether known pitfalls and perils from other domains have analogues in the assessment of IT-based solutions. From a formal point of view, the present study is itself subject to a number of pitfalls, and this has to be discussed.

First, the outcome is based on a (subjective) interpretation and conversion of the pitfalls found from the source domains to a completely different professional arena. As Fraser and Smith (1992) discuss, *"researchers should use caution in referring to well known biases"*. In this respect, there might be a difference between methodical, cognitive and action-oriented biases. All of these types are included in the present part. Fraser and Smith (1992) focus on the cognitive biases and they themselves point out that question marks have been put at some of them within the literature. However, as they also state, these cognitive biases, *"can clearly be used to identify task conditions under which undesirable behaviours could arise in principle. Such an alert would be of value in calling these conditions to the attention of the designers of computer aids, for example"* so that these biases can be avoided. As the biases in question constitute cognitive biases, they might primarily be relevant at the assessment of marginal effects, like in comparing knowledge-based decision-support systems with the performance of a domain expert or perhaps also when using a questionnaire to quantify an effect because of the judgmental nature.

Second, there may actually be a danger of a *hypothesis fixation* as the framework and its contents have developed gradually over the period 1999 to 2002 with successive cycles of interim applications and refinements without thorough verification by independent third parties. This is primarily of relevance for the SWOT concepts as a means for structuring and organizing the experimental pitfalls and perils, as the pitfalls and perils in general are adopted directly from the literature sources. It should be remembered at this point that the framework itself is primarily used for structuring and grouping the information to cope with the volume and to present it in a more comprehensible fashion. Nevertheless, the structuring principle will inevitably influence the transfer and adaptation of literature examples of biases.

Third, the outcome of the transfer and adaptation of biases reported within the literature was applied by the same person as the one in charge of the transfer itself, with the purpose of accomplishing a (first) verification of the validity of the outcome. Hence, the same eyes that designed the characteristics to look for also identified the sample cases within the literature. Consequently, from a strictly scientific point of view, both an *insight bias* as well as a *circular inference* may be present. The eyes looking for the sample cases are biased by the understanding already achieved and thus are able to compensate for potential problems within both the clarity and construct validity of the descriptions. The circular inference may arise as given cases within the literature are used both to identify additional biases and to extend the framework, while at the same time serving as illustrations of these problems.

The paper of Southon et al. (1999) stresses that results are based on (human) interpretation and thus should be taken only as indicative, not conclusive. This viewpoint is strongly supported by the scary number of perils and pitfalls in experimental assessments of IT-based systems and by the fact that so few cases escape them all. Their statement is valid for the present report on perils and pitfalls as well, and in several places it has been necessary to stress that an example used may be included for indicative or illustrative purposes only, while it has (still) not been feasible to verify and conclude on the actual presence or absence of a given bias.

In conclusion, the only way to verify the framework (structure and contents) at this stage of its development is to have other scientists apply it, to elicit a second opinion on the cases found, and to find more or better examples.

List of Abbreviations

The following abbreviations are generally used abbreviations, while those that are used exclusively within a given context where it is described are not included below. Examples of the latter type are an abbreviation for a method used within the description of the method.

EHR	Electronic Healthcare Record
HTA	Health Technology Assessment
ID	Identity
IT	Information Technology
IT system	(also called IT-based system) is the actual technical construction consisting of hardware, software, basic system software, and so forth
IT-based solution	The overall solution consisting of an IT system and its surrounding organization, including work procedures, organizational structure, and so on.
LIS	Laboratory Information System
QA	Quality Assurance
QC	Quality Control
QI	Quality Inspection
QM	Quality Management
RCT	Randomized Controlled Trial

List of References

Please note that the appendix with the description of methods has its own list of references, including an extensive list of references to websites.

Allan J, Englebright J. Patient-centered documentation: an effective and efficient use of clinical information systems. J Nurs Adm 2000;30(2):90-5.

Altman DG, Schultz KF, Moher D, Egger M, et al. The revised CONSORT statement for reporting randomized trials: explanation and elaboration. Ann Intern Med 2001;134(8):663-94.

Ammenwerth E, Brender J, Nykänen P, Prokosch H-U, Rigby M, Talmon J. Visions and strategies to improve evaluation of health information systems – reflections and lessons based on the HIS-EVAL workshop in Innsbruck. Int J Med Informatics 2004;73(6):479-91.

Ammenwerth E, Iller C, Mansmann U. Can evaluation studies benefit from triangulation?. Int J Med Inform 2003;70:237-48.

Andersen I, Enderud H. Preparation and use of questionnaires and interview guides. In: Andersen I, editor. Selection of organization sociological methods - a combinatorial perspective. Copenhagen: Samfundslitteratur; 1990. p. 261-81 (in Danish).

Anderson JG, Aydin CE. Evaluating the impact of health care information systems. Int J Technol Assess Health Care 1997;13(2):380-93.

Arbnor I, Bjerke B. Methodology for creating business knowledge. Thousand Oaks: Sage Publications; 1997.

Assmann SF, Pocock SJ, Enos LE, Kasten LE. Subgroup analysis and other (mis)uses of baseline data in clinical trials. Lancet 2000;355:1064-9.

Bansler JP, Havn E. The nature of software work: systems development as a labor process. In: van den Besselaar P, Clement A, Järvinen P, editors. Information system, work and organization design. Proceedings of the IFIP TC9/WG9.1 Working Conference on Information System, Work and Organization Design; 1989 Jul; Berlin, GDR. Amsterdam: Elsevier Science Publishers B.V.; 1991. p. 145-53.

Barry CA. Critical issues in evaluating the impact of IT on information activity in academic research: developing a qualitative research solution. Libr Inf Sci Res 1995;17(2):107-34.

Berg M. Implementing information systems in health care organizations: myths and challenges. Int J Med Inform 2001;64:143-56.

Beuscart-Zéphir MC, Anceaux F, Renard J.M. Integrating users' activity analysis in the design and assessment of medical software applications: the example of anesthesia. In: Hasman A, Blobel B, Dudeck J, Engelbrecht R, Gell G, Prokosch H-U, editors. Medical Infobahn for Europe. Proceedings of the Sixteenth European Congress in Medical Informatics; Aug 2000; Hannover, Germany. Amsterdam: IOS Press. Stud in Health Technol Inform 2000;77:234-8.

Beuscart-Zéphir MC, Brender J, Beuscart R, Ménager-Depriester I. Cognitive evaluation: how to assess the usability of information technology in healthcare. Comput Methods Programs Biomed 1997;54(1-2):19-28.

Beuschel W. What will impact assessment tell us about expert systems design? In: van den Besselaar P, Clement A, Järvinen P, editors. Information system, work and organization design. Proceedings of the IFIP TC9/WG9.1 Working Conference on Information System, Work and Organization Design; 1989 Jul; Berlin, GDR. Amsterdam: Elsevier Science Publishers B.V.; 1991. p. 63-72.

BIPM, IEC, IFCC, ISO, IUPAC, IUPAP, OILM. International vocabulary of basic and general terms in metrology. Geneva: ISO; 1993.

Bjerregaard B, Brynitz S, Holst-Christensen J, Kalaja E, Lund-Christensen J, Hilden J, et al. Computer-aided diagnosis of the acute abdomen: a system from Leeds used on Copenhagen patients. In: De Dombal FT, Gremy F, editors. Decision making and medical care. North-Holland Publishing Company; 1976. p. 165-74.

Boy O, Ohmann C, Aust B, Eich HP, Koller M, Knode O, Nolte U. Systematische evaluierung der Anwenderzufriedenheit von Ärzten mit einem Krankenhausinformationssystem – erste ergebnisse. In: Hasman A, Blobel B, Dudeck J, Engelbrecht R, Gell G, Prokosch H-U, editors. Medical infobahn for Europe. Proceedings of the Sixteenth European Congress on Medical Informatics and GMDS2000; Aug 2000; Hannover, Germany. Amsterdam: IOS Press. Stud Health Technol Inform 2000;77:518-22.

Brender J. Methodology for assessment of medical IT-based systems - in an organizational context. Amsterdam: IOS Press, Stud Health Technol Inform 1997a; vol. 42.

Brender J. Medical Informatics: Does the healthcare domain have special features? [Letter]. Methods Inf Med 1997b;36(1):59-60.

Brender J. Trends in assessment of IT-based solutions in healthcare and recommendations for the future. Int J Med Inform 1998;52(1-3):217-27.

Brender J. Methodology for constructive assessment of IT-based systems in an organizational context. Int J of Med Inform 1999;56:67-86.

Brender J. Project assessment. Project internal report. Copenhagen: CANTOR (HC 4003) Healthcare Telematics Project; 2001 Mar. Report No.: D-10.2 v1.1.

Brender J. Methodological and methodical perils and pitfalls within assessment studies performed on IT-based solutions in healthcare. Aalborg: Virtual Centre for Health Informatics; 2003 May. Report No.: 03-1 (ISSN 1397-9507).

Brender J, Ammenwerth E, Nykänen P, Talmon J. Factors influencing success and failure of health informatics systems, a pilot Delphi study. Methods Inf Med 2006; (in press).

Brender J, McNair P. Tools for constructive assessment of bids to a call for tender - some experiences. In: Surján G, Engelbrecht R, McNair P, editors. Health data in the information society. Proceedings of the MIE2002 Congress; 2002; Budapest, Hungary. Amsterdam: IOS Press. Stud Health Technol Inform 2002;90:527-32.

Brender J, Mouritsen TB, Magdal U, McNair P. Enterprise viewpoint. In: Brender J, Grimson W, Yearworth M, Grimson J, McNair P, editors. Specification of the architecture for an open clinical laboratory information systems environment. Public report. Copenhagen: OpenLabs (A2028) AIM Project; 1995 Jan. Report No.: ARCH-3.

Brender J, Schou-Christensen J, McNair P. A case study on constructive assessment of bids to a call for tender. In: Surján G, Engelbrecht R, McNair P, editors. Health data in the information society. Proceedings of the MIE2002 Congress; 2002; Budapest, Hungary. Amsterdam: IOS Press. Stud Health Technol Inform 2002;90:533-8.

Brookes ST, Whitley E, Peters TJ, Mulheran PA, Egger M, Davey Smith G. Subgroup analyses in randomized controlled trials: quantifying the risks of false-positives and false-negatives. Health Technol Assess 2001;5(33). *(Also available from: http://www.ncchta.org, last visited 31.05.2005.)*

Bryan S, Keen J, Muris N, Weatherburn G, Buxton M. Issues in the evaluation of picture archiving and communication systems. Health Policy 1995;33:31-42.

Cabrera Á, Cabrera EF, Barajas S. The key role of organizational culture in a multi-system view of technology-driven change. Int J Inf Manag 2001;21:245-61.

Celli M, Ryberg DE, Leaderman AV. Supporting CPR development with the commercial off-the-shelf systems evaluation technique: defining requirements, setting priorities, and evaluating choices. J Healthc Inf Manag 1998;12:11-9.

Chilingerian J. Evaluating quality outcomes against best practice: a new frontier. In: Kimberly JR, Minvielle E, editors. The quality imperative, measurement and management of quality in healthcare. London: Imperial College Press; 2000. p. 141-67.

Chin L, Haughton DM. A study of users' perceptions on the benefits of information systems in hospitals. J Healthc Inf Manag Sys Soc 1995;9:37-46.

Collins English Dictionary, third updated edition. Glasgow: HarperCollins Publishers; 1995.

Coolican H. Introduction to research methods and statistics in psychology. 2nd ed. London: Hodder & Stoughton; 1999.

Crist-Grundman D, Douglas K, Kern V, Gregory J, Switzer V. Evaluating the impact of structured text and templates in ambulatory nursing. Proc Annu Symp Comput Appl Med Care 1995:712-6.

Cunningham RJ, Finkelstein A, Goldsack S, Maibaum T, Potts C. Formal requirements specification – the forest project. In: Proceedings of the Third International Workshop on Software Specification and Design1985 Aug; London, UK. Washington DC: IEEE Computer Society Press; 1985. p. 186-91.

Demeester M. Adaptation of KAVAS to the cultural components of a medical domain. Public report. Brussels: KAVAS-2 (A2019) AIM Project; 1995 Apr. Report No.: TELE-2.1.

DeMets DL. Distinctions between fraud, bias, errors, misunderstanding, and incompetence. Control Clin Trials 1997;18:637-50.

de Verdier C-H, Aronsson T, Nyberg A. Quality control in clinical chemistry – efforts to Find an Efficient Strategy. Helsinki: Nordkem; 1984. (reprinted in: Scand J Clin Lab Invest 1984;53 (Suppl 172))

Dreyfus HL. Intuitive, deliberative and calculative models of expert performance. In: Zsambok CE, Klein G, editors. Naturalistic decision making. Mahwah: Lawrence Erlbaum Associates, Publishers; 1997. p. 17-28.

Dreyfus HL, Dreyfus SE. Mind over machine, the power and expertise in the era of the computer. New York: The Free Press; 1986.

Dybkær R, Jordal R, Jørgensen PJ, Hansson P, Hjelm M, Kaihola H-L, et al. A quality manual for the clinical laboratory, including the elements of a quality system – proposed guidelines. Esbo: Nordtest; 1992. Report No.: 187. (reprinted in: Scand J Clin Lab Invest 1993;53 (Suppl 212)).

Egger M, Smith GD, Sterne JAC. Uses and abuses of meta-analysis. Clin Med 2001;1(6):478-84.

Einbinder LH, Remz JB, Cochran D. Mapping clinical scenarios to functional requirements: a tool for evaluating clinical information systems. Proc AMIA Annu Fall Symp 1996:747-51.

Feinstein AR. The problem of cogent subgroups: a clinicostatistical tragedy. J Clin Epidemiol 1998;51(4): 297-9.

Fernandez AM, Schrogie JJ, Wilson WW, Nash DB. A review and description of a "best practice" technology assessment process. Best Practices and Benchmarking in Healthcare 1997;2(6):240-53.

Fineberg HV. Technology assessment – motivation, capability, and future directions. Med Care 1985;23:663-71.

Fivelsdal E. Some problems at the interview of persons occupying leading positions. In: Andersen I, editor. Selection of organisation sociological methods – a combinatorial perspective. Copenhagen: Samfundslitteratur; 1990. p. 283-293 (in Danish).

Fraser JM, Smith PJ. A catalogue of errors. Int J Man-Machine Stud 1992;37:265-307.

Friedman CP, Wyatt JC. Evaluation methods in medical informatics. New York: Springer-Verlag; 1997.

Fröhlich D, Gill C, Krieger H. Workplace involvement in technological innovation in the European Community, vol I: Roads to participation. Dublin: European Foundation for the Improvement of Living and Working Conditions; 1993.

Galfalvy HC, Reddy SM, Niewiadomska-Bugaj M, Friedman S, Merkin B. Evaluation of community care network (CCN) system in a rural health care setting. Proc Annu Symp Comput Appl Med Care 1995:698-702.

Gamm LD, Barsukiewicz CK, Dansky KH, Vasey JJ. Investigating changes in end-user satisfaction with installation of an electronic medical record in ambulatory care settings. J Healthc Inf Manag 1998a;12:53-65.

Gamm LD, Barsukiewicz CK, Dansky KH, Vasey JJ, Bisordi JE, Thompson PC. Pre- and post-control model research on end-users' satisfaction with an electronic medical record: preliminary results. Proc AMIA Symp; 1998b:225-9.

Gluud LL. Bias in intervention research, methodological studies of systematic errors in randomized trial and observational studies [Doctoral dissertation]. Copenhagen: Faculty of Health Sciences, University of Copenhagen; 2005. (ISBN 87-990924-0-9)

Goodman C. It's time to rethink health care technology assessment. Int J Technol Assess Health Care 1992;8:335-58.

Goodman G. Group processes of decision making for hospital-based technology assessment committees, improving operating parameters can enhance committee effectiveness. Biomed Instrum Technol 1995;Sept/Oct:410-5.

Gordon D, Geiger G. Strategic management of an electronic patient record project using the balanced scorecard. J Healthc Inf Manag 1999;13:113-23.

Gremy F, Fessler JM, Bonnin M. Information systems evaluation and subjectivity. Int J Med Inform 1999;56:13-23.

Gruding J. Groupware and social dynamics: eight challenges for developers. Scientific American 1991;September:762-74.

Haimes YY, Schneiter C. Covey's seven habits and the systems approach: a comparative approach. IEEE Trans Syst, Man Cybern 1996;26(4):483-7.

Hall EM. Managing risk: methods for software systems development. Reading: Addison-Wesley; 1998.

Hampden-Turner C, Trompenaars F. The seven cultures of capitalism. New York: Doubleday; 1993.

Hampden-Turner C, Trompenaars F. Mastering the infinite game – how East Asian values are transforming business practices. Oxford: Capstone Publishing Ltd; 1997.

Handbook for objectives-oriented planning. 2nd ed. Oslo: Norwegian Agency for Development Cooperation; 1992. *(Commentary: this book can be difficult to get a hold of. You could ask the Norwegian Aid organization. Alternatively, find a résumé in Brender 1997a).*

Heathfield H, Clamp S, Felton D. PROBE project review and objective evaluation for electronic patient and health record projects. UK Institute of Health Informatics; 2001. Report No.: 2001-IA-611.

Herbst K, Littlejohns P, Rawlinson J, Collinson M, Wyatt JC. Evaluating computerized health information systems: hardware, software and human ware: experiences from the Northern Province, South Africa. J Public Health Med 1999;21:305-10.

Hetlevik I, Holmen J, Krüger Ø, Kristensen P, Iversen H, Furuseth K. Implementing clinical guidelines in the treatment of diabetes mellitus in general practice; evaluation of effort, process, and patient outcome related to implementation of a computer-based decision support system. Int J Technol Assess Health Care 2000;16(1):210-27.

Hoppe T, Meseguer P. VVT terminology: a proposal. IEEE Expert 1993:48-55.

Hornby AS, Gatenby EV, Wakefield H. The advanced learner's dictionary of current English. 2nd ed. London: Oxford University Press; 1963.

ISO. Quality-vocabulary. 1st ed. Geneva: ISO; 1986 Jun. Report No.: ISO 8402-1986.

ISO. Quality management systems – fundamentals and vocabulary. 1st ed. Geneva: ISO; 2000; Report No.: ISO 9000:2000.

ISO. Quality management and quality assurance standards - part 3: guidelines for the application of ISO 9001 to the development, supply and maintenance of software. 1st ed., corrected and reprinted. Geneva: ISO. 1993 May; Report No.: ISO 9000-3-1991 (E).

Jaeschke R, Sackett DL. Research methods for obtaining primary evidence. Int J Technol Assess 1989;5:503-19.

Kaplan B. Culture counts: how institutional values affect computer use. MD Comput 2000;17(1):23-6.

Kaplan B, Lundsgaarde HP. Toward an evaluation of an integrated clinical imaging system: identifying clinical benefits. Methods Inf Med 1996;35:221-9.

Keen J, Bryan S, Muris N, Weatherburn G, Buxton M. Evaluation of diffuse technologies: the case of digital imaging networks. Health Policy 1995;34:153-66.

Krogstrup HK. Evalueringsmodeller. Århus: Systime; 2003.

Kukla CD, Clemes EA, Morse RS, Cash D. Designing effective systems: a tool approach. In: Adler PS, Winograd TA, editors. Usability: Turning Technologies into Tools. New York: Oxford Press; 1992. p. 41-65.

Kuperman GJ, Teich JM, Tanasjevic MJ, Ma'luf N, Rittenberg E, Jha A, Fiskio J, Winkelman J, Bates DW. Improving response to critical laboratory results with automation: results of a randomized controlled trial. JAMIA 1999;6(6):512-22.

Kushniruk AW, Patel VL. Cognitive computer-based video analysis: its application in assessing the usability of medical systems. In: Greenes RA, Peterson HE, Protti DJ, editors. Medinfo'95. Proceedings of the Eighth World Congress on Medical Informatics; 1995 July 23-27; Vanvouver, Canada. Edmonton: Healthcare Computing & Communications Canada Inc; 1995. p. 1566-9.

Kushniruk AW, Patel VL. Cognitive and usability engineering methods for the evaluation of clinical information systems. J Biomed Inform 2004;37:56-76.

Kushniruk AW, Patel VL, Cimino JJ. Usability testing in medical informatics: cognitive approaches to evaluation of information systems and user interfaces. Proc AMIA Annu Fall Symp 1997:218-22.

Lauer TW, Joshi K, Browdy T. Use of the equity implementation model to review clinical system implementation efforts: a case report. J Am Med Inform Assoc 2000;7(1):91-102.

Leavitt HJ. Applied organizational change in industry: structural, technological and humanistic approaches. In: March JG, editor. Handbook of organizations. Chicago: Rand MacNally & Co; 1970.

Lindberg G. Studies on diagnostic decision making in jaundice [Doctoral thesis]. Stockholm: Kongl. Carolinska Medico Chirurgiska Institutet; 1982.

Malling P. Implementation of information technology in Thailand [Master thesis, Organizational Psychology]. Copenhagen: Psychology Laboratory at Copenhagen University; 1992 (in Danish).

Marcelo A, Fontelo P, Farolan M, Cualing H. Effect of image compression on telepathology: a randomized clinical trial. Arch Pathol Lab Med 2000;124(11):1653-56. *(Reprinted in Yearbook 2002).*

Mathiassen L. Reflective systems development [Doctoral thesis]. Aalborg: Aalborg University; 1998 Jun. Report No.: R-98-5006, ISSN 1397-8640.

Mathiassen L, Munk-Madsen A. Formalizations in systems development. Behavior Inf Technol 1986;5(2):145-55.

McKay J, Marshall P. Action research: a guide to process and procedure. In: Remenyi D, editor. Proceedings of the European Conference on Research Methodology for Business and Management Studies; 2002 Apr; Reading, UK. Reading: MCIL; 2002. p. 219-27.

McNair P. Bone mineral metabolism in human type 1 (insulin dependent) diabetes mellitus [Doctoral thesis]. Dan Med Bull 1988;35(2):109-21.

Moehr JR. Evaluation: salvation or nemesis of medical informatics? Comput Biol Med 2002;32:113-25.

Murphy CA, Maynard M, Morgan G. Pretest and post-test attitudes of nursing personnel toward a patient care information system. Comput Nurs 1994;12:239-44.

Nolan J, McNair P, Brender J. Factors influencing transferability of knowledge-based systems. Int J Biomed Comput 1991;27:7-26.

Nowlan WA. Clinical workstations: identifying clinical requirements and understanding clinical information. Int J Biomed Comput 1994;34:85-94.

Nykänen P, editor. Issues in evaluation of computer-based support to clinical decision making. Oslo: Oslo University Research Reports; 1990. Report No.: 127.

Ohmann C, Boy O, Yang O. A systematic approach to the assessment of user satisfaction with health care systems: constructs, models and instruments. In: Cappas C, Maglavera N, Scherrer J-R, editors. Medical Informatics Europe '97. Proceedings of the Thirteenth European Congress on Medical Informatics; 1996 Aug; Copenhagen, Denmark, Amsterdam: IOS Press. Stud Health Technol Inform 1997;43:781-5.

O'Moore R, Clarke K, Brender J, McNair P, Nykänen P, Smeets R, et al. Methodology for evaluation of knowledge based systems. Public Report. Dublin: KAVAS (A1021) AIM Project; 1990a May. Report No.: EM-1.2.

O'Moore R, Clarke K, Smeets R, Brender J, Nykänen P, McNair P, et al. Items of relevance for evaluation of knowledge-based systems and influence from domain characteristics. Public Report. KAVAS (A1021) AIM Project; 1990b March. Report No.: EM-1.1.

Patel VL, Kushniruk AW. Understanding, navigating and communicating knowledge: issues and challenges. Methods Inform Med 1998;37:460-70.

Preece J, Rombach HD. A taxonomy for combining software engineering and human-computer interaction measurement approaches: towards a common framework. Int J Human-Comput Stud 1994;41:553-83.

Rector AL. Editorial commentary: art and science – problems and solutions. Methods Inf Med 1996;35(3):181-4.

Rosenthal R. Experimenter effects in behavioral research. Enlarged edition. New York: Irvington Publishers Inc.; 1976.

Royle P, Waugh N. Literature searching for clinical and cost-effectiveness studies used in health technology assessment reports carried out for the National Institute for clinical excellence appraisal system. Health Technol Assess 2003;7(34). *(Also available from: http://www.ncchta.org. last visited 31.05.2005.)*

Sackett DL, Wennberg JE. Choosing the best research design for each question. BMJ 1997;315:1636.

Schneider SC, Barsoux J-L. Managing across cultures. Harlow: FT Prentice Hall, 2003.

Sher KJ, Trull TJ. Methodological issues in psychopathology research. Ann Rev Psychol 1996;47:371-400.

ShojaniaKG, Yokoe D, Platt R, Fiskio J, Ma'luf N, Bates DW. Reducing Vancomycin use utilizing a computer guideline: Results of a randomized controlled trial. JAMIA 1998;5(6):554-62.

Silverman D. Interpreting qualitative data, methods for analysing talk, text and interaction. 2nd ed. London: Sage Publications; 2001.

Smith GD, Egger M. Incommunicable knowledge? interpreting and applying the results of clinical trials and meta-analyses [Commentary]. J Clin Epidemiol 1998;51(4): 287-95.

Southon G, Sauer C, Dampney K. Lessons from a failed information systems initiative: issues for complex organizations. Int J Med Inform 1999;55:33-46.

Stage J. The use of descriptions in analysis and design of information systems. In: Stamper RK, Kerola P, Lee R, Lyytinen K, editors. Proceedings of the IFIP TC8 Working Conference on Collaborative Work, Social Communications and Information Systems, COSCIS '91; 1991 Aug; Helsinki, Finland. Amsterdam: Elsevier Science Publications B.V.; 1991. p. 237-60.

Swartz E, Remenyi D. Action Research: The researcher-intervener or consultancy approach. In: Remenyi D, editor. Proceedings of the European Conference on Research Methodology for Business and Management Studies; 2002 Apr; Reading, UK. Reading: MCIL; 2002. p. 335-44.

Symons V, Walsham G. Evaluation of information systems: a social perspective. In: Bullinger HJ, Protonotarios EN, Bouwhuis D, Reim F, editors. Information technology for organizational systems, concepts for increased competitiveness. Proceedings of the 1st European Conference – EURINFO '88; 1988 May; Athens, Greece. Amsterdam: North-Holland. 1988:204-11.

Talmon J, van der Loo R. Literature on assessment of information technology and medical KBS evaluation: Studies and methodologies. In: van Gennip EMSJ, Talmon J, editors. Assessment and evaluation of information technologies. Amsterdam: IOS Press. Stud Health Technol Inform 1995;17:283-327.

Timpka T, Sjöberg C. Development of systems for support of collaboration in health care: the design arenas. Artif Intell Med 1998;12:125-36.

Trompenaars F, Hampden-Turner C. Riding the waves of culture – understanding cultural diversity in business. 2nd ed. London: Nicholas Brealey Publishing Ltd; 1997.

Truex DP, Klein HK. A rejection of structure as a basis for information systems development. In: Stamper RK, Kerola P, Lee R, Lyytinen K, editors. Proceedings of the IFIP TC8 Working Conference on Collaborative Work, Social Communications and Information Systems, COSCIS '91; 1991 Aug; Helsinki, Finland. Amsterdam: Elsevier Science Publications B.V.; 1991. p. 213-35.

van der Lei J. Critiquing based on computer-stored medical records [PhD thesis]. Rotterdam: Erasmus University; 1991.

van Gennip EM, Bakker AR: Assessment of effects and costs of information systems. Int J Biomed Comput 1995;39:67-72.

van Gennip EMSJ, Talmon J, editors. Assessment and evaluation of information technologies. Amsterdam: IOS Press. Stud Health Technol Inform 1995;17:283-327.

Wall R. Computer Rx: more harm than good? J Med Syst 1991;15:321-34.

Wiik A, Lam K. On the usability of Extended DOORS for education and training, quality assurance and consensus formation. Public report. Copenhagen: CANTOR (HC4003) Healthcare Telematics Project; 2000 Nov. Report No.: D09.1 v2.1.

Without change there is no progress – coping with chaos, a global survey. Price-Waterhouse; 1997.

Wyatt J, Spiegelhalter D. Field trials of medical decision-aids: potential problems and solutions. In: Clayton P, editor. Proc Ann Symp Comput Appl Med Care 1991:3-7.

Østbye T, Moen A, Erikssen G, Hurlen P. Introducing a module for laboratory test order entry and reporting of results at a hospital ward: an evaluation study using a multi-method approach. J Med Syst 1997;21:107-17.

Annotated, Generally Useful References, Including Case Studies

Ammenwerth E, de Keizer N. An inventory of evaluation studies of information technology in health care, trends in evaluation research 1982-2002. Methods Inf Med 2005;44:44-56.

If you are one of those who feel that very few studies have been made of this or that topic, please refer to this paper. Furthermore, it refers to an inventory of evaluation publications; see http://evaldb.umit.at.

Ammenwerth E, Iller C, Mansmann U. Can evaluation studies benefit from triangulation? Int J Med Inform 2003;70:237-48.

This case study aims at demonstrating the value of triangulation through application of multiple methods, quantitative as well as qualitative ones,

Ammenwerth E, Shaw NT. Bad health informatics can kill – is evaluation the answer? Methods Inf Med 2005;44:1-3.

A discussion of hazards associated with information technology in healthcare, and justification of evaluation activities to prevent such hazards. The authors refer to a home page presenting examples of such hazards (see http://www.iig.umit.at/efmi).

Anderson JG, Aydin CE. Evaluating the impact of health care information systems. Int J Technol Assess Health Care 1997;13(2):380-93.

Together with (Fernandez et al. 1997), this article is particularly relevant when one needs to find out the connection between purpose and applicable methods and to get inspiration to find one's own assessment focus.

Anderson JG, Aydin CE, Jay SJ, editors. Evaluating health care information systems, methods and applications. Thousand Oaks: Sage Publications; 1994. p. 69-115.

The book contains a lot of practical and theoretical advice, methods, and case studies, as well as guidelines on how to assess IT-based systems within the healthcare sector.

Bindels R, Winkens RAG, Pop P, van Wersch JWJ, Talmon J, Hasman A. Validation of a knowledge based reminder system for diagnostic test ordering in general practice. Int J Med Inform 2001;64:341-54.

A case study of the validity of feed-back from a knowledge-based system. The validation is executed as a peer-review method, with the majority-evaluation of a panel of experts acting as the frame of reference.

BIPM, IEC, IFCC, ISO, IUPAC, IUPAP, OILM. International vocabulary of basic and general terms in metrology. Geneva: ISO; 1993.

This reference can be quite useful should you need a down-to-earth definition of the key expressions in metrology ('the science of measurement').

BIPM, IEC, IFCC, ISO, IUPAC, IUPAP, OILM. Guide to the expression of uncertainty in measurement. Geneva: ISO; 1993.

This reference can be quite useful should you need concepts and calculations that indicate uncertainties.

Brown SH, Coney RD. Changes in physicians' computer anxiety and attitudes related to clinical information system use. JAMIA 1994;1(5):381-94.

In a case study the authors investigate physicians' fears of new IT technology in a before-and-after study.

Dahler-Larsen P, Krogstrup HK. Nye veje i evaluering. Århus: Systime; 2003 (in Danish).

The book goes through assessment methods and the principles for evaluation within the social sector.

Feeny D, Guyatt G, Tugwell P, editors. Health care technology: effectiveness, efficiency & public policy. Quebec: The Institute for Research and Public Policy; 1986.

This is a good overall book on medical technology assessments. It describes principles and guidelines for different types of technologies (diagnostic, therapeutic) and different aspects for assessment (economic, clinical) with case stories, while also discussing difficulties and typical problems.

Fernandez AM, Schrogie JJ, Wilson WW, Nash DB. Technology assessment in healthcare: a review and description of a "best practice" technology assessment process. Best Practices and Benchmarking in Healthcare 1997;Nov.-Dec.:240-53.

A review of American technology assessment activities. It discusses different types of requirements analysis. This article and (Anderson and Aydin 1997) are particularly relevant when you need to find the relationship between an objective and the relevant methods and to get inspiration to find one's own assessment focus.

Fraser JM, Smith PJ. A catalogue of errors. Int J Man-Machine Stud 1992;37:265-307.

This article thoroughly discusses various biases and errors described in the literature. These biases and errors concern people's (lack of) ability to express themselves correctly on the probabilities of events observed, causal relations, and logical conclusions.

Friedman CP, Wyatt JC. Evaluation methods in medical informatics. New York: Springer-Verlag; 1996.

Contains a very good introduction to the assessment of IT-based systems, knowledge-based as well as others. The book spans most assessment designs and discusses aspects of planning as well as sources of bias.

General principles of software validation; final guidance for industry and FDA staff. Food and Drug Administration, U.S. Department of Health and Human Services. 2002.

The report describes the overall verification principles that FDA considers necessary when assessing medical equipment. (Available from www.fda.gov/cdrh/comp/guidance/938.html. Last visited 31.05.2005.)

Goodman C. It's time to rethink health care technology assessment. Int J Technol Assess Health Care 1992;8:335-58.

The author puts medical technology assessment into a larger perspective, discusses its concepts, role, and a number of key problem areas, including that of RCT and the difference between measuring efficacy, effectiveness, and efficiency.

Harrison MI. Diagnosing organizations: methods, models, and processes. 2nd ed. Thousand Oaks: Sage Publications. Applied Social Research Methods Series 1994. vol. 8.

The book discusses evaluation (diagnosis) of a number of aspects in an organization, such as investigation of power structures and differences between official and actual ways of doing things. Appendix B of the book contains a number of references to standard questionnaires.

Heathfield H, Clamp S, Felton D. PROBE project review and objective evaluation for electronic patient and health record projects. Technical Report of the UK Institute of Health Informatics 2001;2001-IA-611.

The objective of the report is to give practical guidelines for those who are involved in assessing an EHR. It does give sound advice and a number of guidelines, but not far enough to give the reader guidelines and references to methods. However, Appendix C contains a list of potential measures and where they are available. Appendix D contains a list of designs and tools with a short résumé of their pitfalls.

Jaeschke R, Sackett DL. Research methods for obtaining primary evidence. Int J Technol Assess 1989;5:503-19.

Some of the methods (and the rationale for their use) for evaluation studies of therapeutic and diagnostic technologies are discussed with regard to the handling of the placebo effect, confounders, and biases. Advantages and risk in using RCT, case control and cohort studies are discussed.

Kaplan B, Shaw NT. Review, people, organizational, and social issues: evaluation as an examplar. In: Haux R, Kulikowski C, editors. Yearbook of Medical Informatics 2002:91-102.

A relatively complete review of assessment studies for IT-based systems in the healthcare sector.

Kelly JR, McGrath JE. On time and method. Newbury Park: Sage Publications. Applied Social Research Methods Series 1988. vol. 13.

The book thoroughly and stringently (and with a philosophical background) discusses a number of aspects concerning time and the influence of time on experimental studies. Additionally and beyond the problems and pitfalls of time studies, it discusses, for instance, changes in the observer and problems at causal analysis of phenomena of a cyclic nature.

Kimberly JR, Minvielle E. The quality imperative, measurement and management of quality in healthcare. London: Imperial College Press; 2000.

The book is an anthology of the handling of quality in the healthcare sector. Therefore, it touches on many methods and problems in connection with quality measurement.

Krogstrup HK. Evalueringsmodeller. Århus: Systime; 2003. (in Danish)

The book runs through assessment methods and principles of evaluation within the social sector.

Kushniruk AW, Patel C, Patel VL, Cimino JJ. 'Televaluation' of clinical information systems: an integrative approach to assessing Web-based systems. Int J Med Inform 2001;61:45-70.

This article does not really contain a lot of new material compared to other articles by the same author (see under 'Cognitive Assessment', 'Cognitive Walkthrough', and 'Videorecordings'), but it summarizes quite well how the methods, described earlier, can be used for remote testing by means of telecommunication technology.

Kushniruk AW, Patel VL, Cimino JJ. Usability testing in medical informatics: cognitive approaches to evaluation of information systems and user interfaces. Proc AMIA Annu Fall Symp 1997:218-22.

With the aid of method triangulation the authors demonstrate convincingly the problems of people's biased evaluations of events measured through questionnaires.

Love AJ. Internal evaluation: building organizations from within. Newbury Park: Sage Publications. Applied Social Research Methods Series 1991. vol. 24.

Internal evaluation deals with staff's commitment to evaluate programs, projects or problems with direct relevance to the management in an organization that is, it is often a risky affair for the one carrying out the assessment task. The book is concerned with how to get the most from using internal resources to assess internal problems, evaluation of a needs assessment, objectives, user satisfaction, or effectiveness, for example.

Mair F, Whitten P. Systematic reviews of studies of patient satisfaction with telemedicine. BMJ 2000;320:1517-20.

A review of investigations of patient satisfaction within telemedicine, with a discussion of error sources and potential for generalization.

McKillip J. Need analysis: tools for the human services and education. Newbury Park: Sage Publications. Applied Social Research Methods Series 1987. vol. 10.

The book outlines a number of methods to identify and analyze needs, although 'needs' in the book are correlated to problems that can be solved.

McLinden DJ, Jinkerson DL. Picture this! multivariate analysis in organizational development. Evaluation and Program Planning 1994;17(1):19-24.

This little article may give some inspiration as to how one can manipulate and present data in an information carrying way, when the ordinary mean and standard deviation are of no use.

Mitchell E, Sullivan F. A descriptive feast but an evaluative famine: systematic review of published articles on primary care computing during 1980-97. BMJ 2001;322:279-82.

One of the very few systematic reviews of the impact of IT in the primary healthcare sector. It is particularly valuable because it is critical and contains many impact measures and references to studies, which have good case studies with precisely these impact measures. And another plus: The authors do it without automatically leaving out non-RCT studies; instead they score the quality by means of a Delphi method.

Murphy CA, Maynard M, Morgan G. Pretest and post-test attitudes of nursing personnel toward a patient care information system. Comput Nurs 1994;12:239-44.

A very good case study with questionnaires in a before-and-after study. Recommended for studying because they make a real effort to verify the internal validity of the elements in the questionnaire.

Murphy E, Dingwall R, Greatbatch D, Parker S, Watson P. Qualitative research methods in health technology assessment: a review of the literature. Health Technol Assess 1998;2(16). *(Available from http://www.ncchta.org. Last visited 31.05.2005.)*

This extensive literature review of qualitative assessment methods from social science deals with their potential to study health informatics applications. Beyond the known methods like interview and questionnaire, there are also methods like conversation analysis, interactionist, and ethnomethodological approaches.

Rosenthal R. Experimenter effects in behavioral research, enlarged edition. New York: Irvington Publishers, Inc.; 1976.

This somewhat unsettling book reviews the impact of the experimenters on their test objects, including biosocial attributes, psychosocial factors, and situational factors (the context of the study).

Rosenthal R. Meta-analytic procedures for social research. Newbury Park: Sage Publications. Applied Social Research Methods Series 1984;6.

This book is primarily of relevance as concerns quantitative studies, and it is mainly of interest to those who need to analyze the value of the evaluation studies reported by others. It looks into what information is needed and which conditions need to be fulfilled in order to compare or aggregate study results from the literature.

Smith AE, Nugent CD, McClean SI. Evaluation of inherent performance of intelligent medical decision support systems: utilizing neural networks as an example. Int J Med Inform 2003;27:1-27.

Contains a thorough investigation of measures and metrics (primarily statistical tools) regarding precision and accuracy of neural networks from binary to multiple categories and continuous decision problems. Thus, it is also relevant where the diagnostic problem involves more than two diagnoses or when the diagnoses are on a continuous scale.

Thomas P, editor. CSCW Requirements and evaluation. London: Springer-Verlag; 1996.

This book is a collection of different authors' contributions and contains many useful thoughts and angles of relevance in overall assessment work. It is particularly relevant in assessing constraints and consequences of an IT-based system on the interaction in a social context. The book is probably too longwinded in some contexts, but for dialogue-intensive systems like an electronic healthcare record system, it may be inspirational for those who want to dig deeper into the consequences of the IT technology or into the assumptions for using it optimally.

van Gennip EM, Bakker AR. Assessment of effects and costs of information systems. Int J Biomed Comput 1995;39:67-72.

A case control study evaluating an IT-based solution where the handling of differences and similarities between the intervention group and control group are carefully taken into consideration during the design of the evaluation study and the interpretation of the study results – including the resulting secondary impacts.

van Gennip EMSJ, Willemsen W, Nieman HBJ, Bakker A, van der Loo RP. How to assess cost-effectiveness of HIS-applications. In: Lun KC, Degoulet P, Piemme TE, Rienhof O, editors. Medinfo 92. Proceedings of the Seventh World Congress on Medical Informatics; 1992 Sep; Geneva, Switzerland. Amsterdam: North-Holland; 1992. p. 1209-15.

The article discusses alternative method for assessing cost-effectiveness.

Wyatt J, Spiegelhalter D. Field trials of medical decision-aids: potential problems and solutions. In: Clayton P, editor. Proc Annu Symp Comput Appl Med Care 1991:3-7.

Based on the literature, the authors describe and illustrate a number of biases related to the assessment of medical decision-support systems.

Yamaguchi K. Event history analysis. Newbury Park: Sage Publications. Applied Social Research Methods Series 1991. vol. 28.

A book for those who want to conduct studies over time in an organization.

Yin RK. Case study research: design and methods. 2nd ed. Thousand Oaks: Sage Publications. Applied Social Research Methods Series 1994. vol. 5.

Describes concepts and aspect of a case study and how to organize a case study. At the same time the book gives an elaborated explanation of the concepts of 'construct validity', 'internal validity', 'external validity', and 'reliability', which is useful to understand when planning an assessment study.

Zoë Stavri P, Ash JS. Does failure breed success: narrative analysis of stories about computerized provider order entry. Int J Med Inform 2003;70:9-15.

Uses a narrative analysis approach to retrospectively elicit aspects of success and failure for an IT-based solution.

Annotated World Wide Web Links

http://www.ahfmr.ab.ca/hta/

This link is to the home page of Alberta Heritage Foundation for Medical Research, and it has several interesting reports such as an overview and meta-analysis of evaluation studies of telemedicine projects (Last visited 31.05.2005).

http://www.ahic.org.au/evaluation/index.htm

This website contains a set of guidelines developed to assist novices at evaluation of electronic decision-support systems (EDSS). The aim of the guidelines is to raise understanding of the topic areas and stimulate thinking around key techniques, with pointers to useful journal references, books, and websites for those seeking more information (last visited 01.03.2005).

http://evaldb.umit.at

A fairly complete inventory of evaluation publications. The search engine allows you to search author name, year, topic, type of system, and so on (last visited 31.05.2005).

http://www.evalueringsmodeller.dk

This home page describes the content and results of a big evaluation project carried out by Institute for Political Science and Public Management at the University of Southern Denmark and Institute for Social Studies and Organization at Aalborg University. Among other things it contains a number of very useful recommendations ('good evaluation practice'), a couple of links and a list of the literature dealing primarily with the social sector (last visited 31.05.2005).

http://www.icbl.hw.ac.uk/ltdi/cookbook/contents.html

The home page aimed at teachers contains a number of descriptions of methods for evaluation. Nevertheless, it may be inspirational (last visited 31.05.2005).

http://www.icmje.org/index.html

Describes the Vancouver Rules for scientific manuscripts. The reference is quite instructive for everybody who has to put the results of a study in writing, regardless of whether it is a scientific article or a technical report (last visited 31.05.2005).

http://www.iea.cc

Home page of IEA (International Ergonomics Association) with various information and links (last visited 31.05.2005).

http://www.infodesign.com.au/usabilityresources/general/readinglist.asp

Contains a list of references to books on usability assessment (last visited 31.05.2005).

http://iig.umit.at/efmi/ (previously: http://www.umit.at/efmi)

Home page of the Working Group for 'Assessment of Health Information Systems' under the European Federation for Medical Informatics (EFMI). The Working Group and its results are openly accessible to anyone interested in evaluation of IT-based solution in the healthcare sector. The home page contains an annotated bibliography and some links (last visited 31.05.2005).

http://www.inria.fr/publications/index.en.html

The report on Usability is of particular interest, and it is relevant in connection with assessment of IT systems: Click on 'Research Reports & Thesis", type "ergonomic criteria" in the search engine text field, and press 'Enter'. Find the report RT0156, mentioned under the description of 'Usability' assessment. By clicking on 'pour obtenir la version papier' you get the e-mail address of the person concerned, and you may request the report (last visited 31.05.2005).

http://jthom.best.vwh.net/usability/

Lots of method overviews, links, and references, including many books. The method descriptions are only summaries but perhaps good for getting a feel for the possibilities of the references and links.. A disadvantage of the home page is that it only contains a few references to European websites and literature (last visited 31.05.2005).

http://www.lboro.ac.uk/research/husat/eusc/index.html

Is a website of a research center dealing with human-centered design, including the ergonomic aspects. The home page gives access to a whole range of technical reports on evaluation, but not all of them are relevant to the health informatics area. Nevertheless it may be inspirational and an opening to other relevant pages (last visited 31.05.2005).

http://www.ncchta.org

NHS R&D Health Technology Assessment Programme, which contains a number of reports of relevance for assessing IT-based systems (last visited 31.05.2005). It is possible to go straight to the list of publications at http://www.ncchta.org/ProjectData/3_publication_listings_ALL.asp.

http://qpool.umit.at

The aim of this website, which is still under construction, is to collect a series of more or less validated questionnaires from the literature (last visited 31.05.2005).

http://www.ucl.ac.uk/kmc/evaluation.html

Contains lists of articles on assessments of different types of IT systems that the Knowledge Management Centre at University College London has carried out, including case studies and a number of 'commentaries' (last visited 31.05.2005).

http://www.umit.at/efmi

(See http://iig.umit.at/efmi/.)

www.usableweb.com

A number of links to documents and information regarding the use of interface design and evaluation and more – specifically for www (last visited 31.05.2005).

www.usabilityfirst.com

A number of links to documents and information regarding usability – among other things, the terminology (last visited 31.05.2005).

http://www-vatam.unimaas.nl

This link is the home page for an EU Healthcare Telematics Project on evaluation of IT-based systems in the healthcare sector. The home page contains the project's technical reports, proceedings from its conferences and a comprehensive terminology (last visited 31.05.2005).

www.vineyard.net/biz/drdeb/

Contains a short description of the model on which the method in (Mayhew 1999) is built and may therefore be a good introduction before one chooses to order the book (last visited 31.05.2005).

Index